Working With Parents of Noncompliant Children

SCHOOL PSYCHOLOGY BOOK SERIES

Working With Parents of Noncompliant Children

A Guide to Evidence-Based Parent Training for Practitioners and Students

Mark D. Shriver and Keith D. Allen

American Psychological Association • Washington, DC

Published by
American Psychological Association
750 First Street, NE
Washington, DC 20002
www.apa.org

To order
APA Order Department
P.O. Box 92984
Washington, DC 20090-2984
Tel: (800) 374-2721; Direct: (202) 336-5510
Fax: (202) 336-5502; TDD/TTY: (202) 336-6123
Online: www.apa.org/books/
E-mail: order@apa.org

In the U.K., Europe, Africa, and the Middle East, copies may be ordered from
American Psychological Association
3 Henrietta Street
Covent Garden, London
WC2E 8LU England

Typeset in Goudy by Circle Graphics, Columbia, MD

Printer: Maple-Vail Manufacturing Group, Binghamton, NY
Cover Designer: Mercury Publishing Services, Rockville, MD
Technical/Production Editor: Devon Bourexis

The opinions and statements published are the responsibility of the authors, and such opinions and statements do not necessarily represent the policies of the American Psychological Association.

Library of Congress Cataloging-in-Publication Data

Shriver, Mark D.
  Working with parents of noncompliant children : a guide to evidence-based parent training for practitioners and students / Mark D. Shriver and Keith D. Allen.—1st ed.
    p. ; cm.—(School psychology book series)
  Includes bibliographical references and index.
  ISBN-13: 978-1-4338-0344-4
  ISBN-10: 1-4338-0344-5
  1. Behavior disorders in children—Treatment. 2. Child psychotherapy—Parent participation.
3. Parenting—Study and teaching. 4. Evidence-based psychiatry. I. Allen, Keith D.
II. American Psychological Association. III. Title. IV. Series.
  [DNLM: 1. Parent-Child Relations. 2. Parents—education. 3. Behavior Control—methods. 4. Child Rearing. 5. Child. WS 105.5.F2 S561w 2008]
  RJ506.B44S47 2008
  618.92'8914—dc22
                                                                                    2007043835

British Library Cataloguing-in-Publication Data

A CIP record is available from the British Library.

Printed in the United States of America
First Edition

CONTENTS

LIST OF TABLES AND EXHIBITS

TABLES

EXHIBITS

PREFACE

In most cases, a parent is the single most influential person in a child's life. Parents are instrumental in teaching children to walk, talk, and ride bikes. Parents can be equally instrumental in solving a child's problems, not because the parents are the cause of those problems but because they can provide their children with so many learning opportunities through their day-to-day interactions. This is true for everyday common problems as well as problems of more clinical significance. As a result, for those of us who train current or future behavioral and mental health practitioners, both in the classroom and in the clinic, ensuring their competence in parent training is necessary.

Over the years, we have found that training practitioners to train parents can be a particular challenge. Consistent with the tenets of an evidence-based practice, we train practitioners to identify the best available treatment research regarding what to teach parents and integrate that research with an understanding of why those treatments work and how to teach parents to implement those treatments. To accomplish this feat, we also strive to teach our future practitioners to take interventions developed under tightly controlled research conditions and adapt them to the conditions of day-to-day practice, in which resources are more limited, presenting problems are more complex, and practitioner skills are often less developed.

The challenge for us is that none of this information has previously been available in a single source. With this book, we hope to change that. We intend to provide practitioners, both current and future, with a resource on which they can rely to find the best available evidence regarding the what, why, and how of parent training. From the vast array of professional resources on helping parents, we have distilled those that we believe are the necessary components for practitioners who want their interventions to be based on good science but are unsure how best to translate research into practice.

The result is a book that is designed for any practitioner interested in an evidence-based approach to training parents to resolve a myriad of child problems. The book is likely to appeal to both students and practitioners who provide or would like to provide parent training in clinics, schools, or community agencies. The combination of empirical, conceptual, and practical recommendations about parent training should provide any practitioner—professional or student—with the tools to address even the more complex and difficult problems encountered in everyday practice.

As with any writing endeavor of this magnitude, we found the process to be challenging and stimulating. Our discussions about how best to accomplish this task were at times provocative and at other times disquieting, but always inspiring. Of course, sacrifices were made to accomplish the task. We thank the Munroe-Meyer Institute—Joe Evans, in particular—for support of not only our writing but also our teaching, research, and clinical experiences that have served as our inspiration. Joe is a remarkable and visionary leader who is unmatched in his ability to attract resources and then distribute them to others so that they can pursue their own visions. This book was one of ours. We also thank the Maternal and Child Health Bureau and the Administration on Developmental Disabilities for financial support.

We are, of course, indebted to many other individuals for their assistance in the development of this book. We are grateful to our series editors, Christopher H. Skinner and R. Steve McCallum, and to several anonymous reviewers whose comments were invaluable in focusing our efforts. We know we have a better product as a result of their feedback. Ultimately, we are also deeply indebted to the community of scientists dedicated to the science of training parents and to the treatment and prevention of childhood problems. These intellectual colleagues and forebears are too numerous to name, but we hope this book serves to help translate their efforts to everyday practice.

Finally, we offer sincere appreciation to our families, who gave up time with us to allow us to pursue this vision. Without the love and support of our wives, Kathy Shriver and Paula Allen, we would not have been able to complete this book.

Working With Parents of Noncompliant Children

INTRODUCTION

Working with parents is a fact of life for many mental health practitioners who work with children, and it is a worthwhile endeavor not only because many parents want the help but because parenting affects all areas of a child's development. Effective parenting has been found to predict positive behavioral, social, emotional, and academic adjustment, whereas ineffective parenting has been found to be predictive of later dysfunction and antisocial behavior (Borkowski, Landesman Ramey, & Bristol-Power, 2002; Patterson, Reid, & Dishion, 1992; Wade, 2004). Parents are a logical vehicle for many types of preventive and remedial interventions. Consequently, practitioners in schools, clinics, and other community agencies who are concerned about children's well-being find working with parents to be essential.

Although working with parents may be essential, knowing exactly what to do with parents to have a positive effect on child behavior and development can be difficult. Many, if not most, mental health practitioners working with children have not been trained to work with parents. For those practitioners who want to work with parents, finding helpful, research-based information can be challenging. Paradoxically, finding useful information is not difficult because little information is available but because there is so much available. A vast array of professional resources about parenting is available, and it spans the fields of medicine, law, religion, education, philosophy, and biology. The literature within psychology alone can be mind numbing. A recent search on PsycINFO, an electronic research database, found more than 7,000 articles on parenting in scholarly journals, almost 2,000 books and monographs, and some 3,000 other abstracts, dissertations, and encyclopedias. Efforts to understand and predict the impact of parents on their children have led to the publication of entire volumes on the myriad variables that influence child outcomes, such as *The Handbook of Parenting* (Bornstein, 2002), which condenses the professional literature on parenting into a mere five volumes!

In addition to the vast research identifying parenting variables that may predict child outcomes, hundreds of research investigations have explored which skills to teach parents to help prevent and solve child problems. Although the number of actual well-controlled empirical investigations is much smaller, the magnitude of research in this area can be overwhelming. In addition to this vast literature base, there are also manuals, workshops, seminars, and conferences on effective parenting. All of these sources of information and resources come from professionals across the mental health spectrum, including psychologists, physicians, nurses, social workers, and counselors. For any practitioner, the process of trying to discern helpful information on parenting from hyperbole can be daunting.

In the chapters that follow, we provide guidance for students and practitioners on how to separate helpful from less helpful information regarding evidence-based practice in parent training. *Parent training* is defined as the active, targeted teaching of specific parenting skills with the goal of positively affecting child behavior. Our use of the term *active, targeted teaching* is important because it means that the practitioner is not just a conveyor of information to a passive parent. Instead, both the practitioner and the parent are actively interacting within a dynamic teaching process. We refer to specific parenting skill because we believe it is important that parent training not only impart knowledge but also change parent behavior. Finally, *positively affecting child behavior* is important because ultimately the goal of parent training, at least from our perspective, is actually to change child behavior for the better.

For practitioners interested in an evidence-based practice, the ability to discern helpful information is particularly critical. Evidence-based practice involves the conscientious, explicit, and judicious use of the best available research in making decisions about the care of individual patients or clients. Thus, practitioners must be able to evaluate the quality of available research so that they select methods that are known to work—or at least the best available methods. After the best available research has been discerned, an evidence-based practice involves integrating that research with clinical expertise and client values. This allows the practitioner to tailor treatments to the unique social, cultural, economic, and developmental needs of individual clients.

Maintaining an evidence-based practice with respect to parent training is not easy. First, it requires considerable effort to stay abreast of the latest and best research on parent training and to separate the wheat from the chaff. Second, for students in particular, it may be overwhelming to try to combine research information with clinical skills that are perhaps still developing. Finally, more seasoned practitioners may find it particularly challenging to try to take the evidence from published research and translate it to meet the unique needs of their clients in everyday practice. In sum, an evidence-based approach to parent training challenges all practitioners to know what and how to teach parents to improve child outcomes. This book was written to help practitioners overcome that challenge.

ORGANIZATION OF THE BOOK

This book is informally organized in three parts. The first helps the practitioner or student discern the best available research—that is, it helps identify what to teach parents. It presents information about why parent training is used to solve child problems and the research that supports this approach; it also provides the criteria for evaluating research in parent training and describes how to use these criteria to identify the best available research support. The reader is then provided with detailed information on parent training programs. Finally, the criteria for evaluating research are applied to a variety of other popular parent training programs to help the reader practice the discernment necessary to maintain an evidence-based practice.

The second part describes the clinical expertise necessary for an evidence-based practice—that is, how to teach parents. It provides the reader with the clinical expertise to teach the relevant parent skills identified during the research review. This part begins by describing the theoretical framework that underlies evidence-based parent training programs. On the basis of behavior theory, the framework helps demonstrate why the empirically supported parent training programs are effective in solving many child problems. This part also provides information about how best to train parents to do what it is they have been asked to do. The underlying behavior theory helps refine the clinical expertise necessary to overcome the many obstacles to parent training success. This portion of the text also provides practical information about the ways in which practitioners can adapt to various parent characteristics, preferences, and cultures.

The third part describes the integration of research with clinical expertise and client values. It describes how to translate parent training research to address the myriad child problems seen in everyday practice. In addition, this part addresses more broadly how to use evidence-based parent training as part of a problem-solving process in daily practice. This portion of the text concludes with information about recent efforts to apply parent training in prevention efforts and suggests some directions for future research that may affect practice. Specific chapters are detailed in the sections that follow.

PART I: SEARCHING FOR THE BEST AVAILABLE EVIDENCE

Part I begins with a brief historical context for parent training. Chapters 2 and 3 then provide guidance for the reader on identifying parent training programs with the best available research support.

Chapter 1: Parenting and Parent Training

It is certainly possible to conduct parent training without any knowledge of history, basic philosophical or theoretical assumptions on human behavior, and parenting research in general. However, a practitioner who is knowledgeable of the vast amount of research on parenting can make better decisions when reading research about what would be useful in practice. Keeping abreast of research is part of an evidence-based practice.

Likewise, all practitioners have basic assumptions about human behavior corresponding to their respective theoretical and philosophical orientations in the science of psychology. Being aware of these assumptions can help practitioners make decisions about which practices best fit with their assumptions and, more important, acknowledge the lens through which the practitioner interprets research and makes decisions. A practitioner's clinical expertise and decision making as part of an evidence-based practice is certainly influenced by his or her theoretical orientation.

This chapter provides an overview of the historical roots of parenting and parent training research and theory. Although it is beyond the scope of the chapter to provide a comprehensive history of parent training, a summary of the historical influences with regard to theory and research in parenting and parent training can provide an important context for readers about the basic assumptions underlying parent training today. This chapter includes a discussion of the contemporary development of parent training as a practice.

Chapter 2: Empirically Supported Parent Training Programs

In an evidence-based practice, the identification of "best available research" is paramount, and this chapter presents information on four programs identified as meeting the criteria for empirically supported treatments. *Empirically supported treatments* are defined as programs or interventions that meet specific criteria for research support as developed by professional or scientific organizations. Emphasis is placed on describing what each program teaches parents and how the parent training is conducted. A brief review of the history of each program, as well as the empirical support for it, are provided. Similarities across programs are discussed, and unique aspects of each are described. Specific impressions about the programs' practical aspects are included as a part of the reviews, and the chapter concludes with a summary of their relative strengths and weaknesses.

This chapter provides the reader with a clear description of the best available research in parent training and a clear description of which skills are taught in these empirically supported parent training programs. The tools provided in this chapter for evaluating research are then used and expanded in chapter 3 to evaluate alternative parent training programs, and the program descriptions in this chapter supply essential groundwork for discussions about why the programs work (chap. 4) and how to go about training parents (chaps. 5 and 6). The parent training programs described in this chapter largely address problems of child noncompliance. However, these programs can also provide practitioners with a strong foundation for developing their own evidence-based parent training interventions for other child problems as described in chapters 7 and 8.

Chapter 3: Evaluating the Scientific Merit of Parent Training Alternatives

For practitioners and students trying to establish an evidence-based practice in parent training, discerning what is "best" in the available research requires also discerning what is not. Numerous alternatives exist, many with considerable popular appeal but with varying degrees of empirical support. This chapter describes more fully the process involved in evaluating the scientific merit of the available research support for other parent training programs. The chapter provides many examples for using criteria for evaluating the scientific merit of other parent training programs. The ability to apply these criteria is important for readers because practitioners are so often assaulted with a wide variety of claims of "evidence." In addition, these criteria provide an important foundation for later chapters when translating research to practice in parent training. Together, chapters 2 and 3 provide the reader with an excellent foundation for critically examining the best available research regarding treatment in general and parent training programs in particular.

PART II: DEVELOPING CLINICAL EXPERTISE

Part II begins with a description of the conceptual foundation of the empirically supported parent training programs. This foundation is important for understanding how to train parents, as described in chapter 5. Chapter 6 then discusses considerations for training parents of different cultures.

Chapter 4: Conceptual Foundations of the Empirically Supported Parent Training Programs

Although it may be possible to implement an empirically supported parent training program without understanding the conceptual foundation on which the program elements lie, maintaining an evidence-based practice requires otherwise. Simply put, the expertise required to teach parents skills and to translate the research into practice requires a clearly delineated conceptual foundation. This foundation provides a basis on which a practitioner can make sound clinical judgments when faced with unique challenges to implementation of standardized programs.

The conceptual foundation presented in this chapter is that of behavior analysis. The decision to focus on behavior analysis follows logically from the evidence reviewed in the first part of the book. The empirically supported parent training programs each come from a decidedly behavioral tradition. Thus, this chapter reviews the principles that are the foundation of that orientation. The chapter is a basic primer on behavioral principles of reinforcement, extinction, stimulus control, and punishment, and it describes how each of these scientific principles is consistently revealed in the empirically supported parent training programs. This conceptual foundation describes why parent training works. Many of the remaining chapters in this book on how to train parents to increase adherence to treatment recommendations or extend parent training to address other child problems are dependent on an understanding of these behavioral principles. The chapter serves as the conceptual link between the empirical research and the implementation issues that are presented in later chapters.

Chapter 5: How to Teach Parents

It is one thing to know what to teach parents to do to solve child problems and to know why we teach parents certain skills to solve child problems. It is still another thing to know how to train parents so that they are likely to do what is necessary to solve child problems. This chapter describes how the components of behavioral skills training are commonly used in the empirically supported behavioral parent training programs (see also chap. 2). The components of behavioral skills training include instruction, modeling, practice, and feedback. It is the inclusion of an active behavioral skills training component that distinguishes parent training from parent education. Yet even after skills training, there are many possible barriers to parents' actual application of these skills in everyday life. Strategies to prevent or overcome these barriers to parental adherence are presented in this chapter. The chapter highlights how the conceptual knowledge gained in chapter 4 informs the techniques used in developing and maintaining new skills in parents. Examples are provided throughout this chapter on the basis of our own clinical practice with parents. In addition, the stages of behavioral skills training described are applied in developing evidence-based parent training treatments to address other types of child problems in chapters 7 and 8.

Chapter 6: Cultural Issues in Parent Training

Practitioners pursuing an evidence-based approach must understand how culture affects both the research and the practice of parent training. In an increasingly diverse society, practitioners will likely work with children and parents who identify with cultural traditions and values that are different from those of the practitioner and the parent training programs they use. This chapter reviews and discusses five major cultural influences on parenting practices and on parenting programs in the United States today. These cultural influences include European American, African American, Latino American, Asian American, and Native American cultures. Guidelines are provided to readers to encourage culturally sensitive approaches to parent training with all parents and children. Awareness of these issues can help the practitioner develop ways to introduce interventions that increase parents' motivation in learning and implementing parenting skills.

PART III: INTEGRATING AND TRANSLATING RESEARCH INTO EVERYDAY PRACTICE

Part III begins by pulling together information from previous chapters to describe how to implement parent training to address other types of child problems. Chapter 8 discusses how to use parent training as part of a problem-solving model in day-to-day practice. Finally, the volume concludes with a review of prevention programs that incorporate parent training and a discussion of directions in research in parent training that may help inform practice.

Chapter 7: Beyond Noncompliance: Developing Evidence-Based Parent Training Interventions

Chapter 7 takes information from previous chapters on the empirical, conceptual, and practical foundations of training parents and integrates it into a framework for practitioners to address various child problems that the practitioner may encounter. The framework can be particularly valuable as a tool to guide practitioners when the literature does not provide empirically supported manuals and protocols to follow when treating problems other than noncompliance. Strategies learned in Part I for evaluating the scientific merit of research are used in developing parent training interventions to address more complex, unique, or health-related problems. In addition, information presented in chapter 4 on the conceptual foundations of parent training and chapter 5 on how to train parents are core components in developing interventions using the parent training framework described in this chapter. The chapter includes examples of applying this parent training framework to sleep, toileting, and feeding problems, as well as school behavior issues, academic challenges, and adolescent–parent conflict.

Chapter 8: Delivering Evidence-Based Parent Training: From Research to Practice

Chapter 8 covers additional practical issues in translating parent training research to everyday practice. In particular, key issues in examining the match between research and practice and implications for parent training are discussed. The chapter then outlines practical steps for integrating parent training into a problem-solving model of psychological service delivery. Parent training is then seen to fall within a larger process that includes conducting a comprehensive assessment, defining and then monitoring target behaviors, developing interventions, training parents, collecting data on parent adherence and child outcomes, and engaging in data-based decision making. Three case examples are provided to illustrate how these steps may be implemented in actual practice.

Chapter 9: Parent Training: Prevention and Future Research

The final chapter discusses the potential application of parent training to prevent child problems. It examines several promising prevention programs with parent training components. The chapter also examines current research trends with regard to parent training and identifies needed and promising directions for research important to future practice in parent training.

I

SEARCHING FOR THE BEST AVAILABLE EVIDENCE

1

PARENTING AND PARENT TRAINING

Although humans are likely social by nature, socialization also requires nurturing. As the human social milieu has increased in complexity because of increasing human numbers, decreasing resources, technological advances, and worldwide instantaneous communications capabilities, so, too, has the seeming complexity of raising children so that they will be successfully socialized. What constitutes successful or at least acceptable or sufficient socialization is difficult to define but is largely determined by an individual's immediate and extended family as well as the larger societal and cultural context within which the family lives. It is the community in which we live and work that determines whether we have been sufficiently socialized. The adults responsible for that care and socialization represent a diverse group. Extended family, teachers, clergy, physicians, and neighbors all have a role to play in helping children develop and learn. To varying degrees across sociocultural contexts, it is typically the biological mother and father of a child who are assigned the primary responsibility for his or her care and socialization. They are the parents. Sometimes, however, when the biological mother and father are incapable of providing these to the child, others may take on these responsibilities. For example, grandparents, aunts, uncles, and foster or adoptive parents may be legally, professionally, or communally charged with the parental care of a child. For our purposes, *parent* is used to refer to any adult charged as the primary person responsible for the socialization and care of a child. *Parenting* refers to the actions of parents that compose the socialization and care of a child.

The actions of parents that promote the socialization of children are referred to as *effective* parenting behaviors, whereas those actions by parents that delay or disrupt the socialization of children are *ineffective* parenting behaviors. Parents who demonstrate effective parenting behaviors or practices are more likely to have children considered to be well adapted, socially functioning adolescents and adults. However, ineffective parenting practices are predictive of delinquency, school failure, antisocial behavior, and adult psychopathology (Borkowski, Landesman Ramey, & Bristol-Power, 2002; Patterson, Reid, & Dishion, 1992; Wade, 2004). The circular or interdependent nature of this conceptualization of effective parenting is clear in that parenting practices are largely defined by their correlations with later child or adolescent and adult outcomes. For better or for worse, few of us can look back on our lives and say that our parents did not have some influence over who we are today. What is more difficult to determine is how exactly our parents influenced our development. This is a question that has captured the imagination of a vast and diverse number of individuals and scientists to the extent that the study of parents and parenting has almost evolved into a discipline in its own right (e.g., see Bornstein, 2002; Hoghughi & Long, 2004).

In fact, ideas about human behavior and particularly how parents treat or should treat children have been expressed through writings in religion, philosophy, law, and science throughout history (French, 2002). For example, some of the earliest known systematic theorizing about parenting and parent training occurred in the 4th century BC with Plato and Aristotle. In particular, Plato wrote that children begin to learn the concepts of right and wrong or good and evil in infancy through their subjective experiences of pain and pleasure and the associated events related to those experiences. As such, he believed it important that parents attend closely to the care of infants so that the child experienced pleasure in activities and behaviors that should be maintained over time (French, 2002). In addition, as children grew, Plato believed that their games and the socialization skills they learned during play were important to later governing abilities necessary for a stable state. He therefore advocated that parents be involved in structuring children's play activities to encourage the most positive or useful social traits (French, 2002).

To a large extent, early writings about principles of child development and parenting were based on philosophical or religious theory and opinion or matters of political law, but not science. Parenting advice throughout history was dominated primarily by philosophers, religious leaders, and physicians (Holden, 1997). With the advent of psychology as a science and as a discipline distinct from philosophy in the late 19th and early 20th centuries, more systematic study of parenting and recommendations for addressing child and parent problems began to occur. Psychology developed as a science of behavior and psychologists developed theories and literature on human behavior that directly affect how we study parenting. Theory and research in psychology have directly influenced current conceptualizations of and subsequent recommendations for what is considered effective parenting.

THEORIES OF HUMAN BEHAVIOR AND PARENTING

Theories in psychology, as well as science in general, help guide empirical and experimental studies and explain data and observations from these studies. Theories also provide explanation and guidance for psychological practice founded on scientific findings. Early psychological science was largely based on naturalistic observations of human behavior. These observations led to hypotheses and theories about how and why individuals do what they do. Theories about behavior abound in psychology, but several have dominated psychological science and practice.

The more dominant theories in psychology are now summarized with particular attention to how they informed scientific inquiry regarding parenting, child development, and parent training. It should be noted that the following descriptions of theories unavoidably provide superficial treatment of rich traditions in psychology. Each theoretical tradition has produced a large and complex literature related to the study of human behavior. We necessarily ignore many contributors and contributions within each theoretical tradition and highlight only some of the primary contributors and contributions specific to parenting and parent training.

Psychodynamic Theory

One of the first systematic theories of child development that included hypotheses regarding parenting effects is the psychodynamic theory developed by Sigmund Freud (1856–1939). Psychodynamic theory was proposed to describe the development of personality. Freud's theory of personality received immense early professional attention and has inspired much writing in the popular press over the years. The dynamic processes of ego, id, and superego integration proposed by Freud are still presented in many introductory psychology courses today.

Freud proposed a psychosexual stage theory of child development that had implications for child behavior and later adult dysfunction. According to this theory, an understanding of an individual's psychosexual stage of development, in conjunction with development of the ego, id, and superego dynamic processes, is facilitated by examination of an individual's relationship with his or her parents and other life events (Hall, 1979). The development of the superego, in particular, which is the moral compass of the personality, is proposed to be largely determined by the morals and values impressed on the child by his or her parents. For example, toilet training is said to occur during the anal stage of child development and to have potential implications for later adult functioning. A mother who is overly punitive may have a child who intentionally soils himself and grows up to be irresponsible and wasteful. A mother who is overly strict may have a child who grows up to be compulsively concerned with order or cleanliness (Hall, 1979). In essence, psychodynamic theory proposes that the development of the dynamic processes of the personality across the various stages of child development is largely determined by the child's interaction with parents.

Other theories regarding the role of parents in the development of a child's personality have evolved out of the psychodynamic tradition. For example, Alfred Adler (1870–1937) proposed that all human behavior is purposive and goal directed (Croake, 1983) and that children's problems result from feelings of inferiority with respect to their idealized goals. These feelings of inferiority are thought to be influenced by a child's physical limitations, family dynamics, and societal influences (Stein & Edwards, 1998). Children's problem behaviors are categorized as representing (a) attention getting, (b) power, (c) power with revenge, and (d) display of inadequacy (Croake, 1983). How a parent feels or responds when a child's problem behavior occurs determines how the child's behavior will be characterized. Corrective measures, such as the use of logical and natural consequences, are used to change how a parent responds to misbehavior (Croake, 1983). Adlerian theory has led to the development of one contemporary and popular approach to parenting called Systematic Training for Effective Parenting (Croake, 1983; Dinkmeyer & McKay, 1977; Stein & Edwards, 1998). This particular parent training program is discussed in more detail in chapter 3 of this volume.

Humanistic Theory

Humanism has been described by its proponents as the "third force" in psychology relative to psychoanalysis and behaviorism (discussed subsequently; Aanstoos, Serlin, & Greening, 2000). The major theorists involved in the founding of this approach were Abraham Maslow (1908–1970), Carl Rogers (1902–1987), and Rollo May (1909–1994; Aanstoos et al., 2000). There are five basic postulates of humanistic psychology:

1. Human beings, as human, are more than merely the sum of their parts. They cannot be reduced to component parts or functions.
2. Human beings exist in a uniquely human context, as well as in a cosmic ecology.

3. Human beings are aware and aware of being aware—that is, they are conscious. Human consciousness potentially includes an awareness of oneself in the context of other people and the cosmos.
4. Human beings have some choice, and with that, responsibility.
5. Human beings are intentional; aim at goals; are aware that they cause future events; and seek meaning, value, and creativity (Bugental, 1964, pp. 19–25, as cited in Aanstoos et al., 2000).

One practical implication derived from humanism centers on the notion that by creating a context of genuine acceptance and trust, a therapist may provide clients with the ability to solve their own problems. Although this approach to psychology has had minimal impact on theory and research regarding parenting and child development, the Parent Effectiveness Training program was developed out of this approach (Gordon, 1970). Further discussion of this program is provided in chapter 3 of this volume.

Developmental and Cognitive Theories

Freud's theory of personality development incorporates a view of childhood that includes stages of development or maturation and describes parental influences on children's developmental progression (Hall, 1979). Examination of parent behavior and child problems within a developmental perspective has continued this tradition. Developmental and cognitive theorists differ from early psychodynamic theorists in that the stages of child development represent differences in cognitive structures and cognitive or information processing, rather than psychodynamic conflicts.

Jean Piaget (1896–1980) was an early developmental theorist. On the basis of extensive observations of infants and young children, he extrapolated universal stages of intellectual development (Piaget, 1976). Piaget proposed that a child's development and maturation occurs naturally as the child actively interacts with his or her surroundings. Subsequently, children's behavior was thought to be largely determined by their level of maturation, cognitive processes, or both.

The developmental perspective has broadened considerably since Piaget and encompasses many diverse theories and research literatures (Holden, 1997; Lerner, Rothbaum, Boulos, & Castellino, 2002). A common aspect across many theories within a developmental and cognitive theoretical approach is the identification or development of hypothesized child characteristics, developmental stages, or cognitive constructs. These variables are correlated with parental characteristics, traits, behaviors, or attributes to identify possible relationships between child and parent variables.

Lev Vygotsky (1896–1934) postulated a specific heuristic to describe how a child's environment, including the parents, might affect a child's cognitive development (Wertsch, 1985). Vygotsky described a "zone of proximal development," meaning that a child's development is largely dependent on interaction with an environment that provides for small challenges in learning to promote cognitive development (Wertsch, 1985). Parents and teachers can be important agents in setting up an effective learning environment, or zone of proximal development, for children. Although this theory has been described as influential in subsequent developmental theories (Holden, 1997), specific mechanisms for how the environment or zone of proximal development interacts with the child to influence behavior and outcomes are not identified in this heuristic. Specific causative mechanisms for how parents and children interact and affect each others' behavior typically have not been explored experimentally in the child developmental and cognitive literature (Larzelere, 1999; Patterson & Fisher, 2002).

One theory that developed from the psychodynamic tradition but currently may be more consistent with the developmental and cognitive approach is attachment theory (Van Dijken, Van Der Veer, Van Ijzendoorn, & Kuipers, 1998). Attachment theory explores how parent behaviors affect child feelings of security, trust, efficacy, and subsequent child developmental outcomes related to successful socialization in adolescence and adulthood. Attachment theory stresses the importance of

> parental sensitivity and warmth in infancy and early childhood for shaping parent–child relationships in which both partners are invested in and committed to the relationship and to each other. Indeed, achieving such a relationship appears to be one of the most important goals of early socialization, not only because it fosters an early internalization of parental values, but because it smoothes the way for later socialization success (Teti & Candelaria, 2002, p. 165).

Likewise, the infant and child's behavior and temperament affect the parent or caregiver's behavior toward the child (Ainsworth & Bowlby, 1991). John Bowlby (1907–1990) was one of the originators of attachment theory. Theory about parent–child attachment has served to inform research and practical recommendations of at least one current parent training program, namely, Parent–Child Interaction Therapy (Eyberg & Boggs, 1998). This parent training program is discussed in more detail in chapter 2 of this volume.

Behavioral Theory

The psychodynamic and developmental–cognitive theoretical approaches to the study of human behavior infer that behavior is, in large part, a product of variables and processes internal to the child. Dynamic conflicts between the id and the ego, the development of cognitive structures, and information processing that occurs during particular stages of child maturation and during a child's active interaction with the environment are examples of variables or processes that occur largely unseen within the child. Although the child's behavior or interaction with the environment is proposed to affect the development of internal cognitive structures or dynamic processes, the emphasis of research and literature within these theoretical traditions is largely on the internal child variables. Within these explanatory frameworks for human behavior, there is an active hypothesized internal variable that resides within the individual and is necessary to explain his or her behavior.

Relative to the other theoretical approaches, behaviorism emphasizes the study of environmental variables as causes of behavior. Behaviorism is a philosophy of science, or an approach to the study of human behavior, that seeks to understand and explain behavior by examining the *interaction* between an individual and his or her environment. B. F. Skinner (1904–1990) is the most well-known scientist associated with this approach to human behavior. From a behavioral perspective, internal variables related to cognitive processes or emotions are included in the study of behavior. The term *behavior* encompasses not just observable motor responses but also cognitive and emotional responses. In other words, cognitions, cognitive processes, and emotions are dependent variables, or things to be studied, not necessarily independent variables, or causes of other behavior (Skinner, 1953, 1974). It is the interaction between the individual and his or her environment that is the object of study in explaining human behavior, not internal processes.

The implication of a behavioral approach for studying parenting is that the researcher or practitioner is interested in parent behaviors and environmental events that affect child behavior. Likewise, if one is studying parent behavior, then the practitioner or researcher would be interested in child behaviors and environmental events that affect parent behavior. If one is interested in why a parent has a particular belief about child rearing, then the behavioral researcher would look to that parent's learning history and the contingencies in the parent's environment that shaped and maintain that belief. The term *contingency* is defined by environmental variables that function to affect human behavior. A contingency exists when the occurrence of an event is dependent on the occurrence of another event.

Behavioral contingencies may be further defined as contingencies of reinforcement or punishment depending on whether behavior is seen to increase or decrease respective to an observed contingency between the behavior and environmental event. A learning history is an individual's respective history of interaction with his or her specific environment. Environmental variables that interact and function to affect human behavior are difficult to identify, and a behavioral approach to the study of human behavior tends to focus on reliable and accurate measurable behavior and environmental events (Johnston & Pennypacker, 1993).

Behaviorism, as a philosophy of science, has developed two overlapping research traditions: experimental analysis of behavior and applied analysis of behavior. The former has identified specific principles of behavior that describe or explain the effects of the environment on human behavior; the latter seeks to understand, describe, and demonstrate the application of principles of behavior in natural human situations. Principles regarding contingencies of reinforcement (Ferster & Skinner, 1957) are particularly well developed in this theoretical and research approach, and it is this approach that has led most directly to development of effective parent training programs, as described in greater detail throughout this book. Although largely overshadowed by developmental and cognitive approaches, behavioral theory and research continues as a strong vein within psychological science (Friman, Allen, Kerwin, & Larzelere, 1993). Other, more recent theories of human behavior such as social learning, ecological, and cognitive–behavioral theories largely developed from a behavioral approach to the study of human behavior.

RESEARCH ON PARENTING

All of the theoretical approaches briefly presented in this section acknowledge the importance of parenting on child development. However, each theoretical tradition emphasizes a different aspect of child development and has different basic assumptions about human behavior and how parents may influence children. For example, behavioral approaches have tended to focus on observable behavior and behavior–environment relations to describe parenting. However, psychodynamic, humanistic, and developmental–cognitive theories have tended to rely heavily on a large number of inferred constructs to describe and explain how people parent. Constructs are labels used to describe categories, groups, or classes of behavior. Indeed, the appeal to constructs is a mainstay of many areas of psychological theory and has been a driving force in much of the research on parenting. For example, since the 1930s more than 30 parent traits or characteristics and attributes have been created by researchers (Holden, 1997).

Parenting Attributes, Characteristics, and Styles

Much of the early research on parenting has attempted to label or categorize classes or groups of parent behaviors that appear to have similar effects or are correlated with specific child outcomes. These constructs have been labeled as attributes or characteristics of the parent, such as intelligence, health, education, or inclination to substance abuse. These attributes are often considered to be a part of the parent's biological or personality makeup. These parent characteristics or attributes typically fall along a continuum but are often categorized for research purposes. Correlations with child outcomes between various categories of parents presenting with these attributes are examined in much of the parenting research to date. As might be expected, parents with lower intellectual ability, substance abuse problems, and physical or mental health problems are more likely to have children with poor outcomes (Conley, Caldwell, Flynn, Dupre, & Rudolph, 2004).

Parenting style also represents a construct that describes a class or grouping of parenting behaviors that are given a categorical name. Here the focus is less on describing the parent and more about describing parent behaviors. Perhaps the most well-known parenting styles are the authoritarian, authoritative, and permissive categories (Baumrind, 1971). These are defined along a continuum of nurturance and control behaviors that parents exhibit toward their children. These styles are then correlated with various types of child outcomes. Better child outcomes are typically correlated positively with the authoritative parent who demonstrates a high and balanced degree of control and nurturance toward a child (Holden, 1997; Teti & Candelaria, 2002). The permissive parenting style has been further delineated to include a permissive–indulgent parenting style and a permissive–negligent parenting style. Children of parents rated as demonstrating a permissive–negligent style appear to have the worst outcomes (Teti & Candelaria, 2002).

More recent research on parenting style has addressed parent responsiveness. Responsiveness has been defined as the degree to which a parent responds with positive regard to a child's positive behavior (Patterson & Fisher, 2002). Exploration of parent responsiveness has resulted in an interesting coalescing of two theoretical approaches in psychology, behavioral and developmental. Behavioral theory and research on principles of reinforcement would predict that positive parent responses to positive infant behaviors would increase the probability of continued positive child behavior, as well as positive child socialization. Developmental theory also stresses the importance of parental sensitivity and warmth (i.e., responsiveness) with respect to attachment (e.g., see Teti & Candelaria, 2002). Both are reminiscent of Plato's ancient proposal that parents should attend closely to the care of infants so that they may be responsive to appropriate child behavior.

Environmental Variables

Although much of the research in psychology has explored parent characteristics, environmental variables have certainly not been ignored. All of the theoretical approaches to the study of human behavior and parenting acknowledge the role of the environment on human behavior and parenting and child development, although to differing degrees.

The concept of environment is exceedingly broad and complex, and research on the effect of the environment on parenting encompasses a number of potential variables (Bradley, 2002). For purposes of this chapter, research on environmental variables and parenting is categorized on the basis of the level of direct influence that environmental variables might be hypothesized to have on parent and child behavior (e.g., see Bronfenbrenner, 1986). Research is described under the categories of sociocultural variables, family variables, and variables specific in direct parent–child interaction.

Sociocultural Variables

Sociocultural aspects of the environment refer to variables such as culture, ethnicity, socioeconomic status, educational attainment, religion, and community setting (e.g., rural, urban). These variables describe where families live, the resources that are available to them, opportunities for employment, type of employment, and educational attainment. They are hypothesized to have a distal or indirect effect on parent or child behavior (or both).

The effects of variables specific to culture, ethnicity, socioeconomic status (SES), and religion on parenting style and practice have been examined (Frosh, 2004; Harkness & Super, 2002; Hoff, Laursen, & Tardif, 2002; Puckering, 2004; see also chap. 5, this volume). For example, parents in higher SES homes have been found to be more likely to demonstrate an authoritative parenting style relative to parents in low SES homes, who are more likely to use an authoritarian parenting style. Also, parents in higher SES homes engage in more verbal interaction with their children relative to parents in lower SES homes. Finally, high SES parents' verbal interactions with their children contain more conversation and less directive comments relative to parents in lower SES homes (Hoff et al., 2002). Sociocultural variables may help predict certain types of parenting practices (e.g., see Bradley, 2002; Pachter & Dumont-Mathieu, 2004), and some are correlated with children's development (Hart & Risley, 1995). Further discussion of cultural issues and parenting and parent training is provided in chapter 6 of this volume.

Family Variables

Family variables include aspects of the structure of the family, such as whether the family is headed by a single parent or a married couple. Family variables can include the size of the family or the inclusion and involvement of extended family members, such as aunts, uncles, or grandparents. Family variables may also include family types such as same gender parents or foster parents.

There is overlap with sociocultural variables and family variables, but family variables seem likely to have a more direct influence on parent and child behavior and interaction. Parents' marital status (Weinraub, Horvath, & Gringlas, 2002), family size (Bradley, 2002), involvement of extended family (Smith & Drew, 2002), and the type of family (e.g., foster parents; Haugaard & Hazan, 2002) are all examples of family variables that can affect parenting and child outcomes. For example, it is more difficult for a single parent, usually a mother, to provide as much verbal interaction and parental monitoring as may be found in a two-parent family. A single parent has fewer opportunities relative to two parents to interact with a child. Likewise, a single-parent family will be more likely to have lower economic status, which will affect financial resources that can be devoted to child development and learning. Cultural variables may influence family dynamics, and there may be higher prevalence of mother-headed single-parent households in some cultures relative to others.

Parent–Child Interaction

Not only sociocultural and family variables but also the parent–child interactions have a significant impact on parenting (Wahler & Hann, 1986). Researchers investigating parent–child interactions have largely examined how parents directly affect child behavior, but researchers are also beginning to examine how children affect parental behavior (Patterson & Fisher, 2002). Much of the research on parent–child interaction has occurred within a behavioral framework (Patterson, Reid, & Dishion, 1992; J. B. Reid, Patterson, & Snyder, 2002; Wahler & Hann, 1986). In particular, mechanisms of human behavior specific to contingencies of reinforcement have been explored as causal variables in parent–child interaction. With consideration for ecological and family variables, as well as parent and child characteristics, it is the behavioral research on parent–child interaction that most directly forms the empirical basis for parent training. Application of behavioral research to parent training is described in the section on the history of parent training, and the principles of human behavior specific to parenting and parent–child interaction are discussed in more detail in chapter 4 of this volume.

HISTORY OF PARENT TRAINING

Psychology began emerging as a scientific discipline that incorporated systematic theory and research in the latter half of the 19th century and early 20th century. As psychology developed as a scientific discipline, it also began to inform the work of practitioners working with children and families. These practitioners often were medical professionals or social workers. Psychology as a distinct profession applied for the benefit of children, adults, and families began to emerge at this time.

The first psychology clinic for children in the United States was started by Lightner Witmer at the University of Pennsylvania in 1896. The clinic provided services for children with learning and behavioral difficulties and their families. There was a substantial emphasis on working with teachers and schools to improve children's education, particularly children with disabilities. In addition, the clinic worked with parents to assist with child problems at home. The clinic was a training ground for students interested in applied psychology (Levine & Levine, 1992). This psychological training and service clinic led to the development of other university-based psychology clinics. Similar university-based clinics are in operation today where many psychologists, counselors, and social workers receive their training.

There was increased attention in the early 20th century within the federal government and local and national social agencies to the idea that problems in childhood may progress to even more severe problems in adulthood. As such, an increased awareness of the need to treat child problems early to prevent later problems emerged. This recognition that mental illness and maladjustment in children may be treated and perhaps even prevented led to the creation of child guidance clinics as part of the Commonwealth Fund's Program for the Prevention of Delinquency in 1922. These clinics were created to treat mild behavior and emotional problems in school-age children of normal intelligence (Horn, 1989). Throughout the next several decades, child guidance clinics were opened throughout the country to provide psychological, social, and health services to children and their families (Horn, 1989; VandenBos, Cummings, & DeLeon, 1992). In addition to the university-based and child guidance clinics, psychologists were also beginning to work in residential and in-patient facilities and start their own private practices (VandenBos et al., 1992).

The importance of the family and the school system were clearly acknowledged in early efforts to provide psychological services to children. Witmer worked extensively with parents and schools (Levine & Levine, 1992). Adolf Meyer, a well-known psychiatrist and a member of the National Committee on Mental Hygiene, recommended in 1922 that psychiatrists be placed in school systems to work with teachers to prevent child problems (Donohue, Hersen, & Ammerman, 2000). Social workers in the child guidance clinics also typically worked with parents and schools in efforts to solve child problems (Horn, 1989). However, although there was emphasis on working with parents to help address child issues, there was little or no systematic training provided to them. Rather, parents largely received advice or information about child development and education.

The theoretical influences on psychological practice at that time were primarily early behavioral and psychodynamic theories. Neither behavioral nor psychodynamic approaches had yet acquired an empirical database of treatment techniques that could be shown to be effective in remediating or preventing child problems. Psychoanalysts, however, were publishing case studies of work with children and adults, and over time, psychoanalytic approaches to treating children and families became most common in practice (Donohue et al., 2000; Horn, 1989; VandenBos et al., 1992). The psychoanalytic approach to treating child problems acknowledged the role parents play in child development and involved parents in the treatment process (e.g., see Freud, 1909/1955). However, much of the treatment focused on working directly with the child to bring unconscious psychodynamic conflicts into consciousness, often through the use of drawing, art, and play therapy techniques (Donohue et al., 2000). As before, parents may have been provided information and advice, but they did not receive systematic training in specific parenting skills or treatment to help their children. Although not necessarily psychoanalytically based, this child-focused approach to the psychological treatment of children is still common today.

After decades of providing psychological services for children and their families, there was still a dearth of scientific evidence to support the efficacy of psychoanalytic and play therapy approaches to treating child problems. Although parents reported that their children appeared to have improved, there were no direct observations of child behavior. Later, observations of child behavior conducted in home settings revealed no differences pre- and posttreatment in child behavior following traditional psychoanalytic or play therapy (e.g., see Patterson & Narrett, 1990).

At the same time, behavior theory was becoming more sophisticated in explaining how environmental contingencies could shape animal and human behavior. Application of behavioral theory to the psychological treatment of child problems indicated that manipulation of environmental variables could be useful in changing child behavior. Although it had long been acknowledged but not yet carefully or systematically examined, parents were thought to be the key environmental variable in treating child problems. However, changing parent behavior to have a positive impact on child behavior required better understanding of how parents affect child development and outcomes.

In the early 1960s researchers and clinicians at several university centers in the United States, notably Gerald Patterson and his colleagues at the University of Oregon, began to study parent–child interaction and, at the same time, to develop treatment programs for child behavior problems; these programs were primarily based on training parents to change child behavior. Patterson and colleagues began to conduct home observations in an attempt to determine which variables might be maintaining oppositional and aggressive child behavior (R. R. Jones, Reid, & Patterson, 1975). They initially hypothesized that parental attention or access to preferred items and activities could positively reinforce negative child behavior (J. B. Reid, Patterson, & Snyder, 2002). Over time, however, they realized that many parent–child interactions were best represented by a model of negative reinforcement in which escalating negative behavior of both the parent and the child is reinforced by escaping the demands the other has imposed. Patterson and colleagues described this as a "coercive cycle" and used this as a core concept in a complex and comprehensive research-based theory of problematic parent–child interaction (Patterson, 1982; see also chap. 4, this volume).

During the 1970s and 1980s parent training for the purpose of providing treatment for child problems began to be more systematically developed. Researchers and clinicians at university clinics developed specific treatment manuals for parent training based on an empirical foundation of systematic research rooted in behavior theory (Hembree-Kigin & McNeil, 1995; McMahon & Forehand, 2003; Patterson, Reid, Jones, & Conger, 1975; Webster-Stratton, 1992). These empirically supported parent training programs are reviewed in detail in chapter 2 of this volume. Parent training was initially developed to treat child problems of noncompliance, oppositional behavior, tantrums, and aggression, and thus it has been evaluated as a specific treatment for child conduct concerns (Brestan & Eyberg, 1998; Patterson, 1979).

Given that the bulk of attention and empirical support for parent training has addressed child problems of noncompliance, it has sometimes been referred to as a "treatment" for noncompliance and conduct problems (Biglan, Mrazek, Carnine, & Flay, 2003; Brestan & Eyberg, 1998; Kumpfer, 1999). This is partially true. Parents are an essential part of the treatment for child noncompliance through parent training. They are taught specific skills, and implementation of these constitutes treatment. Together with the practitioner, parents are the behavior change agents. As such, parent training may also be described as a service delivery model. This is an *indirect* service delivery in that the practitioner trains parents to apply treatment to children (Shriver, 1998). This method of service delivery stands in contrast to a *direct* service delivery model in which practitioners work directly with children to deliver treatment components. As an indirect service delivery model, parents may be trained to provide treatment for a variety of child problems beyond child noncompliance and conduct disorders (Briesmeister & Schaefer, 1998). In a parent training service delivery model, changing parent behavior becomes a primary target of the practitioner's treatment of child problems.

More recently, it has been recognized that there are a substantial number of parents who either could not or did not want to follow through with this type of treatment approach. Mothers with depression, parents of lower socioeconomic status, single parents, parents with lower cognitive skills, and those with marital problems have difficulty adhering to treatment recommendations in parent training (Chamberlain & Baldwin, 1988; McMahon, 1999). In the 1980s and 1990s, clinical researchers in parent training began to examine the addition of adjunctive treatments combined with parent training to improve success for treatment of child behavior problems (McMahon & Forehand, 2003). These treatments often address parent-specific problems to reduce barriers to success in parent training. These expanded parent training approaches have been termed *behavioral family interventions* because they incorporate a package of behavioral interventions that may be tailored for use with an individual family to improve its functioning (Sanders & Dadds, 1993). The core of most of these interventions remains parent training. The research for behavioral family interventions is relatively recent but appears promising at this time.

SUMMARY

Parenting is an essential aspect of effective child socialization, and the fact that parents have an effect on child development and behavior is indisputable. Parenting is a complex topic that can encompass a wide range of skills, behaviors, attitudes, cognitions, and emotions. Theories and research on the topic of parenting can be overwhelming at first glance. For practitioners who wish to make sense of this literature so that they can have an immediate and direct impact on child behavior, turning the focus to parent training makes sense. It is in this literature that practitioners can find both the principles and the procedures that describe how positively and effectively to teach parents to change child behavior.

The therapeutic techniques and principles of parent training were largely derived from behavioral theory and research that was developing in the mid-20th century. Several teams of clinical researchers developed parent training programs that now have extensive empirical support. These parent training programs, or components of them, are now beginning to be incorporated into larger treatment packages to address family concerns beyond child compliance and to prevent future child problems. For the practitioner interested in an evidence-based practice that includes parent training, a clear understanding of these empirically supported parent training programs is necessary. In the next chapter, we review these programs.

2

EMPIRICALLY SUPPORTED PARENT TRAINING PROGRAMS

A competent practitioner interested in an evidence-based practice in parent training begins with a review of the best available research. Doing so promotes effective practice, improves patient outcomes, and enhances public health (American Psychological Association, 2005). However, evaluating the best available research in parent training is not as easy as it might seem. The process begins with a search for empirical support in peer-reviewed published research that focuses on the training of parents with children who have behavior problems. Not all outcome studies are the same, however, and *empirically supported* can be defined in many ways.

There has been a significant amount of effort devoted to defining what good empirical support looks like, but the standards vary among professional organizations. Scholars from professional organizations such as the Institute of Medicine (Mrazek & Haggerty, 1994), the American Psychological Association (Chambless & Hollon, 1998), and the U.S. Department of Justice (e.g., see Kumpfer, 1999) have all weighed in on the discussion. How good does empirical support need to be? Although there is no consensus standard, empirically supported interventions, treatments, or programs have generally been defined as those that have been shown to have a significant impact in two or more well-designed, randomized, controlled trials or in three or more interrupted time-series experiments (e.g., see Chambless & Hollon, 1998). This level of evidence offers the practitioner confidence that the effects found in any one study are representative and "real." In addition, empirically supported interventions are typically required to have been described and standardized in treatment manuals that specify what is to be done in each session and how many sessions should be implemented. Finally, the research must have been conducted by two or more independent investigators (Biglan, Mrazek, Carnine, & Flay, 2003), which provides the practitioner with some confidence that the program's efficacy is not dependent on it being implemented by one specific scientist or research team.

Programs that meet these criteria are often described by terms such as *empirically supported* or *well-established,* or even *exemplary.* Some organizations have begun generating their own lists of parent training programs that meet the most rigorous criteria (e.g., see Brestan & Eyberg, 1998), and practitioners can refer to these lists to expedite the process of identifying the best available research. However, these lists can become dated as new research is published, and it is important for practitioners not to rely on published lists alone. As a result, our interest centers on parent training programs that meet the criteria of empirically supported programs both by their inclusion in published lists of empirically supported parent training programs and by our own review of published research and use of the criteria for "empirically supported" described earlier. These empirical reviews are included in each of the program descriptions that follow.

In reviews of the treatment literature for children with behavior problems, four parent training programs consistently stand out as meeting the criteria for empirical support (see Table 2.1). First, Patterson's Living With Children program (Patterson, 1976) is the oldest of the parent training programs. It is designed primarily to teach individual families basic operant principles of behavior change and how to use these in the home. Living With Children, as pioneered by Patterson and his colleagues at the Oregon Research Institute, is backed by extensive research and has been judged to have a robust effect on parent and child behavior (Brestan & Eyberg, 1998).

Second, Webster-Stratton's The Incredible Years (Webster-Stratton, 1984) is a group-based parent training program that relies on videotaped mod-

TABLE 2.1
Empirically Supported Parent Training Programs

Program name	Principal developer(s)	Year
Living With Children	Gerald Patterson	1968
The Incredible Years	Carolyn Webster-Stratton	1984
Helping the Noncompliant Child	Rex Forehand and Robert McMahon	1981
Parent–Child Interaction Therapy	Sheila Eyberg	1982

eling and therapist-led discussions about the videotapes. It also has an extensive research base and is part of a family prevention and intervention program that is considered exemplary by the U.S. Department of Justice (Kumpfer, 1999).

Finally, the third and fourth programs described are McMahon and Forehand's (2003) Helping the Noncompliant Child, also considered exemplary by the U.S. Department of Justice (Kumpfer, 1999), and Eyberg's Parent–Child Interaction Therapy (Hembree-Kigin & McNeil, 1995). Although Eyberg's program was originally identified as falling just short of the empirically supported criteria when reviewed earlier (Brestan & Eyberg, 1998), recent publications by independent researchers have established it as an empirically supported parent training program. These last two parent training programs emphasize individualized skill teaching in interactions between parents and children. Both programs have been investigated extensively in well-designed research studies, have easily accessible treatment manuals, and offer what are considered to be effective skills training approaches in the prevention and treatment of problem behaviors (Kumpfer & Alvarado, 2003).

These four empirically supported programs represent the best available research in parent training. As a result, our discussion of programs that practitioners should consider for use in their work settings focuses on describing and reviewing these programs. Of course, this list should not replace a practitioner's own decisions about what is most appropriate for an individual family or situation. Even though these programs all offer manuals that guide implementation of treatment, evidence-based practice requires more than slavish adherence to treatment manuals. It requires that clinical expertise is integrated with the best available research to allow flexibility and adaptation to the unique requirements of each situation. One of the dangers of treatment manuals is that the programs they describe have the potential to become hammers in the hands of those who see every child disruptive behavior problem as a nail. Thus, in subsequent chapters, we address how to integrate clinical expertise and when and whether it is appropriate to adapt or flex published research programs to meet situational needs.

What follows is a descriptive overview of each of the four empirically supported parent training programs, including their history, the populations they have served, and the length and structure of the intervention. The unique features of each program are highlighted. Specific program components are described, emphasizing what skills are taught and how best to teach them. Finally, the empirical support for each program is reviewed, as are the more recent research activities associated with the program.

LIVING WITH CHILDREN

Gerald Patterson (1976), a founder of the Oregon Social Learning Center (OSLC), is widely recognized for his original work related to exploring how coercive family processes influence child behavior problems. He and his associates from the Oregon Research Institute (ORI) helped pioneer behavioral parent training in the late 1960s and early 1970s. At that time, strategies regarding how parents could or should be used effectively as agents of change for children with conduct problems had not been empirically developed. However, extensive observational data collected in the natural home settings of disruptive children by the clinicians at ORI demonstrated that the ways in which parents respond to disruptive behavior have a significant influence on that behavior. Indeed, their observations defined a *coercive* process in which some child problem behaviors were learned through inadvertent modeling and reinforcement by parents. Furthermore, they found that, over time, parents and children inadvertently reinforced each other for escalating cycles of intense and noxious behavior (see chap. 4, this volume, for more details on this process).

Perhaps most important, Patterson and his colleagues conducted treatment research that began showing that parents could be taught to track important behavior and consistently deliver consequences that would reinforce more appropriate behavior. By combining reinforcement for appropriate behavior with punishment for inappropriate behavior, parents could produce positive changes in the problem child's behavior with corresponding improvements in parental perceptions of their children.

Although Patterson and colleagues' is the first parent training program, theirs is the most difficult to clearly describe. By all accounts, the Living With Children parent training program that came out of the ORI was never intended to be a treatment package that would be disseminated in a "cookbook" fashion. The ORI scientists were interested in disseminating the basic notion that parents could and should be trained in understanding and applying basic behavioral technology. However, disseminating a specific program manual of standard procedures was not a priority. The developers did publish a practitioner manual in 1975, describing the procedures that were used in the early research (Patterson, Reid, Jones, & Conger, 1975), but it was never revised or published for general dissemination. It can still be accessed with some difficulty, but the authors themselves considered the program to be a work in progress—little more than a snapshot of the treatment process. Patterson and his associates appeared to have a strong sense that standard procedures were rather limited in their applicability. Indeed, they wrote that the successful practitioner must be innovative with the standard procedures (Patterson et al., 1975, p. 80). Even recent reviews of the program by contemporary OSLC researchers emphasize that the parent training program is flexible in format (Forgatch & Martinez, 1999). In fact, they provide no specific descriptions of the actual intervention procedures other than general acknowledgment that parents are taught through instruction, role-play, and homework to respond contingently to their child's behavior.

The program "manuals" appear to be the parent guidebooks that have been published over the years. First published by Patterson in 1968 (and revised in 1976), *Living With Children: New Methods for Parents and Teachers* served primarily as a primer of basic behavior principles while providing basic guidance for parents on how to implement behavior programs. However, it provided no specific guidance to practitioners about how to train parents. A gradual evolution and refinement of this original book can be seen in the publication of *Families* (Patterson, 1975) and *Parents and Adolescents: Living Together* (Forgatch & Patterson, 1987, 2005; Patterson & Forgatch, 1987, 2005), but these, too, are parent guidebooks, not practitioner manuals. As a result, some aspects of current parent training program implementation remain elusive. Nevertheless, the core elements of the program can be clearly identified, and the evidence to support it is rather substantial.

Program Specifics

Target Population

Children who were included in the original studies were typically between ages 3 and 14 years, referred for significant "social aggression." *Social aggression* was defined as behavior that included noncompliance, temper tantrums, crying, arguing, hitting, teasing, and stealing.

Treatment Setting

The treatment was typically delivered with individual families in a clinic setting, but some of the early research also provided individual consultation in a group format. Parents were typically contacted before the initial sessions to ensure that home observations and frequent telephone contact were acceptable.

Program Materials

The practitioner manual, *A Social Learning Approach to Family Intervention*, was published in 1975 (Patterson et al., 1975). It has not been revised since then and is not currently in print. The manual includes appendices that contain the original referral form used during the initial parent interview to gather basic information about family demographics, past treatment efforts, and description of the current problem. There is a referral problem checklist included in the form to identify potential problems ranging from whining, pouting, and irritability to fire setting, stealing, and destructiveness. The manual also includes several checklists to assess parent perceptions of the quality and frequency of various potential problem behaviors. These forms guide practitioners in conducting assessment phone calls with parents, who are asked to report daily (using the Parent Daily Report form) on the frequency of problem behaviors in baseline during treatment and at follow-up. Finally, the manual includes forms to remind the practitioner of critical elements to include during treatment sessions and to assist the practitioner and parents in setting up point systems and behavior contracts.

In addition to the manual, the treatment program relied heavily on the use of a guidebook for parents to read before practitioner-led sessions began. The book, *Living With Children* (Patterson, 1976), was first published in 1968 and then revised, most recently in 1976. It includes chapters on basic concepts of learning and on specific strategies for managing problems such as noncompliance, teasing, stealing, whining, toileting, and bed-wetting. An appendix includes a simple sample of a "star chart" that could be used as part of a reinforcement program for young children. Patterson published *Families* in 1975 in an effort to provide more details about child management. Then, along with Forgatch, he published the two-part *Parents and Adolescents: Living Together* in 1987 (revised in 2005). These two parent books provide information about specific behavioral principles and management techniques and the steps to successful implementation with adolescents, including numerous charts and examples. However, the original supporting research relied primarily on the *Living With Children* book, which is the focus here.

Program Length

The program typically began with a 90-minute intake session and then was followed by 6 to 10 brief 25-minute observations in the home over a 2-week period to establish baseline rates of problem behaviors. In the manual, the authors emphasize that the initial assessment and Parent Daily Reports are helpful but often not representative of actual behavior in the home, especially after treatment completion, so in-home observations are important. The manual and the supporting research are unclear about the number of treatment sessions that are required after treatment begins, apparently averaging about 12 sessions across anywhere from 5 to 12 weeks. The practitioner can reportedly expect to average more than 30 hours in direct contact with parents during treatment, excluding home observations during baseline and intervention.

Program Content (What to Teach)

At the heart of this program is the *Living With Children* (Patterson, 1976) book, which provides an introductory course for parents in behavioral theory and contingency management. The authors discuss how children and parents learn, emphasizing the importance of consequences and how they can be used to change behavior in a positive way. Parents are taught to view themselves as agents of that change.

Parents first learn the importance of observing and counting behaviors and selecting behaviors for intervention. They then learn about the importance of rewarding more appropriate ways of behaving using both social (e.g., praise) and nonsocial (e.g., privileges) reinforcers. Point systems, also called token reinforcement programs, in which children earn points that are later exchanged for nonsocial privileges, activities, and prizes are emphasized as effective ways to reinforce appropriate behavior. Point systems are encouraged on the basis of evidence that children with a history of coercive interactions with parents are often not as responsive to social reinforcers.

Finally, parents read about how to use discipline in the form of response cost (i.e., loss of points) and time-out for problem behaviors. The book contains numerous examples of scenarios in which various parenting skills are used, and it includes, in the appendix, a sample of what a point system chart might look like. The premise of the book is that after parents understand the basic principles of changing behavior, they will eventually be able to design their own programs when problems arise. Assistance with applying the principles that have been learned is provided in the form of specific program recommendations for how to deal with 10 problems (e.g., noncompliance, teasing, toilet training, tantrums, stealing).

Before any teaching begins, the practitioner conducts an initial intake to identify problem behaviors, using the referral form and checklists provided in the manual. The practitioner then confirms conclusions about potential behaviors to target with follow-up observations in the home and with separate phone assessments in which parents report on pretreatment frequencies of problem behaviors. The practitioner then teaches parents a "pinpointing" process in which parents learn to select specific behaviors and then observe and count them daily.

After parents have pinpointed specific behaviors to target, they are taught how to develop a contingency contract that specifies the rewards and punishments a child will experience for two or three selected (i.e., pinpointed) behaviors. The behavior contract typically involves children earning or losing points that can later be traded for rewards. For example, parents might pinpoint "asking before going outside," "completing chores," and "hitting" as target behaviors. Their child might be rewarded with 3 points each time he or she asks before going outside and 5 points for successful completion of each chore each day, whereas their child might lose 5 points each time he or she hits. The practitioner works with the parent and the child together to develop a list of "backup" rewards and their assigned point value, such as staying up 30 minutes late (10 points), choosing a special snack (7 points), or 15 minutes of computer games (5 points). These elements are recorded in a formal, written contract that specifies the behaviors targeted, points earned or lost for each behavior, the backup reinforcers that will be available, and the cost, in points, of each reinforcer. Parents are taught how to deliver points using labeled praise, eye contact, and enthusiasm, as well as how to label problem behaviors and remove points as required by the program. Charts are used for tracking behaviors and the points that have been earned or lost (see Exhibit 2.1).

Parents are also taught "time-out" from positive reinforcement, typically meaning isolation from people and fun things to do. Time-out is used in addition to point losses required by the contingency contract and is used for only one or two problem behaviors. The authors recommend using a bathroom as the location in which a time-out is served and not using a chair in the corner or hallway. Time-outs are recommended to be brief (2–3 minutes); however, parents are taught to enforce going to time-out with the addition of more time in 5-minute increments up to 30 minutes. Following 30 minutes of time-out, parents remove a privilege.

Although the program specifically teaches parents to use contingent punishment of target behaviors such as point losses and time-out, the emphasis of the program is on reinforcing appropriate behavior and keeping rewards small and immediate. Subsequent sessions involve pinpointing new target behaviors for addition to the token reinforcement program.

Program Content (How to Teach)

In the practitioner manual, the authors describe step-by-step guidelines for conducting assessment and therapy sessions and for teaching parents effective child management skills. The program is designed primarily to be implemented in individual sessions with parents and their children. Perhaps it is not surprising that practitioners are encouraged to use contingency management to promote behavior change in parents. Indeed, there is heavy reliance on delivering treatment components contingently. From the outset, parents

EXHIBIT 2.1
Sample Point Chart

Name: William	Dates: 8/7–8/14						
Behaviors	Mon	Tues	Wed	Thurs	Fri	Sat	Sun
Asks to go out (3)	3, 3	3	0	3, 3			
Does two chores (5 points each)	10	10	10	5			
Hits (−5)	No	−5	No	No			
Totals	16	8	10	11			

Menu: May stay up 30 minutes late (10 points), special snack (7 points), 15 minutes of computer time (5 points)

are required to read *Living With Children* (Patterson, 1976) before scheduling of the next appointment. On arrival at the next session, a test is given to verify that parents have read and understand the basic principles of contingency management before treatment can proceed.

To help parents make difficult changes, practitioners are encouraged to use prompts and cues, such as wrist counters, to assist with recording behavior. Practitioners are also asked to provide daily phone contact to prompt parents to observe and record behavior. The use of the Parent Daily Report helps prompt practitioners to assess child progress and helps parents to monitor child behavior.

In session, parent training involves well-established teaching strategies that include instruction, modeling role-playing, and feedback. Practitioners model and role-play how to set up and implement contracts with children, and they are prompted by the manual to use specific scripts to describe things to parents. The manual prompts practitioners initially to maintain daily phone contact, in addition to the Parent Daily Report, to enhance adherence and improve the quality of implementation. It is suggested that practitioners phone parents 3 days a week throughout treatment and weekly during a 6-month follow-up posttreatment.

The manual recommends that practitioners assume that the program will always work if implemented properly and that any program failure is linked to poor parental implementation (i.e., treatment resistance). Practitioners are cautioned that parents will reinterpret, misunderstand, or simply not comply with program requirements and that it is the job of the practitioner to develop contingencies necessary to change parent behavior. The manual recommends praising parents more for successes relative to corrective feedback for failures, using videotapes of parent–child interactions to guide the provision of feedback, asking the child to report on how the program is being implemented, and working to recruit each parent to monitor and provide feedback to the other parent regarding implementation of program components. Finally, practitioners are provided with examples of how to set up behavior contracts addressing marital conflict and how to address school-based social and academic problems.

Unique Program Features

Compared with the other three programs reviewed in this chapter, the Living With Children program places a much stronger emphasis on teaching parents to understand the behavior theory behind the techniques, requiring parents to read the *Living With Children* (Patterson, 1976) book before treatment can begin. Underlying this emphasis is the notion that parents who understand the basic principles of behavior change may be able to develop their own programs in response to new problems. In addition, parents who understand the basic principles of behavior change may be better equipped to modify behavior change techniques when the techniques are not working well. For example, if a parent understands that immediate reinforcement is more potent than delayed reinforcement, a point that is emphasized in the *Living With Children* book, then parents may deduce, when a point system flounders, that allowing their child to exchange points twice a day rather than at the end of the day might strengthen the program and improve the outcome. Finally, parents who can apply basic principles may be more likely to develop an appropriate response to any problem behavior that arises, even if related to children who were not originally targeted in treatment. Although there have been independent investigations suggesting possible merit to this approach (e.g., see Glogower & Sloop, 1976), it is not a widely used practice in the other empirically supported parent training programs.

The Living With Children program also places relatively greater emphasis on parents observing and recording child behavior compared with the other parent training programs reviewed in this chapter. The program places a strong emphasis on this aspect of behavior change because (a) some change occurs simply by virtue of observing and counting; (b) behavior change is slow, and observation helps to delineate small changes; and (c) it prompts parents to respond consistently to behaviors that have been pinpointed. The program not only emphasizes teaching parents to observe and count, there is considerable emphasis on helping the practitioner know how to help parents remember to observe and count (i.e., dispensing wrist counters and making phone calls).

This program is unique in its emphasis on maintaining a high level of contact between practitioners and parents, requiring frequent contact. These contacts begin immediately with the pinpointing process and continue with high frequency throughout the program. Although this certainly increases the response effort on the part of the practitioner, it also serves as ongoing prompting that may increase the integrity of program implementation. Unfortunately, for those in private practice, insurance companies are unlikely to reimburse a practitioner for this indirect contact, and the volume of weekly contacts could become prohibitive for an active, full-time practitioner.

Finally, the program places a relatively strong emphasis on use of point systems as the primary means of behavior change in children. Point systems offer a significant degree of flexibility in addressing a variety of behaviors in children across a wide age range. In addition, the presence of the charts for monitoring the point system serves as a prompt to parents for implementation.

Empirical Support

The Living With Children parent training program was first evaluated in a nicely controlled study in which it was compared with a placebo control group. Parents in the treatment group first read the *Living With Children* (Patterson, 1976) book. The practitioner then helped parents implement what they had learned, including observing and recording, pinpointing, and developing a point system. Practitioners modeled skills and role-played with parents as needed. The placebo group met with other parents regularly to discuss problems but did not read the book or meet with practitioners. Both groups reported that they thought they were obtaining useful treatment, but only the children in the parent training group evidenced actual positive behavior change. There was no change in the observed behavior of the placebo treatment group (Walter & Gilmore, 1973).

Subsequent studies have also showed that the Living with Children program produced significantly greater reductions in observed rates of disruptive behavior compared with wait-list control groups (Patterson, Chamberlain, & Reid, 1982; Wiltz & Patterson, 1974). Follow-up studies with the families participating in these early studies indicated that the treatment benefits persisted up to 12 months posttreatment (DeGarmo, Patterson, & Forgatch, 2004; Patterson et al., 1982). In addition, positive outcomes of the parent training program were supported in research by other investigators (e.g., see Firestone, Kelly, & Fike, 1980), some of whom did not use the practitioner manual to guide treatment but who did adhere to the core components of the Living With Children treatment program. Alexander and Parsons (1973) developed their own manual to guide their research practitioners but still showed that parents who read the *Living With Children* (Patterson, 1976) book, then received coaching on observing and recording behavior, and then used social reinforcement, effective commands, and contingency contracting experienced significantly greater positive changes in child behavior compared with parents who received client-centered or psychodynamic counseling.

Not all of the early research demonstrated a clear benefit to using the Living With Children program, at least not with inexperienced providers. Bernal, Klinnert, and Schultz (1980) used students as therapists in their research comparing the Living With Children program with a client-centered approach and a wait-list control. Although the students were thoroughly trained and supervised, they were less experienced than the treatment providers in previous studies, and the investigators did not find any improvements in child outcomes relative to the client-centered treatment approach or the wait-list control group. However, they found that parents in the Living With Children group reported significant improvements in child behavior. This type of finding underscores the propensity for parents to report positive outcomes in response to treatment regardless of actual child behavior change. This supports Patterson and colleagues' emphasis on the need for direct observations of child behavior (Patterson & Narrett, 1990).

Over the past 20 years, research efforts have been directed less at refining and disseminating the original program for parents with young children and more at extending the concepts and applying the basic principles with different populations and in various settings. Researchers have continued to explore the mechanisms of parent–child interaction (Schrepferman & Snyder, 2002) and the variables that contribute to antisocial behavior (Patterson, Reid, & Dishion, 1992). In addition, the core elements of the original parent training program are being incorporated into treatment packages for children in foster care (Chamberlain, Fisher, & Moore, 2002), for divorced mothers (Forgatch & DeGarmo, 2002), for school prevention programs (J. B. Reid & Eddy, 2002), and for use with adolescents (Dishion & Kavanagh, 2003). Finally, having helped clearly establish the foundations of what to teach parents during parent training sessions, Patterson and colleagues have focused recent efforts on trying to understand better the clinical skills involved in training parents and the foundations of how to teach parents to manage child behavior effectively (Moore & Patterson, 2003).

Impressions and Recommendations

The Living With Children program represents the first of four outstanding, empirically supported parent training programs (see Table 2.2). With the emphasis on teaching parents behavior theory and then to observe, record, and use contingency management to shape new behaviors, Patterson and his colleagues in effect taught parents to be behavior therapists. Their efforts have reached far beyond the parents and children who participated in the original program.

TABLE 2.2
Program Features of Living With Children

Program domain	Program features
Ages	3–14
Problems	Noncompliance, tantrums, arguing, hitting, stealing
Materials	Parent Book: *Living With Children* Manual: *A Social Learning Approach to Family Intervention* (Patterson, Reid, Jones, & Conger, 1975)
Format	Predominantly individual
Length	12 sessions
What to teach	Behavior theory, observing and counting, praising and rewarding, points systems, response cost, time-out, contingency contracts
How to teach	Individual sessions, contingent delivery of treatment components, lots of cues and prompts, Parent Daily Report, behavioral skills training, videotape feedback, frequent phone follow-up

The evolution of the Living With Children parent training program can be traced through the publication of the three parent books *Living With Children* (Patterson, 1976), *Families* (Patterson, 1975), and *Parents and Adolescents: Living Together* (Forgatch & Patterson, 1987, 2005; Patterson & Forgatch, 1987, 2005). Each deals with core behavior concepts, but the recent guidebooks provide the most detailed information for training parents. The principles and technology are well established and empirically supported; by themselves, they offer considerable flexibility in addressing everyday problems that parents might encounter in children of just about any age. A practitioner could easily purchase the books and use them as a guide in helping parents learn and implement basic concepts and techniques.

However, a practitioner looking for equally well-established, refined, and easy-to-follow guidance regarding how to teach parents basic concepts and skills will find the program lacking. The original practitioner manual is dated, difficult to find, and not user-friendly like some of the manuals found in more contemporary empirically supported parent training programs. Although Patterson and his colleagues were and still are clearly interested in the clinical skills associated with how to teach parents, the only practical evidence of this interest is the 1975 manual. This is somewhat surprising because some of their own early research suggested that the clinical skills of the practitioner could be critical to overall outcome.

In addition to problems with accessibility, the 1975 program requires a relatively high level of contact between the practitioner and the parents that many parents may find intrusive and many practitioners may find prohibitive. In addition, the original program required that parents read the *Living With Children* (Patterson, 1976) book before treatment could begin. Adherence to this requirement could result in a selection bias against parents who cannot read yet would find the program attractive and beneficial. Also, the requirement might result in a selection bias against parents who are initially poorly motivated or who find a behavioral approach to be unacceptable. These types of resistance can often be overcome with practitioner clinical skills that are sensitive to how as well as what to teach parents, skills that are addressed in chapters 5 through 7 of this volume. However, requiring that parents read the book before continuing treatment does help to ensure a basic level of commitment to improvement.

In sum, this program is strong on what to teach parents but relatively weak on how to teach them. Many practitioners may find this attractive, preferring to blend the core concepts and techniques of a sound behavior parent training program into an individualized, flexible approach to structuring sessions, motivating adherence, and overcoming resistance to change. For others who prefer a more structured and even standardized approach to parent training, any one of the following three alternative empirically supported programs may prove more appealing.

THE INCREDIBLE YEARS—BASIC PROGRAM

Given that Patterson and colleagues virtually led the way to parent training, it should come as no surprise that subsequent programs were highly influenced by their pioneering work. Carolyn Webster-Stratton (1987, 1992), director of the Parenting Clinic at the University of Washington, developed The Incredible Years and was strongly influenced by Patterson and the social learning model, which emphasizes the critical role that parent–child interactions play in the development and maintenance of child deviant and parental coercive behaviors (Webster-Stratton & Hancock, 1998). Webster-Stratton was also heavily influenced by the modeling literature and by the unpublished work of Constance Hanf, who emphasized teaching parents interactive play skills, as well as reinforcement skills and nonviolent discipline (Hanf, 1969).

Initially developed by Webster-Stratton in the early 1980s as a video-taped modeling education program for groups of parents with children presenting conduct problems, the goals of the program are to strengthen parent competencies by training parents in positive communication and child-directed play skills, consistent and clear limit setting and nonviolent discipline strategies. The program has expanded over the years to target teachers and to emphasize prevention as well as treatment. It has also been expanded to address broader topics such as self-confidence, academic work habits, homework completion, and advocacy. Nevertheless, at the heart of the program is training for parents of young children who have conduct problems or are at risk for conduct problems.

Program Specifics

Target Population

The BASIC Early Childhood program targets young children ages 2 to 8 years with behavior problems, defined broadly to include issues such as dawdling, disobedience, bedtime problems, stealing, lying, bed-wetting, meal-time problems, and sibling rivalry. There are advanced versions for parents of school-age children (ages 5–12 years); however, the Early Childhood program is considered a prerequisite to the advanced programs.

Treatment Setting

Treatment delivery typically occurs with groups of parents in a clinic setting. Children are not included in group sessions with parents; however, the program advocates that practitioners provide child care so that parents can more easily attend sessions.

Program Materials

A practitioner can purchase program materials online (http://www.incredibleyears.com), including a manual for practitioners, videotapes, handouts, and a parent book. These materials can be purchased for about $1,300. The practitioner's manual, which can only be purchased as a part of the entire program materials, includes specific questions to be asked during discussions (e.g., "How does this encourage his son's imaginary play and independent ideas?") and provides suggested interpretations of the videotape vignettes to be used during discussions (e.g., "Notice that with this approach the boy is intensely involved and interested in the play activity"). The videotapes include more than 250 videotaped vignettes depicting parent and child models engaged in a variety of situations portraying both positive and negative examples of the skills that parents need to acquire. The videotapes come in Spanish, Norwegian, and English languages.

A parent book (Webster-Stratton, 1992) describes all of the content included in the BASIC program and is also the foundation of each of the subsequent advanced programs that teach parents communication, problem solving, and academic support skills and teach children problem solving and social skills. The book can be purchased separately in bookstores and online. A practitioner can also go online to purchase a newly developed group-leader manual (see http://www.incredibleyears.com/). The manual is purported to go "beyond the basics" to help group leaders deal with process issues that arise in all small groups, including how to handle multiple roles and how to deal with resistance. The group-leader manual comes with accompanying videotapes that reportedly provide examples of process issues and guidance regarding how to handle them.

Program Length

This is a 10- to 14-week program. Parents meet weekly in groups of 8 to 12, for 2-hour training sessions.

Program Content (What to Teach)

The program content centers initially on teaching parents how to play with their children in ways that will strengthen the parent–child relationship. The program teaches parents that this can be accomplished by letting children take the lead in play. Parents are asked to focus on their child and to follow their child's play by describing and commenting on what they see, by praising and approving of creative and appropriate actions, and by imitating what their child does. Parents are asked to resist urges to direct, command, organize, teach, and question. Parents are also taught, independent of play, to "catch 'em being good," to use specific and immediate contingent praise and touch, and to model self-praise.

Much like the Living With Children program, The Incredible Years also teaches parents to use an incentive program or point system, arguing that praise alone may not be enough to change behavior. These programs typically deliver stickers or points to children for appropriate or desired behavior, with the idea that the stickers or points can later be exchanged for other rewards, such as treats, privileges, or tangibles. Parents are encouraged to use the incentive programs to help a child to achieve specific large behavior goals, such as completing all chores each day, and using praise for small steps along the way, such as completing just one chore. Practitioners also encourage parents to use surprise rewards to increase already frequent behavior and planned rewards from the incentive program to increase low-frequency behavior. For example, a parent might surprise a child and let him or her stay up late and watch a movie with dad because the child was good about including a brother during play. As another example, a parent may use a sticker or give points for each aisle the mom and child complete together at the grocery store. Parents are encouraged not to remove points or stickers for misbehavior; instead, they are encouraged to use the rewards exclusively for reinforcing rewarding new or appropriate behaviors.

Subsequent sessions involve teaching parents how to set effective limits by using simple, direct, "do" commands and by offering choices. Groups discuss and prepare for limit testing that will occur. Parents also observe, discuss, and practice consistent use of selective ignoring for inappropriate behavior combined with praise for appropriate behavior.

Spanking is clearly discouraged as a method of discipline, with time-out being the preferred means of dealing with behaviors that cannot be ignored. Parents are instructed to use a dull corner or room for the time-out location and to keep the duration to 5 minutes or less. Parents are permitted to hold a door shut or even lock a door if a child is uncooperative with staying in a room for time-out. Release is contingent on 2 minutes of quiet, and then the child must comply with the original command if the time-out was for noncompliance. Although parents are taught time-out, several alternative discipline methods are taught as well. Parents are taught that natural and logical consequences (see Table 2.3) can also be effective, as long as they are not degrading, harmful, or painful. Natural consequences are considered to be those that would have occurred anyway, without adult supervision, such as being late for school as a result of sleeping in. Alternatively, logical consequences are those that are designed by a parent as a punishment that "fits the crime," such as having gum taken away if the parent sees it out of the child's mouth.

In addition to these child management skills, parents are taught to teach their children classic problem-solving skills. Children as young as 3 years are

TABLE 2.3
Natural and Logical Consequences

Type of consequence	Examples
Natural: That which would have occurred without parent intervention.	If late for dinner, food will be cold.
	If clothes are not in hamper, clothes are dirty.
	If one jumps in puddles, he or she wears wet shoes.
	If ball glove is left outside, it is stolen.
Logical: That which has been designed by the parent to "fit the crime."	If crayons are used on the table, they are taken away.
	If child won't stay in the backyard, he or she must play inside.
	If child is throwing blocks, the blocks are put away.
	If child refuses to eat dinner, there is no dessert.

encouraged to define problems, brainstorm solutions, appraise consequences, implement alternatives, and evaluate outcomes. The emphasis is focused more on learning the process of problem solving than on coming up with "correct" solutions.

Finally, parents are taught self-management skills to aid them in becoming more effective parents. These skills include using calming, coping thoughts; self-praise; humor; and "thought stopping" to interrupt negative thoughts. Parents also learn to take "time-out" from stressful and upsetting situations to relax, calm themselves, and use the self-management skills. Parents learn to improve their own communication skills through active listening and "I" messages (i.e., parents' describing how they feel, "I feel . . . ," rather than using accusatory statements that start with "You didn't . . ." or "You are . . .") and to use these skills in conducting their own problem solving regarding their interactions with adults.

Program Content (How to Teach)

Webster-Stratton has given significant attention to the issue of how to teach parents; she has developed separate manuals and videotapes to help practitioners in this regard and authored an entire book on the process of parent training (Webster-Stratton & Herbert, 1994). Central to the process is the idea, consistent with other parent training models, that parents can assume responsibility for solving their own problems if they are given the specific skills necessary to do so. However, divergent from other parent training models, this program embraces a more nondirective approach. The practitioner is viewed not as an expert but as a facilitator who establishes a collaborative relationship in which parents set agendas, share experiences, discuss ideas, and problem solve to adapt techniques to their own situation. This process is thought to be best facilitated through a group format, in part because groups offer an important source of diverse experiences to consider in collaborative problem solving. Groups are also thought to foster a sense of community support, reducing isolation, normalizing parents' experiences, and offering a less threatening environment than more individualized parent training programs. Of course, groups also can be more cost-effective because practitioners can potentially meet the needs of four or five families at once rather than one at a time (Webster-Stratton & Taylor, 1998).

The process also relies heavily on videotaped modeling as a means of teaching parenting skills. Hundreds of videotaped vignettes depict parents and children of different sex, ages, cultures, and socioeconomic backgrounds in a wide variety of common situations that parents encounter with children, such as play, eating, dressing, toileting, and bedtime. The videotapes depict both "correct" and "incorrect" interactions and are thought to be more accessible to less verbally oriented parents and to promote better generalization because of the variety of models and situations depicted (Webster-Stratton & Hancock, 1998). The videotaped modeling is also thought to provide benefits to practitioners because the videos may stimulate group discussion. The training format also includes role-playing and rehearsal of the skills that have been discussed and observed, with each session typically involving three or four brief role-plays in which parents pair up, with one pretending to be the child and the other the parent. Weekly homework assignments and handouts are used to enhance learning and promote use of the skills at home or in the classroom.

Finally, the program is attentive not only to what practitioners do but also to what they say and how they say it. An important component of the how-to process is assumed to involve translating concepts into words and behaviors that parents can readily apply. This might involve using metaphors and analogies to convey important concepts or even reframing concepts and ideas in ways that will reshape parents' perceptions about their children. Practitioners are also advised on how to identify resistance and, rather than confront it, to use collaborative problem solving to open parents to new ideas and to encourage parents to experiment with new techniques.

Unique Program Features

The Incredible Years is most unique in its training format, a combined use of videotaped modeling within groups of parents. Although other programs, especially the Helping the Noncompliant Child program, promote the use of videotaped vignettes as a means of depicting specific skill sequences, no other program relies on videotapes to play such a central role in the teaching process (see Table 2.4).

Equally unique to this program is the group format itself, given that the other programs all involve teaching of skills primarily in individual family ses-

TABLE 2.4
Program Features of The Incredible Years

Program domain	Program features
Ages	2–8
Problems	Dawdling, disobedience, bedtime problems, stealing, lying, bed-wetting, mealtime problems, sibling rivalry
Materials	Parent book: *The Incredible Years: A Trouble-Shooting Guide for Parents of Children Aged 3–8* (Webster-Stratton, 1992) Manual: Available for purchase online
Format	Group
Length	10–14 weeks, 120-minute sessions
What to teach	Child-directed play, praising and imitation, "catch 'em being good," incentive systems, time-out, natural and logical consequences, problem solving, self-management
How to teach	Nondirective, collaborative, group sessions; behavioral skills training; videotaped modeling; role-playing and rehearsal; translating concepts; normalizing parent experiences; encouraging experimentation with new techniques

sions. Perhaps as a result of teaching in a group format, the program is also unique in that children do not typically attend the group sessions with their parents. Teaching relies on role-playing between parents rather than direct rehearsal with children. Indeed, practitioners are encouraged to offer child care to allow both parents to attend the group sessions.

The training philosophy is also distinctive in that a much greater emphasis is placed on a collaborative model of parent training compared with the other evidence-based programs. Practitioners are not viewed as experts who train parents. Rather, the practitioner is considered to be a source of support and knowledge that is available to facilitate the process of parents using their own knowledge and perspective to set goals and treatment agendas.

The content of the program is largely consistent with the other supported programs, with some minor variations. For example, The Incredible Years does incorporate incentive programming, a feature that is central to the Patterson program, but it emphasizes the separation of reward and discipline features. That is, the incentive programs focus only on rewarding desirable behaviors. Ignoring, time-out, or natural consequences are recommended for discipline. The program content also includes units on teaching parents self-management strategies such as controlling negative self-statements, taking breaks, and using problem-solving and communication skills to become more effective parents.

The program content seems entirely unique in its reliance on teaching parents to teach problem-solving strategies to children as young as 3 years. This appears somewhat unusual, particularly in light of the fact that parents are encouraged, from the outset, to not view the family as a democracy or partnership and to recognize that children feel secure when parents provide behavioral control and decision making, especially in the early years. However, this is probably more consistent with the collaborative philosophy of The Incredible Years treatment process.

Finally, the program is alone in the training and costs necessary to deliver the program. At a minimum, the cost for the program materials as this book was going to press, including the manual and the videotapes, is approximately $1,300. In addition, program advisors recommend that practitioners become trained before implementing the program, requiring a 3-day workshop in Seattle, costing an additional $400, not including travel expenses. Even advanced practitioners are encouraged to complete an intensive 1-day workshop provided by Webster-Stratton or program staff.

The complete training program for practitioners covers basic program components and also issues related to therapeutic group process, such as cultural sensitivity, collaboration, empowerment, reframing, and self-management. Program promotional materials suggest that the training is important for leader effectiveness and that effectiveness is linked largely to an individual practitioner's comfort level with the collaborative process. The training leads to certification as a group leader, and only certified trainers can offer authorized workshops; however, no empirical evidence is available indicating whether certification is linked to improved outcomes by trainers.

Empirical Support

Extensive empirical evaluation of this program began in the early 1980s. Initial investigations showed that a therapist-led discussion group format using videotaped modeling (i.e., tapes depicting parents interacting with children using operant techniques such as praise, effective commands, and time-out) was effective as a parent training program (e.g., Webster-Stratton, 1981). Subsequently, a randomized, controlled comparison of the videotaped modeling discussion group approach showed that noncompliance and deviant behaviors could be significantly reduced when compared with an untreated wait-list control group (Webster-Stratton, 1984). Perhaps more important, the same study showed that the group videotape modeling format, with no rehearsal or direct feedback for parents, was as effective as an individualized treatment approach teaching the same parenting skills using role-plays, rehearsal, and direct feedback during practice of the skills with the child.

Since then, in numerous investigations conducted across the next 20 years with hundreds of children and families, well-controlled, peer-reviewed studies have demonstrated that The Incredible Years BASIC program has consistently resulted in (a) improved parent–child interactions, (b) less violent discipline, and (c) fewer child conduct problems. Much of this research has been conducted by Webster-Stratton herself (e.g., see Webster-Stratton, 1990, 1994) or with her colleagues (e.g., see Webster-Stratton, Kolpacoff, & Hollingsworth, 1988); however, positive results have also been found by other groups of researchers (e.g., see Spaccarelli, Cotler, & Penman, 1992; Stewart-Brown et al., 2004). More recently, investigations with multiethnic families have demonstrated that the program is also effective for and accepted by diverse populations (e.g., see Gross et al., 2003; M. J. Reid, Webster-Stratton, & Beauchaine, 2001).

The videotaped modeling and therapist-led discussions have not always been found to be necessary components of the treatment program. Webster-Stratton and colleagues (1988), in a component analysis of their program, found that when the content and number of sessions were held constant, significant improvements were noted in both children and parents, regardless of whether the parents participated in a self-administered treatment with videotapes, a therapist-led discussion with videotapes, or only a therapist-led discussion without videotapes. Although the parents who had a therapist generally found the treatment to be easier to implement, this did not significantly affect outcome. In addition, the parent self-management components of the program have been found to improve parent communication, problem-solving, and satisfaction with treatment but not to provide significant benefit in terms of child behavior outcomes (Webster-Stratton, 1994).

More recently, Webster-Stratton and her colleagues have continued to expand the scope of the program by investigating to what extent the teacher training and child training components add to program outcomes. These investigations have found, for example, that training teachers to understand and use the same concepts and skills as parents is important to produce changes in child behavior at school but only in long-term follow-up and with no immediate or long-term benefit on child behavior at home (M. J. Reid, Webster-Stratton, & Hammond, 2003). This is consistent with other research showing that clinic-based changes produced by parent training do generalize to the home setting but not reliably to the school setting (T. K. Taylor & Biglan, 1998).

Webster-Stratton has also initiated extensive efforts to evaluate the preventive benefits of the program. Studies have shown that The Incredible Years can, when offered as a prevention program to all parents in Head Start programs, produce significant improvements in positive parent behavior but somewhat weaker results for child behavior (e.g., see Webster-Stratton, 1998). Perhaps it is not surprising that preventive efforts have been found to produce more significant improvements when baseline rates of parent and child negative behaviors are higher (e.g., see M. J. Reid, Webster-Stratton, & Baydar, 2004). Selected prevention studies are also being conducted by some independent researchers who have demonstrated that The Incredible Years can significantly increase positive parent behaviors of parents referred to Child Protective Services (Hughes & Gottlieb, 2004).

Impressions and Recommendations

For many practitioners, the training methods of this program will hold much appeal. The videotapes are commercially available, and the manual provides specific guidance about how to use the videos and lead the discussions that follow (see Table 2.4). In addition, the group format likely improves treatment efficiency by increasing the number of families that can access treatment at one time. Indeed, many parents may find the group format more inviting and less threatening than the more intensive individualized treatment formats. Furthermore, Webster-Stratton has gone to great lengths to take a behavioral program and to repackage it in language that will have broad appeal to many parents, reframing treatment components as skills that build warm relationships, enhance self-worth, create stability and security, and help children internalize responsibility. Finally, the group-oriented program may hold particular appeal to school-based practitioners, where assessment and consultation demands can make individualized approaches to prevention or treatment rather impractical.

Unfortunately, the program is not inexpensive for the practitioner. Even without the recommended training, which itself is expensive in terms of cost, travel, and time, the program manual and tapes are expensive to procure relative to other programs that work. In addition, The Incredible Years advocates trainers to offer child care, dinners, and transportation to increase attendance, but this would prove prohibitive for many practitioners. Cost issues aside, The Incredible Years is the only one of the four empirically supported programs for which training opportunities are easily identified via its Web site and are widely available. Consultation services are also offered, and practitioners can host workshops on site, if desired.

Overall, the BASIC program, as a treatment package, has extensive empirical support and has great potential to be used as both a prevention and a treatment program. There is considerable assistance regarding how and what to teach, and the program offers unparalleled technical support in developing the skills and competencies necessary to implement the program. As a result, it may be the program of choice for practitioners seeking training opportunities in parent training.

HELPING THE NONCOMPLIANT CHILD

The Helping the Noncompliant Child program (HNC; McMahon & Forehand, 2003) was first described in the early 1980s in what was one of the first behaviorally oriented parent training manuals (Forehand & McMahon, 1981). Rex Forehand, now at the University of Vermont, was for years the director of the Institute for Behavioral Research at the University of Georgia, where he conducted early studies evaluating critical components of behavioral parent training programs. Eventually he, along with Robert McMahon (currently at the University of Washington), developed, refined, and evaluated a standardized program for training parents in how best to manage and treat noncompliant children.

The program embraces the coercion model, originally described by Patterson (1982), as the foundation of disruptive behavior problems, including noncompliance in children. The program structure is based significantly on the work of Constance Hanf (1969), who emphasized a two-phase training model in which parents are first taught to use differential attention and then to use compliance training to address child noncompliance. The goal is to disrupt coercive parent–child interactions and establish positive, prosocial interaction patterns. The parenting skills are designed to help the parent break out of coercive cycles by increasing positive attention for appropriate child behavior, ignoring minor inappropriate behaviors, providing clear instructions to the child, and providing appropriate consequences for compliance (e.g., positive attention) and noncompliance (e.g., time-out). The basic elements of the HNC program closely resemble the original Hanf model, yet recent adaptations and additions designed to enhance the original program have been included. Some of these adaptations, such as regular phone contact between the practitioner and the parents and teaching parents basic social learning principles, hearken back to the Living With Children program. However, this review focuses on the original two-phase program as described in the revised edition of McMahon and Forehand's (2003) original work.

Program Specifics

Target Population

The program targets children ages 3 to 8 who exhibit noncompliance, which is considered to be a keystone behavior in the path to later conduct problems.

Treatment Setting

Treatment delivery typically occurs with individual families in an intensive, clinic-based format. The target children are included in each of the sessions.

Program Materials

A practitioner can purchase a detailed description of the HNC program in the second edition of the book *Helping the Noncompliant Child: Family-Based Treatment for Oppositional Behavior* (McMahon & Forehand, 2003). The manual provides detailed guidelines for how to conduct the initial assessment, including interviews with the parent and with the child. The manual also specifies how to conduct and code observations of parent–child interaction using the Behavior Coding System. Parents interact with the child in a "free play" situation and then in a "command" situation while the practitioner codes parent and child behaviors.

The manual also recommends specific standardized rating scales for soliciting parent perceptions of their own and their child's adjustment. In addition, the authors have developed an instrument for assessing parent knowledge of behavioral principles that has been found to be sensitive to intervention (McMahon, Forehand, & Griest, 1981). Subsequent chapters describe specifically how to explain the program to parents, how to structure sessions, and, in many cases, exactly what to say to parents when introducing concepts and handling problems that arise.

The authors themselves question whether simply reading the book can adequately prepare a practitioner to implement the program. They suggest that minimum prerequisites include a basic knowledge of learning principles and child development, as well as experience with behavioral counseling. The authors also acknowledge that they typically train practitioners using videotapes, modeling, role-plays, and feedback. A videotape that demonstrates the program procedures is reportedly available to assist with practitioner training (Forehand, Armistead, Neighbors, & Klein, 1994); practitioners must contact the first author to acquire it. In addition, a supplemental self-help book for parents, *Parenting the Strong-Willed Child* (Forehand & Long, 2002), is also available but is not considered necessary to complete the HNC program.

Program Length

The manual describes the HNC as a 12-week program, not including the initial intake interviews and structured behavioral observations assessing parent–child interactions. The length of the program, however, is flexible depending on the speed with which parents acquire the skills being taught. The average number of sessions is 10. Parents and children participate in the weekly 60- to 90-minute sessions.

Program Content (What to Teach)

Phase I of the two-phase program centers on teaching parents how to use their attention as a tool in changing child behavior (Table 2.5 details the two-phase program). During an activity called the Child's Game, a free-play activity in which the child directs and leads all activities, parents are instructed to become a constant source of attention by providing a running

TABLE 2.5
Helping the Noncompliant Child: Two-Phase Program

Phase	Specific skills
Phase I: Differential attention	Parents learn to attend.
	Parents learn to reward.
	Parents learn to ignore.
	Parents learn to combine attend, reward, and ignore.
	Parents practice skills in clinic and then at home.
Phase II: Compliance training	Parents learn to give clear instructions.
	Parents learn to praise compliance.
	Parents practice clear instructions at home.
	Parents learn to give warnings.
	Parents learn to use time-out.
	Parents practice in clinic, then at home.
Extending skills	Parents learn to use standing rules.
	Parents learn how to include siblings.
	Parents learn how to handle situations outside of the home.

commentary of their child's activities. During this play-by-play commentary, parents are asked to eliminate questions or commands and to avoid any attempts at teaching the child. Instead, parents learn to use "attends," in which they describe any appropriate play behavior or activity and use immediate and specific praise as well as physical touch to reward improved or desired behavior.

Parents are then taught to ignore minor attention-seeking behavior and to eventually combine all three (i.e., attend, reward, and ignore) during the Child's Game. There are specific behavioral criteria that parents must pass regarding the appropriate use of each skill (e.g., four attends or more per minute during 5-minute observation), and the skills are introduced sequentially contingent on the parent meeting each of the criteria. In addition, practitioners are instructed to engage each child in individual teaching interactions in which the program components are described. Homework requires 10 to 15 minutes of the Child's Game each day, in which the parent practices the skills taught in clinic. The manual includes handouts describing the skills and data sheets for recording home practice.

Phase II involves teaching parents how to conduct compliance training. In compliance training, parents learn how to set up an activity called the Parent's Game in which the parent structures activities that require the child to follow instructions. Parents learn how to give clear "do" commands, how to reward compliance, and how to use time-out for noncompliance.

Time-outs are recommended to last a minimum of 3 minutes, usually located in a chair placed in a boring corner or hallway. Release is contingent on 15 seconds of quiet, and the child must then immediately comply with the original command. Spanking has been rejected as a means of enforcing compliance with the time-out procedure, in part because of acceptability problems but also because there are alternatives that have been found to be effective. These include sending the child to his or her room, removing a privilege, or increasing the amount of time spent in time-out.

Again, the manual provides specific behavioral performance criteria for determining whether parents have mastered the Phase II skills, and ready-to-use handouts in the back of the manual describe each of the Phase II components. Phase II is later supplemented with the use of "standing rules." These are statements that specify a prohibited behavior and the consequence for breaking that rule, usually time-out. These rules usually focus on behaviors that would result in danger to self, others, or property and are typically limited to just one or two behaviors. The HNC program concludes with discussions and practice regarding extension of the program skills from situations in the home to situations outside the home.

Program Content (How to Teach)

The HNC program is direct in its approach with parents. From the outset, parents learn that a child's disruptive behavior is learned and that the purpose of the HNC program is to teach parents effective ways to interact with their child so that the child learns more acceptable ways of behaving. A strong emphasis is placed on the fact that teaching acceptable behavior is at least as important as disciplining inappropriate behavior. Skills are taught in small steps, introduced sequentially, and geared to the parent's own rate of progress to maximize success and to help parents feel comfortable. However, there are specific criteria for parents to meet before training can progress that will help a practitioner know how to evaluate progress and when to advance to the next skill segment. Criteria are included for use of attends, rewards, ignoring, commands, and consequences.

The training model is an expert one in which the practitioner explains, demonstrates, role-plays, and feeds back information to parents about their progress. The developers are careful to direct the practitioner to address parent feelings of guilt about poor parenting or concerns about the awkwardness of intensive skill training but note that these feelings are not the central focus of the parent training program.

The HNC program also makes extensive use of the practitioner playing the role of the child in demonstrating program components to the child. The parent never plays the role of the child in this process. However, the practitioner explains and demonstrates program components to the child and, in some cases, uses the child as a "coach" to the parent, allowing the child to indicate when program components such as ignoring, clear instruction giving, praising, and time-out are necessary.

As with other programs, HNC is also attentive to what practitioners say and how they say it. Specific examples and scripts are provided in the manual to assist practitioners in how to talk to parents and children. In addition, numerous examples are given of how to sell the program rationale to parents using graphs, diagrams, and charts. An important component of the how-to process in this program involves the use of parent handouts. The manual appendix includes more than 17 handouts that briefly describe a skill learned in session. The handouts can be copied and sent home with parents as how-to guides that review all of the basic skills. Practitioners are also advised on likely obstacles to treatment success, including parents' poor adherence or resistance. Of course, skill competence is a clear prerequisite to treatment adherence, and practitioners are advised to make sure that parents can demonstrate the skills in clinic before attempting them in the home. Although the program encourages practitioners to explore other potential barriers to adherence and to problem solve with parents ways to improve follow-thorough, they are also advised to use more direct means if necessary. This might include charging parents for missed sessions, using stipends for homework completion, or even contracting termination contingencies with parents for poor adherence.

Unique Program Features

The HNC program is unique in that the treatment manual is readily available within the context of a scholarly text. In addition to the basics of program implementation, the HNC book provides a conceptual overview of the origins of noncompliance, develops a brief history of parent training, provides extensive discussions of assessment methods and procedures, and delivers a thorough review of the programmatic research over the past 30 years that supports the HNC program.

The HNC program is also somewhat unique in the extent to which the child is included in sessions and participates in training. None of the other programs include the child in every session, and none allow the child such an active role in the training process. Note that although the child might be involved in the training process, including learning about the skills and about how their parents will be implementing them, they are not involved in decision making about how or when the program is implemented. The performance criteria do allow some flexibility in the program, given that the progression from one skill to the next is based on demonstrated proficiency; however, this program is highly directive and structured by the practitioner regarding what, when, and how program components are to be implemented.

Empirical Support

The research support for this program is noteworthy for a number of reasons. First, in the mid-1970s, the HNC developers began systematic research into many of the program's individual components. Thus, the developers were instrumental in demonstrating the efficacy of program components such as labeled praise (Bernhardt & Forehand, 1975), clear instruction giving (Roberts, McMahon, Forehand, & Humphreys, 1978), and contingent release from time-out (Hobbs & Forehand, 1975). They also did initial comparisons of various time-out durations (Hobbs, Forehand, & Murray, 1978).

At the same time that these evaluations of individual parenting strategies were being conducted, Forehand and colleagues were also investigating the systematic application of these components in a parent training program. Results from the initial study, a small, uncontrolled evaluation of the program with eight families, indicated that the two-phase program resulted in parents who used more rewards and had children who were more compliant (Forehand & King, 1974). A subsequent controlled comparison found that not only did the program produce positive changes in both parent and child behavior, but at the conclusion of treatment, the treated children were generally more compliant than the nonreferred "normal" children (Forehand & King, 1977).

Although these initial investigations looked exclusively at clinic-based behavior changes, later studies involved home observations to assess whether improvements generalized to other settings. These studies found that the HNC program produced both short-term efficacy and setting generalization from the clinic to the home for both parent and child behaviors, as well as parents' perceptions of their children (e.g., see Forehand, Griest, & Wells, 1979; Peed, Roberts, & Forehand, 1977). In addition, extensions of the research found that the program was equally effective across socioeconomic levels (Rogers, Forehand, Griest, Wells, & McMahon, 1981) and across children ranging in age from 3 to 8 years (McMahon, Forehand, & Tiedemann, 1985). Finally, in a comparative, randomized controlled investigation of children referred for oppositional behavior problems, HNC produced significantly more positive parent behavior and significantly more compliant child behavior compared with a traditional family systems therapy approach (Wells & Egan, 1988).

More recently, not only have child noncompliance and inappropriate behavior been shown to improve to within the "normal" range by the end of training, but follow-up studies, some done over a decade after training, offer support for the long-term efficacy of the program (e.g., see Long, Forehand, Wierson, & Morgan, 1994). In addition, component analyses have continued to be an ongoing focus of the research program. Investigations of self-control training for parents (Wells, Griest, & Forehand, 1980) and parent training in social learning principles (McMahon et al., 1981) have found that these components can improve child compliance beyond that produced from the HNC program alone.

A study of one of the more unique aspects of the program, the use of verbal rationales and modeling with children before parents implement new skills at home, found that rationales and modeling may improve the effectiveness of some program components (Davies, McMahon, Flessati, & Tiedemann, 1984). However, there have been no subsequent evaluations. Finally, Kotler and McMahon (2004) recently evaluated whether the use of attends alone can have an impact on noncompliance. Early research with nonclinical populations suggests that it may have some benefit for children who are anxious or aggressive, but controlled investigations have yet to be completed.

Currently, the HNC parent training program is reportedly under investigation as a prevention program for at-risk Head Start children (McMahon & Forehand, 2003) and as part of the multicomponent FAST Track program that targets high-risk children and their families. Although the latter program includes numerous other components beyond parent training, such as academic tutoring, home visits, and social skills training, the initial positive outcomes suggest that the HNC program can be successfully adapted for community prevention efforts (Conduct Problems Prevention Research Group, 2002). More information about the FAST Track program is presented in chapter 9 of this volume.

Impressions and Recommendations

The HNC program is based on the most well-developed, systematic program of research of any of the empirically supported programs (see Table 2.6). Research involving individual components was conducted early on, components were combined and studied in a structured treatment program, and then outcomes were followed up over long periods, some as long as 14 years. In addition, the manual is embedded in a scholarly text that is as much a primer on behavioral parent training as it is a how-to handbook. Thus, the HNC book is likely to have wide appeal to graduate students, new practitioners, and

TABLE 2.6
Program Features of Helping the Noncompliant Child

Program domain	Program features
Ages	3–8
Problems	Noncompliance
Materials	Manual: *Helping the Noncompliant Child: Family-Based Treatment for Oppositional Behavior* (McMahon & Forehand, 2003)
Format	Individual family
Length	12 weeks, 60- to 90-minute sessions
What to teach	Child's Game (i.e., attend, reward, ignore), compliance training (i.e., clear instructions, time-out, standing rules)
How to teach	Directive, use of specific performance criteria, geared toward parents' rate of progress, behavioral skills training, practitioner role-plays child, "sell" with graphs and charts, use handouts, address adherence barriers

established clinicians and academics. Nevertheless, the program developers question whether simply reading their book is sufficient to use its contents effectively, and the book is much more detailed in regard to what to teach than how to teach compared with other programs. This program is probably best targeted to practitioners who already have some basic knowledge of behavioral principles and experience with parent training.

PARENT–CHILD INTERACTION THERAPY

Parent–Child Interaction Therapy (PCIT; Eyberg & Robinson, 1982) was first described in the early 1980s by Sheila Eyberg and integrates operant methods with traditional play therapy techniques to restructure parent–child patterns of interaction. The program represents the third empirically supported parent training program to have its origins in the work of Constance Hanf (1969), from the Oregon Health Sciences University, where Eyberg began her program of research on parent–child relationships before moving to the University of Florida.

Much like each of the preceding programs, PCIT espouses social learning theory, emphasizing Patterson's notions that child conduct problems are inadvertently established or maintained by coercive parent–child interactions. However, the PCIT program also embraces attachment theory and the notion that sensitive and responsive parenting will help children develop more secure and effective emotional and behavioral self-regulation. In the PCIT program, play itself is considered to be developmentally therapeutic, offering a child a means of learning problem-solving skills and developing secure attachments.

Similar to the HNC program, the PCIT program uses a two-phase training model in which parents are first taught to use differential reinforcement and then to use effective commands and timeout to manage children's disruptive behavior. Parents are taught to use skills, designed to improve parent–child interactions, individually through didactic sessions using modeling, role-playing, and direct rehearsal and feedback with children. The PCIT program has a dual focus on relationship building and managing disruptive behavior, especially noncompliance.

Program Specifics

Target Population

The program targets children ages 2 to 8 who are exhibiting disruptive behavior, including noncompliance, defiance, verbal and physical aggression, and overactivity. The manual also suggests that the program can be used for children with anxiety, low self-esteem, perfectionism, developmental problems associated with mental retardation, and relationship problems associated with abuse, neglect, divorce, and adoption.

Treatment Setting

Treatment delivery typically occurs with individual families in an intensive, clinic-based, treatment format. Children are included in most, but not all, of the sessions.

Program Materials

A practitioner can purchase a detailed manual of the PCIT program in the book titled *Parent–Child Interaction Therapy* (Hembree-Kigin & McNeil, 1995). The manual provides information about the foundations of the PCIT program and detailed guidelines for conducting each session in the program (see Table 2.7 for a sample session outline).

The manual describes a flexible approach to initial assessment, recommending a number of standardized and widely available rating scales and checklists to evaluate child behavior problems and parent stress. One of the fundamental elements of the assessment involves direct observations of structured parent–child interactions using a Parent–Child Interaction Coding System developed by Eyberg for use with the program. Similar to the HNC assessment protocol, the coding requires observations of parents and children during free play and then during command conditions, but it also adds a situation in which the child must clean up the play area.

The manual includes specific instructions for how to conduct this initial assessment and the observations of parent–child interactions, how to share results with parents, and how to introduce PCIT and various treatment com-

TABLE 2.7
Sample Session Outline in Parent–Child Interaction Therapy:
Steps for Teaching Behavioral Play Therapy Skills

Step	Description	Time allotted (minutes)
1	Describe goals for behavioral play therapy.	<5
2	Discuss 5 minutes of daily home practice.	<5
3	Present and model the "don't" skills.	15
4	Present and model the "do" skills.	20
5	Discuss use of strategic attention.	15
6	Discuss use of selective ignoring.	15
7	Model all skills in combination.	2
8	Coach parents as they role-play skills.	5
9	Discuss logistics of play therapy at home.	15

Note. From *Parent–Child Interaction Therapy* (p. 28, Table 3.1), by T. I. Hembree-Kigin and C. B. McNeil, 1995, New York: Plenum Press. Copyright 1995 by Plenum Press. Adapted with kind permission of Springer Science and Business Media and the authors.

ponents to parents. In many cases, the manual provides specific scripts for how to say things to parents. The manual includes copies of the recommended assessment instruments, homework recording sheets, and parent handouts describing treatment components.

The program also relies heavily on practitioners conducting assessments and coaching from another room, observing through a two-way mirror, and communicating through a "bug-in-the-ear" device, a small radio transmitter that allows the practitioner to talk to parents in another room through a small radio receiver worn in the ear. These observation rooms and radio devices are not necessary, but they are encouraged and described throughout the manual.

Program Length

The manual describes the PCIT program as lasting anywhere from 8 to 14 weeks, with sessions lasting anywhere from 60 to 90 minutes. The average program length is 12 weeks. However, the length of the program is flexible depending on the speed with which a parent acquires the skills being taught.

Program Content (What to Teach)

The PCIT program begins with direct observations in the clinic of parent–child interactions during a free play situation, a parent-directed situation, and a clean-up situation. Specific parent and child behaviors are coded. Videotaping is recommended for less experienced practitioners because coding multiple behaviors at the same time can be difficult. This sets a pattern in which each session begins with a brief, 5-minute period observing and coding parent–child interactions. Results from the assessment are used primarily for tracking progress and to determine whether parents have met criteria for skill mastery and are ready to progress to subsequent treatment components.

The first phase of treatment is dedicated to relationship building, and parents learn to implement what is described as *behavioral play therapy*. Initially, a teaching session is scheduled with the parents, which they attend alone. The behavioral play therapy that parents learn is called child-directed play or sometimes child-directed interactions. As the names indicate, the child is permitted to choose and lead the play. Through discussion, modeling, and role-playing, parents learn skills that will permit them to be nondirective during play. These skills are referred to in the manual using the acronym *DRIP*. Parents are taught to *d*escribe appropriate behavior, *r*eflect appropriate verbalizations, *i*mitate play, and *p*raise desirable behavior observed during their child's play.

In addition, parents learn to avoid giving commands, asking questions, or criticizing play because these each tend to direct play and conversation and add unpleasantness that the practitioner is seeking to avoid. Parents are then taught how to use these skills selectively to encourage good behavior and discourage inappropriate behavior by combining them with systematic ignoring of inappropriate child behavior.

In subsequent sessions of the first phase of treatment, the parents and child are seen together for direct coaching of these same play skills. Parents are requested to practice these child-directed interaction skills at home on a daily basis, and they must meet specific performance criteria before moving on to Phase 2. This first phase typically takes two to four visits.

The second phase of treatment involves the teaching of basic discipline strategies for dealing with noncompliance through the use of "minding exercises." Parents learn that during these parent-directed interactions, children can be taught to comply by breaking compliance down into small steps and overpracticing compliance, first with simple "play" commands and eventually moving toward more difficult, "real-life" commands.

As when teaching child-directed interactions, the therapist and parents meet without the child, and parent-directed interaction skills are discussed, modeled, and role-played. These skills include learning how to give effective instructions, how to set up a good time-out for noncompliance, and how to implement the time-out to maximize effectiveness. Parents learn that effective commands involve not only simple, direct, positively stated directives but also instructions that are developmentally appropriate, supplemented or clarified with gestures, incorporate choices, and give well-timed reasons or explanations for why a command was given. These latter skills reflect the PCIT focus on developmental and operant aspects of behavior change.

Parents then learn how to identify noncompliance and how to implement time-out. Timeouts typically last 3 minutes, with 5 seconds of quiet required before release. Time-out is always followed by a restatement of the original command. If the child is compliant, the parent provides a few minutes of the child-directed interactions before issuing a new command. Time-outs are enforced with spanks (see the subsequent discussion on spanking), restraint, room restriction, or loss of privileges. The manual describes the advantages and disadvantages of each and advises the practitioner to select the appropriate enforcement procedure on the basis of several factors, such as parent comfort and skill levels, child's developmental level, and severity of the child's attempts to escape time-out.

As with the first phase, subsequent sessions involve the parents and child together for direct coaching of the skills involved in parent-directed interactions. Children are given verbal explanations about how they will "practice minding," and then experience role-playing of the time-out procedure. Homework involves conducting minding exercises in the home for 10 minutes each day; however, these are only assigned if the practitioner expects that the parent can be successful with the assignment, on the basis of performance in the clinic. This phase typically lasts four to six visits and may eventually include practicing the skills not only in clinic but also in community settings where problems are likely to occur.

Program Content (How to Teach)

The PCIT program manual provides extensive recommendations about how to teach program components to parents. The manual is formatted such that each treatment phase has one chapter devoted entirely to how to teach the skills to the parents and then a separate chapter about how to "coach" parents when they are actually using the skills with their child. The skill teaching during the parent-alone sessions emphasizes modeling and role-playing of skills by the practitioner and then immediate, direct feedback to the parents about use of each of the skills.

For each treatment component, practitioners are given specific rationales to use with parents in developing their understanding and support for the inclusion of each skill. Then, during actual practice of the skills, particularly the child-directed interaction skills, the practitioner usually plays the role of the child, ensuring that the initial attempts by a parent to use a new skill are met by desirable responses from the "child." During the teaching of parent-directed interaction skills, a doll is used as the "child."

The skill coaching done with parents when the child is present emphasizes the use of the bug-in-the-ear device. This device permits the practitioner to watch closely and provide immediate feedback about the parent–child interactions without actually being present in the room and possibly disrupting the natural flow of parent–child communication and interaction. Practitioners are advised to prepare the teaching environment carefully to enhance the likelihood of success for parents. Indeed, the program is sensitive to the fact that such close supervision and feedback about performance can create a context in which parents are highly self-conscious and anxious, giving rise to numerous recommendations designed to help the practitioner be successful at effective skill coaching. These include general recommendations to keep feedback precise, frequent, and positive, as well as targeting easier skills before harder ones. To help both parents and practitioners be successful at teaching and learning skills, the manual provides extensive discussion of problems that may arise during teaching and learning each of the child-directed and parent-directed skills.

Although practitioners are encouraged during child-directed skill instruction to adjust teaching expectations on the basis of unique aspects of each parent–child dyad, there is little latitude offered during teaching of parent-directed skills. Practitioners are advised to be extremely directive and "to guide nearly every word the parent says." This includes detailed instructions about how a parent should explain timeout to a child and then rehearse the skill. The program advises practitioners to have parents give rather lengthy explanations to their child about time-out and also to have parents use tangible rewards to motivate their child to practice the time-out protocol.

Some descriptions of the program recommend immediately graphing the data from the brief observations conducted during each session and using these graphs to (a) allow parents to review their progress and (b) select the skills they wish to focus on during their daily practice sessions at home (e.g., see Herschell, Calzada, Eyberg, & McNeil, 2002a). These seem clearly designed to enhance parental motivation for follow-through with the skills that are being taught in clinic; however, this particular approach is not emphasized in the manual.

Unique Program Features

The PCIT protocol has a number of components that make it unique when compared with the other empirically supported parent training programs. First, the PCIT program is most unique in its strong appeal to developmental and behavioral elements in conceptualizing effective treatment. The appeal to attachment theory in particular has resulted in the inclusion of "reflection" and "imitation" as parts of child-directed interactions because they are considered important for parents trying to create the sort of secure, responsive, and sensitive environment necessary for emotional self-regulation.

Second, although PCIT is not unique in its use of direct coaching of parent–child dyads, it is unique in the manner in which this coaching occurs. The emphasis on use of the bug-in-the-ear alone has led to this particular feature being labeled the "Cyrano de Bergerac approach" to parent training (Administration for Children and Families, 2002).

In addition, the emphasis on dictating exactly what a parent should say appears to make the PCIT protocol the most directive of the four programs reviewed in this chapter. Perhaps because of this strong directive aspect of the PCIT protocol, the manual offers more specific examples of exactly how to teach each of the skills in the program to both parents and their children. Of course, this has the potential to make the PCIT more intimidating for parents, and it is not unusual for them initially to experience the directive aspects of the program as awkward and contrived. However, the manual is attentive to these issues and offers practitioners strategies to deal with them. Although the protocol is highly directive, practitioners are never instructed to model the skills in direct interaction with the child. Both are modeled and rehearsed only with parents. As noted, parents are then coached from behind a mirror using the bug-in-the-ear.

The PCIT program is also unique in that compliance is treated as a skill that can and should be practiced regularly. Thus, daily minding exercises are arranged in which children overpractice following directions for 5 to 10 minutes each day, first with easy tasks and then with more challenging ones. In this regard, the parenting skills are not only used reactively to manage noncompliance but are also used proactively to practice the skill of "doing what you're told."

It is somewhat surprising that physical punishment, including spanks on the bare bottom and physical restraint, are suggested as means of enforcing acceptance of the time-out routine. We say "surprising" because the modern milieu regarding physical discipline is negative, with many considering it to be unacceptable (e.g., M. L. Jones, Eyberg, & Adams, 1998) or even abusive (e.g., Strauss, 1994). Nevertheless, other teams of investigators have indicated that spanks can be an effective enforcement procedure (Roberts & Powers, 1990). In addition to the spanking enforcement procedure, the manual also discusses a restraint procedure, a room-restriction procedure, and loss of privileges as back-ups for situations in which spanking might not be appropriate to recommend.

Empirical Support

The empirical support for the PCIT program is extensive. Research began in the early 1980s with an uncontrolled evaluation. It demonstrated that the two-phase intervention of child-directed and parent-directed interactions could significantly alter parent–child interactions and produce parents who were more positive and attentive and children who were less demanding and more compliant (Eyberg & Robinson, 1982). Later, in one of the first controlled evaluations of the program, PCIT produced significant improvements in both parent and child behavior; parents who received didactic group training or no training exhibit no changes (Eyberg & Matarazzo, 1980). Parents from the two control groups reported that they perceived improvements, although none were observed, a finding that Patterson and colleagues also have found.

Since these initial studies, research on the PCIT program by Eyberg and many former students has continued into the current decade. Numerous randomized, wait-list controlled research investigations have demonstrated significant improvements in disruptive behavior and noncompliance using the PCIT program (e.g., see McNeil, Capage, Bahl, & Blanc, 1999; Schuhmann, Foote, Eyberg, Boggs, & Algina, 1998). Over the past 20 years, additional research has been conducted demonstrating that these benefits extend into the school setting (McNeil, Eyberg, Eisenstadt, Newcomb, & Funderburk, 1991) and can be maintained well after treatment has terminated (Hood & Eyberg, 2003).

Researchers have attempted to examine issues of cultural sensitivity of the intervention, at least with parents of African American children (Capage, Bennett, & McNeil, 2001). Research has also suggested that the PCIT protocol is equally effective regardless of the order in which the parent-directed or child-directed portions are presented (Eisenstadt, Eyberg, McNeil, Newcomb, & Funderburk 1993; Eyberg et al., 2001). Finally, other groups of researchers have also found significant benefits for behavior-disordered children when comparing those receiving PCIT to wait-list controls or to nondisturbed comparison samples (Nixon, 2001; Nixon, Sweeney, Erickson, & Touyz, 2003).

Although the manual suggests that the PCIT protocol can be implemented in 8 to 12 sessions for most families, those who have participated in the empirical research have averaged nearly 14 sessions to complete treatment (Boggs et al., 2004). This is important to know because parents report slow treatment progression as one reason for dropping out (Boggs et al., 2004).

The manual also suggests that the program can be used for nearly every type of childhood behavior disorder, yet the empirical research to date has focused almost exclusively on noncompliance. In addition, although PCIT includes many treatment components that have independent empirical support, such as praise, time-out, and direct commands, numerous other components have been added, such as reflections, imitation, and providing reasons, despite little empirical support for their inclusion.

Finally, all of the studies supporting PCIT as an empirically supported program appear to have been conducted in clinical settings using master's- or doctoral-level therapists with substantial training in the PCIT protocol (Gallagher, 2003). As a result, the generalizability of findings to less controlled practice settings is uncertain. Nevertheless, a number of PCIT research programs are active and continue the process of exploring diagnostic, cultural, socioeconomic, and therapist variables that may affect outcome and maintenance of outcome (Herschell, Calzada, Eyberg, & McNeil, 2002b).

Impressions and Recommendations

The Parent–Child Interaction Therapy program (see Table 2.8) will be immediately appealing to many practitioners precisely because it is so directive not only in what to teach but also in how to teach. Although other empirically supported programs either require or strongly suggest that practitioners wishing to use their programs should have considerable prerequisite training, the PCIT program seems ideal for practitioners who are just entering into the parent training arena. Perhaps for this reason alone, the PCIT program has been widely disseminated through professional training programs around the country,

TABLE 2.8
Program Features of Parent–Child Interaction Therapy

Program domain	Program features
Ages	2–8
Problems	Noncompliance, defiance, verbal and physical aggression, overactivity
Materials	Manual: *Parent–Child Interaction Therapy* (Hembree-Kigin & McNeil, 1995)
Format	Individual family
Length	8–14 weeks; 60- to 90-minute sessions
What to teach	Behavioral play therapy (using descriptions, reflections, imitation, and praise), minding exercises (using effective and developmentally appropriate commands, time-out)
How to teach	Highly directive; specific performance criteria; teach parents first without child present, then coach skills with child present; behavioral skills training

including University of California—Davis Medical Center, University of Florida, Central Michigan University, and West Virginia University, and through local agencies such as the Oklahoma City-County Health Department. No doubt it is this same directive aspect that will make the program less appealing to others who prefer a more collaborative approach.

Despite the directive nature of the program, there is not uniform agreement about some aspects of its implementation. For example, performance criteria for completion of the child-directed interactions phase have been found to vary widely across authors, and there are some inconsistencies about how and when to use data from direct observations of parent–child interactions. In addition, there are some inconsistencies with respect to philosophy (e.g., using developmentally sensitive interventions) and practice (e.g., engaging in extensive reasoning, explaining of interventions with young children; compare Hembree-Kigin & McNeil, 1995, with Herschell et al., 2002a). However, these may be purely academic debates and are unlikely to bother a practitioner looking to identify a detailed yet practical and accessible program for guiding their parent training.

SUMMARY

Each of the four programs described in this chapter offers considerable empirical support and manuals that can guide effective implementation. As a result, any of the programs must be considered a reasonable choice for the practitioner interested in evidence-based practice. This allows the practitioner to use his or her clinical expertise in deciding which program is most responsive to the unique needs of a given child and family.

In making a choice about which program to use, there may also be practical issues and matters of personal preference. From a practical standpoint, we have described the programs in the order of accessibility to practitioners, whether considering financial costs, training requirements, or the availability of resources. From a philosophical viewpoint, the programs are largely comparable, with the foundation of each program firmly rooted in behavioral and social learning theory and in the pioneering work initially performed at the ORI in the 1960s and 1970s.

From a programmatic viewpoint, the overlap between program content is considerable, as are the numerous similarities (see Table 2.9) in teaching methodology. Each program emphasizes the importance of increasing positive interactions with children by praising, attending, and rewarding and by reducing reactivity to minor problems. Each program highlights the importance of reducing unnecessary demands but being clear when demands are required and when compliance is expected. Each program supports the use of immediate consequences and punishment when necessary, clearly establishing these con-

TABLE 2.9
Empirically Supported Parent Training Program Similarities

Domain	Similarities
Research support	Empirically supported treatments
Philosophy	Rooted in behavioral theory
Teaching methods	Instruction, modeling, practice, feedback
Program emphasis	Developing positive behaviors and interactions through praise, attending, and rewards
Discipline approach	Response cost, time-out

tingencies ahead of time with contracts, practice, or negotiation. Finally, each program uses well-established teaching techniques that include instruction, modeling, and homework to help bring changes into the home.

Despite these many similarities, the programs do have some differences (see Table 2.10). For example, The Incredible Years is distinctly less directive than each of the other programs and the only one that relies on group instruction. Both The Incredible Years and the Helping the Noncompliant

TABLE 2.10
Empirically Supported Parent Training Program Comparisons

Program	Ages	Format	Length	Unique features
Living With Children	3–14	Individual	12 sessions	Parent book test, parents observe and record child behavior, frequent contact between parents and practitioners, point systems
The Incredible Years	2–8	Group	10–14 weeks	Parent book; videotaped modeling; group format; nondirective, collaborative approach; problem solving; extensive technical support; parent self-management; high cost
Helping the Noncompliant Child	3–8	Individual	12 weeks	Manual is a scholarly text; directive; child is included in all sessions; early research involved component analyses; parent self-management
Parent–Child Interaction Therapy	2–8	Individual	8–14 weeks	Developmental considerations, bug-in-the-ear training approach, higher directive manual, daily minding exercises, acceptable time-out enforcement procedures include physical discipline

Child program use videotape as a part of training and offer markedly greater emphasis on parent self-management skills in addition to child management skills. The Parent–Child Interaction Therapy manual seems the most straightforward, accessible, and easily followed; The Incredible Years and the Living With Children program offer a separate parent book.

In sum, the programs are more alike than different. What links them is not only the theoretical underpinnings regarding what new behaviors to teach to parents and children and how to do so but also the extensive body of applied research supporting these parent training approaches. This is distinctly different from a multitude of alternative parent training programs that are widely available. The relative diversity of theoretical approaches and relative lack of empirical support for some alternatives stand in contrast to the uniform conceptual and empirical support underlying the four programs reviewed here. This contrast is easier to detect in the midst of a comparative review, which is provided in the following chapter.

3

EVALUATING THE SCIENTIFIC MERIT OF PARENT TRAINING ALTERNATIVES

The parent training programs described in the previous chapter are considered to be empirically supported treatments, as evidenced by multiple well-designed controlled experimental investigations and accompanying treatment manuals. These programs are endorsed and widely recognized throughout the professional community and are available to both professional and public audiences.

However, the empirically supported programs are not necessarily the most popular. For example, two of the most popular and widely disseminated programs (Ritchie & Partin, 1994) are Parent Effectiveness Training (Gordon, 1975) and Systematic Training for Effective Parenting (Dinkmeyer & McKay, 1983). Indeed, there are numerous other parent training programs from which to choose, and it seems new parenting programs are constantly introduced and promoted. There are programs on active parenting, common-sense parenting, confident parenting, effective parenting, loving parenting, logical parenting, and positive parenting, to name only a few. Many of these pursue dissemination through self-published materials, workshops, and advertising and offer certification through specialized training. Some make rather extraordinary claims about their successes and offer vivid testimonials and anecdotes. Faced with many choices and an abundance of supporting "evidence," practitioners and parents may be left with uncertainties and confusion about which parent training program to choose.

Certainly one strategy that practitioners can use to evaluate the quality of supporting empirical evidence is to limit one's selection to programs that meet criteria for being empirically supported treatments as defined by professional organizations. Criteria often used by professional organizations to identify empirically supported programs and interventions are described in chapter 2. However, not all of the parent training programs available are reviewed by professional organizations. There are literally hundreds of parent training programs available and marketed. In addition, there is a continuously growing research base on parent training, and some lists may not be up-to-date or accurate in describing a program's current research support. Practitioners are likely to come across many parent training programs and must take responsibility to evaluate the scientific merit of the research themselves. The extent of that merit can be determined by consideration of several important criteria derived from the basic criteria many organizations use to identify interventions as empirically supported, as described in chapter 2. These criteria are summarized in Table 3.1. The criteria described in this section are implicit in the criteria for the empirically supported programs described in chapter 2. We explicitly describe them in this chapter to provide more direct guidance for practitioners in reviewing the empirical literature supporting parent training programs.

First, the supporting evidence must have been published in a peer-reviewed journal. *Peer review* refers to a process by which experts in the field read and critique research. This peer-review process is widely considered to be an essential element in maintaining "quality control" in scientific literature (Kazdin, 2003). Supporting evidence that has not undergone the peer-review process has undetermined quality or merit. Through the peer-review process, practitioners allow experts in the field to serve as impartial "gatekeepers of science," making judgments about quality and merit and making decisions about what should and should not be published (Hojat, Gonella, & Caelleigh, 2003). This quality control is so important that online research databases (e.g., PsycINFO) now list whether sources are peer-reviewed journals.

A second criterion requires that the supporting evidence provide some valid demonstration of the effectiveness of the parenting program. This usually requires some element of experimental control. This is important because peer review can help ensure the basic quality of research but provides no guarantee that the publication validates the program as effective. For example, peer-reviewed journals may publish program descriptions that include no actual evaluation of whether the parenting program is effective. More important, not all empirical evaluations provide equal confidence in the validity of a program. For example, pre–post outcome evaluations can help demonstrate

TABLE 3.1

Criteria of Merit in Evaluating Supporting Scientific Evidence

Type of evidence	Evidence continuum			
	Not acceptable	Minimum	Moderate	Strong
Peer review	No peer review	Peer review	—	—
Experimental design	No control group or AB[a] or case study	Wait-list control group or Multiple baseline or comparable small N design[b]	Placebo control group or ABA or comparable small N design	Compare with established treatment or ABAB or comparable small N design
Replication		One between group or Small series of single-case studies (e.g., < 3)	Two or more between group studies or Large series of single-case studies (e.g., ≥ 3)	
Outcomes measured		Parent or child ratings of attitudes, beliefs, perceptions, or satisfaction	Parent or child ratings of child behavior or parent behavior	Direct observation of child or parent behavior

[a]A = baseline; B = treatment.
[b]See Barlow and Hersen (1984) for extended discussion of these designs.

that changes occurred but provide little confidence that they would not have occurred independent of the parenting program. This type of confidence comes only from research designs that arrange for experimental control.

For group research designs, experimental control is generally demonstrated by inclusion of some type of control group—that is, a group that either receives no treatment or receives an established alternative treatment. Researchers using small N research designs generally require some replication of treatment effects within or across (or both) two or more participants. For example, treatment may be introduced sequentially for two or more participants after varying amounts of time in baseline. This type of design is called a multiple baseline. Treatment may also be introduced and then withdrawn, introduced and withdrawn again across several participants (i.e., an ABAB design; e.g., see Barlow & Hersen, 1984, for a more complete discussion of these types of experimental designs). The demonstration of experimental control in control-group designs or in single-subject designs increases confidence that the outcomes were produced by the treatment and not by some other unmeasured or unaccounted-for variable.

Third, the more demonstrations of efficacy that exist, the more confidence a practitioner can have in the merit of the parent training program. A single demonstration of efficacy, regardless of the level of experimental control, simply cannot provide adequate demonstration of the external validity of the treatment and outcomes. *External validity* refers to whether the treatment may be appropriate for a broader sample of children and parents or for use in a broader array of treatment settings. Multiple replications of treatment efficacy help provide increased confidence in the external validity of a treatment, and even more so when those replications are conducted by different investigators.

Finally, it is important for the practitioner to examine the outcomes that were actually measured. Outcomes of interest in parent training programs can include subjective reports of satisfaction by program participants, parent knowledge of the material presented, and parental attitudes and perceptions about parenting. Outcomes that describe attitudes, perceptions, satisfaction, and knowledge can certainly help establish the social validity of a program. However, practitioners should also look for outcomes that measure parent–child relationships and overall child behavior and adjustment. These latter outcomes seem particularly important to measure because we know that parent attitudes, knowledge, and perceptions of change do not always correspond to real changes in child behavior (e.g., Bernal, Klinnert, & Schultz, 1980). For that reason, direct measures and observations of child and parent behavior are listed as stronger examples of evidence for scientific merit in Table 3.1, relative to measures of parental attitudes or indirect ratings of child and parent behavior.

As outlined in Table 3.1, using these four criteria (i.e., peer review, experimental control, replication, and relevant outcomes) can help a practitioner determine how much confidence to place in other parent training programs. These criteria offer a continuum of scientific merit, providing the practitioner with a means to evaluate the merit of a program in which one's confidence in that merit covaries directly with the number and extent to which criteria are met. For example, the more peer-reviewed publications, the better, but this is not independent of experimental control. Likewise, the stronger the demonstration of experimental control, the better, but this is not independent of relevant variables. Finally, the more replications, the better, but this is not independent of whether they have been subject to peer review. Thus, the criteria do offer a continuum of merit for consideration, but the criteria are inextricably linked.

We apply these criteria and adjust our confidence accordingly as we review a representative sample of other popular and prominent parent training programs. The programs selected for review come from a variety of sources. Although there is not a top-ten list of popular parent training programs, the sample of parent training programs selected for this chapter were gathered from a review of the programs most frequently named during online searches of a research database (e.g., PsycINFO) and Web site search engines (e.g., Google, Yahoo). Online searches are probably one of the most common methods to identify interventions and programs practitioners use. We review two of the most frequently cited and widely disseminated large programs in detail and six other programs more briefly. The empirical support for each program is reviewed using the criteria in Table 3.1, and corresponding impressions and recommendations are provided.

Each review also includes an overview of the program, the populations served, and the length of treatment. In addition, the specific and unique program components are described. This information is provided because practitioners should first review program content and parameters to determine whether the program has potential to match their needs in terms of their practice parameters (e.g., resources, time) and client characteristics (e.g., ages served, problems addressed). Additional information on examining the match between research and practice is provided in chapter 8.

PARENT EFFECTIVENESS TRAINING

The Parent Effectiveness Training (PET) program was originally developed by Thomas Gordon in the 1960s (Gordon, 1975). It is based on the premise that parents can be taught to use the same nondirective therapeutic techniques that some counselors and therapists use as they help individuals overcome emotional problems and maladaptive behavior. Gordon, who studied with Carl Rogers at the University of Chicago, was highly influenced by Rogers's humanistic philosophy. Rogers believed that if a therapist could create a context of genuine acceptance and trust, clients would have the ability to solve their own problems.

Consistent with this nondirective approach, Gordon developed a parenting program that does not offer specific advice or principles to follow regarding how to raise children or to solve problems; rather, PET offers a specific set of skills for communicating with a child, thereby helping the child develop his or her own solutions. This approach stands in contrast to the more directive behavioral parenting programs reviewed in chapter 2 in which parents are given specific recommendations about how to promote obedience and cooperative behavior. Indeed, Gordon rejects the notion that parents must insist on obedience from their children, and he is critical of behavioral interventions that, in his view, blame the child for misbehaving.

Instead, Gordon recommends that parents be given skills that allow them to influence, but not control, children, purportedly helping them make choices that allow both child and parent to have their needs met. Although Gordon acknowledges that the use of consequences to control behavior may be appropriate for parents of children with developmental disabilities, he does not believe this is necessary for normally developing children (Gordon, 1975). As a result, Gordon avoids the use of rewards, punishments, and rules to control children, preferring instead the influential use of warmth, acceptance, and effective communication.

Program Specifics

Target Population

The program materials suggest that it is appropriate for children of all ages.

Treatment Setting

The treatment is typically delivered by a certified trainer and may occur with groups of parents, but it may also be administered in individualized sessions. Self-administered program materials are also available. Children under age 12 are not included in group sessions with parents but older children may be included.

Program Materials

A practitioner can purchase the parent program materials online (http://www.gordontraining.com), including the PET book, audiotapes, or CD/DVDs of the Family Effectiveness Training program, as well as related workbooks. The video course is based on PET and intended to be a home-study course for parents and children ages 12 and older. These materials range in cost from \$15 to \$80. There are no specific manuals or materials for practitioners; however, they can participate in a 3-day workshop designed to "train the trainer." These workshops are intended for anyone who has already participated in a PET course or completed the home-video course, which are prerequisites. The training is not limited to individuals with advanced clinical training or experience. The cost is about \$1,100 and results in certification as a PET trainer.

Program Length

This is an 8-week program. Parents meet weekly, typically in groups of 8 to 16, for 3-hour training sessions.

Program Content (What to Teach)

The program content begins with establishing the foundational premise that parents are not perfect, that situational variables such as fatigue, spousal demands, and chores may affect parent behavior and that these influences make it nearly impossible to be consistent. This inability is thought to place significant constraints on behavioral techniques involving management through consequences. Inconsistency may increase the likelihood of problem behaviors in children, cause anxiety, and create power struggles between children and parents. PET techniques focus instead on giving children choices—choices that both the child and the parent must find acceptable. The techniques are thought to increase a child's motivation to comply or cooperate so that enforcement is unnecessary.

At the heart of the program is *active listening*, a skill designed to create a warm relationship between parent and child. This is accomplished by encouraging parents to stop trying to teach, instruct, advise, criticize, control, and solve problems. Rather, parents are encouraged to listen. In particular, active listening involves the parent's reflecting back what he or she feels a child is trying to communicate. This is designed especially for times that a parent wants to encourage a child to communicate more or when a child is trying to express feelings. Because the parent offers no opinion, advice, analysis, or questions in response to something a child says, many parents predictably describe these interactions as feeling unnatural, awkward, and fake. Parents are taught that with practice, the skills become more natural and comfortable.

This emphasis on asking no questions, giving no direction, and reflecting what is said should sound surprisingly familiar to those acquainted with child-directed interactions that several parent training programs discussed in chapter 2 use. Although active listening is strongly encouraged, parents learn that there are times when active listening is simply not appropriate. These situations might arise when a child is not interested in talking, when a parent has limited time to listen, or when the child is really just asking for a specific kind of help or information. Parents are nevertheless encouraged to use active listening with children of all ages, even nonverbal infants, with whom the parent is told to rely on what a child does rather than trying to interpret what the child is trying to communicate.

The PET program also teaches parents that typical styles of communicating with children often involve criticizing, blaming, instructing, and analyzing. This style of communicating is thought to produce children who are defensive and hostile. The PET program asks parents to instead use *"I" messages*, which involve simply explaining to a child how his or her behavior makes the parent feel. This is thought to create an openness and honesty in the parent–child relationship that will reduce conflict and free a child to change in ways that meet his or her own needs but respect the needs of others as well.

Although the PET philosophy is largely focused on helping children find solutions to their own problems and creating opportunity for change, it does advocate direct efforts to change unacceptable behavior. These do not involve altering consequences but changing the environment in ways that alter the probability of children misbehaving. This might include enriching the environment (i.e., adding more things for a child to do), impoverishing the environment (e.g., turning off the TV when it is time for bed), simplifying the environment (e.g., making some tasks easier for children), or even childproofing the environment (e.g., removing breakable objects).

Finally, PET advocates a *no-lose* problem-solving approach to conflict resolution. Rather than imposing control over children, parents are encouraged to let them search for solutions that meet both their own and their parents' needs. The method focuses on choice—not giving a child choices provided by the parents but instead encouraging him or her to identify choices that both parties will find acceptable. Even family rules, which are deemed necessary by program content, are developed by encouraging the child to identify rules that all members of the family will find acceptable. This is believed to increase a child's motivation to comply or cooperate so that enforcement is not necessary. Parents are encouraged to use the technique even with very young children.

No information or training is offered regarding what to do in situations in which a young child offers no solution that is acceptable to the parent. The assumption would appear to be that if a parent persists long enough with problem solving, even into the next day, a solution can eventually be found. Believing that the process itself eliminates conflict, there is little discussion of how to handle children who exhibit defiance and are not willing to participate in the problem-solving process. Again, the program strongly rejects efforts to impose control, believing that these efforts result in children who become "cowed, fearful, and nervous."

Program Content (How to Teach)

There are no resources readily available to a practitioner regarding how to teach the program. A practitioner interested in the how-to aspects must invest in a 3-day train-the-trainer workshop offered by Gordon Training International. The training offers specific insights into how to train and includes videotapes, audiotapes, slide presentations, and handouts to assist the practitioner. The process of teaching involves lecture format, discussions, and practice.

Unique Program Features

This is the only program we could find that offers no age limitations regarding with whom it can be used. Almost all of the empirically supported programs are fairly specific in delineating an age range within which their programs are designed to be used. In contrast, the PET program is encouraged for use with children of any age, including babies and nonverbal infants. This strong emphasis on verbally mediated parenting techniques is particularly unusual in a field that often places considerable import on developmental considerations. Instead, PET encourages that children be "treated as an equal . . . , much as we treat friends or a spouse" (Gordon, 1975, p. 213). In addition, although program materials reject the notion that the program is permissive, the absence of recommendations about how to handle particularly oppositional, defiant, or noncompliant behavior makes this program rather unique among parent training programs. Finally, the 3-hour group sessions are twice as long as typical alternative programs recommend. This is a high expectation for working parents or for those who must find child care for children under 12.

Empirical Support

It is important to note that there have been some efforts to validate important components of the PET program outside its context. Specifically, a small number of controlled investigations have been conducted to study "I" messages and active listening as means of reducing conflict. For example, Peterson (1979) found that teachers who used "I" messages in response to student disruptions in the classroom were able to decrease disruptions and increase study behavior. These results have not been replicated. In addition, Kubany, Richard, and Bauer (1992) found that adult partners rated messages as less aversive and as producing fewer negative emotional responses than typical "you" messages. However, the value of active listening in reducing conflict has been called into question (Gottman, Coan, & Carrere, 1998). In large part, this is because the vast majority of the research on "I" messages and active listening are uncontrolled or unpublished investigations that include

"I" messages and active listening as part of "communication training" so that their independent effects remain unknown.

Research on the PET program itself, conducted since the late 1970s, has resulted in a relatively small number of controlled empirical studies investigating various aspects of PET program effectiveness. Early narrative reviews of this research were critical, suggesting that data did not support the effectiveness of PET (Rinn & Markle, 1977). Another review of the literature, almost a decade later, found that methodological weaknesses (i.e., no control groups and no randomization) severely limited meaningful conclusions about the effectiveness of PET (Dembo, Sweitzer, & Lauritzen, 1985). In addition, studies at that time had shown only that the program produced changes in child-rearing attitudes, with no evidence to support claims that PET could bring about positive effects on children.

Later, a meta-analysis of research conducted through the late 1980s found some support for PET as a means of improving parents' knowledge about PET, as well as attitudes and self-esteem about parenting, but the effects were not overwhelmingly large (Cedar & Levant, 1990). Further, a majority of these studies were dissertations and theses that had not been subjected to peer review, so their scientific merit is unknown. In addition, as with earlier investigations, a vast majority of the investigations used parent-generated ratings of attitudes, perceptions, or behavior, with no controlled investigations providing any direct measures of child behavior or parent–child interactions.

Cedar and Levant (1990) suggested that future researchers should look specifically at the effects of PET on children. Yet reviews of more recent research (C. T. Mueller, Hager, & Heise, 2001) continue to show relatively few well-controlled investigations with a focus on changing attitudes and perceptions of parents. In addition, many of them use different methods for measuring these outcomes, so comparisons across studies are not possible.

Impressions and Recommendations

The PET program (summarized in Table 3.2) is likely to have appeal for some because of its emphasis on communication as the mainspring of effective parenting. In this program, problems are avoided by listening and solved by talking. In addition, some will like its open rejection of more controlling, directive approaches to both parent training and parenting. Although the program does not permit children to do whatever they like, it is relatively more permissive than many other programs in that its materials recommend arranging for children to have their needs met.

Although the program openly rejects interventions that attempt to control child behavior, the PET program clearly promotes altering the environment to change behavior. The program rejects some behavioral methods in part because they are difficult to implement consistently; however, it is difficult to tell

TABLE 3.2
Program Features of Parent Effectiveness Training

Program domain	Program features
Ages	All ages
Problems	Nonclinical
Materials	Available online
	Video: *Family Effectiveness Training* (Gordon, 1997) (http://www.gordontraining.com)
	Manual: None
	Training workshops: Available
Format	Group
Length	Eight sessions, 3 hours each
What to teach	Active listening, "I" messages, enriching and simplifying the environment, childproofing, no-lose problem solving
How to teach	Nondirective, discussions based on videotapes, practice skills, help parents and children find their own solutions
Unique features	No age limits, treatment of children as equals, long group sessions, no-lose problem solving
Empirical support	Peer review: Yes
	Experimental control: Moderate
	Replication: Moderate
	Relevant outcomes: Moderate

how PET techniques would be any easier to implement consistently. All parent training programs require parents to change behavior, and making those changes consistently is difficult, regardless of the specific techniques that are used. Finally, for practitioners who wish to focus on changing attitudes and outlooks about parenting, this program does have some moderate supporting empirical evidence. However, there are no well-controlled, peer-reviewed studies to support the use of PET as a means of actually changing child behavior.

SYSTEMATIC TRAINING FOR EFFECTIVE PARENTING

The Systematic Training for Effective Parenting (STEP) program was developed by Dinkmeyer and McKay (1983) as a structured, formalized approach to disseminating the parenting ideas of Alfred Adler and a former student of his, Rudolf Dreikurs. Central to this approach is the idea that parenting is best approached as a sort of socialistic democracy in which the rights of children are equal to that of parents. As such, parents are encouraged to avoid using planned rewards and punishments, relying instead on letting children learn through natural and logical consequences. According to this approach, by limiting the parent role in correcting children and instead emphasizing active listening and natural consequences, children feel respected and are therefore freed to make decisions and choices and to learn from experience.

Program Specifics

Target Population

The program is directed primarily to parents of children ages 6 to 12. However, related programs are available for parents of children ages 0 to 6 and for parents of teens. The program is not considered to target parents of children with significant behavior problems and is not designed to be group therapy for parents. It is generally considered to target the normal challenges of typical parents.

Treatment Setting

Sessions are conducted in groups without children present. No particular group size is recommended.

Program Materials

The program materials include the *Leader's Resource Guide* (Dinkmeyer & McKay, 1997), which has detailed instructions for running each session. No additional training is required of professional practitioners interested in leading a STEP group, although participation in training workshops is encouraged. Workshops are 1-day sessions that focus on providing practice in leading a STEP parenting program. Materials also include parent handbooks, a video overview, and videotaped examples. The *Leader's Resource Guide* includes questions for group consideration, videos, and activities for practice. The materials are also available in Spanish and all are produced by AGS Publishing; they are available at http://www.agsnet.com/parenting.asp.

Program Length

The program is recommended to last seven sessions, about one per week for 7 weeks. Sessions typically last 1 to 2 hours.

Program Content (What to Teach)

At the heart of this program is the philosophy that parental use of rewards and punishment should be avoided and instead replaced by more democratic procedures for bringing up children. The specific procedures for establishing a more democratic relationship center on (a) improving communication and (b) using natural and logical consequences. The strategies for improving communication are similar to those used in the PET program. Parents learn how to improve listening skills through active listening to use "I" messages to ensure that both children and parents can express their feelings in appropriate ways. A democratic family environment is also thought to be promoted through use of logical and natural consequences, rather than planned artificial consequences involving rewards or punishments that are unrelated to the behavior.

Program Content (How to Teach)

The *Leader's Resource Guide* (Dinkmeyer & McKay, 1997) provides detailed descriptions of the methods involved in effective parenting as well as advice about managing problems that leaders will face in conducting parent training. This includes discussion of the principles of leadership and the problems associated with leading groups, discussion of specific leadership skills, and guidelines for leading discussions with parents. The parent handbook provides review questions, examples of problem situations, an activity for the week, and prompts for goal-setting activities to help plan specific parent behavior change and parenting improvements over the coming week.

Unique Program Features

The notion that children should be treated as little adults and have rights equal to those of parents is consistent with the parenting philosophy of PET but unique from most other parenting programs. However, the STEP program is probably most unique in its melding of behavioral, Adlerian, and Rogerian approaches. Although advocates would deny that there are any behavioral aspects to the program, the programmatic emphasis on the use of logical consequences to change child behavior is behavioral. In addition, parents are encouraged to use ignoring when possible, which is a punitive consequence that, in many cases, is not logical. Parents are also asked to chart behavior and set goals for behavior change, which for many could be considered behavioral strategies.

Empirical Support

Adler believed that true principles of human behavior were best identified through subjective and intuitive evaluations rather than any type of empirical investigation (Hoffman, 1994). As such, he and his students were not particularly interested in subjecting his concepts about parenting to any sort of empirical validation. Others were. Several controlled investigations conducted in the mid-1970s found that Adlerian-type parent training resulted in mothers who self-reported being less controlling and more democratic than untrained mothers (e.g., Berrett, 1975; Freeman, 1975). These initial studies of Adlerian approaches relied on parents' subjective reports of children's attitude and behavior changes (Krebs, 1986).

Since the early 1970s, perhaps because it is such a prominent example of the Adlerian approach, the STEP program has continued to attract considerable interest from researchers. Since the early 1980s, many have pursued objective evaluation of the program, and more than 60 investigations of the STEP program have been conducted. A substantial majority of these are unpublished dissertations, theses, reports, or presentations. This is not to say that these investigations constitute poor research, only that their scientific merit remains unevaluated by formal peer review. As a result, it is difficult to determine whether the Adlerian parenting program works (Kumpfer, 1999).

Of the peer-reviewed, published investigations regarding STEP, a small number have been well-controlled, randomized trials. As with earlier Adlerian research, these controlled investigations have used parent-generated ratings of attitudes, perceptions, or behavior as outcome measures. Some of the results are consistent with previous research on Adlerian approaches, suggesting that STEP does result in parents reporting improved attitudes about their children, improved trust and acceptance of their children, and the use of more democratic parenting practices (e.g., Dembo et al., 1985; Nystul, 1982). However, other researchers have found minimal or no changes in parental attitudes (e.g., Jackson & Brown, 1986), leading some to claim that STEP is ineffective in producing parental attitude changes (Robinson, Robinson, & Dunn, 2003).

In addition, no data suggest that generating changes in attitudes, perceptions, and feelings about parenting translate into meaningful changes in the parent–child relationship or in child behavior, well-being, or psychosocial adjustment (Taylor & Biglan, 1998). For some, this represents a critical void in the literature. Although changes in parental attitudes and perceptions could be involved in changing child behavior and parent–child relationships, simply demonstrating changes in attitudes after training is not enough to warrant conclusions about the effectiveness of the program in changing behavior (Robinson et al., 2003).

Impressions and Recommendations

For practitioners who wish to train parents to feel less controlling and more accepting and positive about their children, STEP may be a reasonable consideration. The scientific data provide moderate empirical support for the conclusion that the STEP program is a reasonable means to accomplish these goals. In addition, the resource materials are well developed and easily accessed, and they provide specific guidance in how as well as what to teach parents (see Table 3.3), an attractive feature for any practitioner. Whether parents who participate in this training actually are (i.e., behave) less controlling and more accepting of their children remains unknown.

As with PET, the STEP program places emphasis on approaching children as equals, an interesting notion in light of decades of developmental,

TABLE 3.3
Program Features of Systematic Training for Effective Parenting

Program domain	Program features
Ages	6–12
Problems	Common nonclinical problems
Materials	Manual: *Leader's Resource Guide* (Dinkmeyer & McKay, 1997)
	Available online and in Spanish
	Training workshops: Recommended
Format	Group
Length	Seven sessions, 1–2 hours each
What to teach	Use of logical and natural consequences, "I" messages, and active listening
How to teach	Discussions, use of leadership skills in leading groups, goal setting, homework
Unique features	Melding of behavioral, Adlerian, and Rogerian approaches
Empirical support	Peer review: Yes
	Experimental control: Moderate
	Replication: Moderate
	Relevant outcomes: Moderate

clinical, and biological literature suggesting that children are not simply little adults. One can value children's worth and dignity, and even equate them with adults', without requiring that children have equal rights and power within the family unit. In fact, although the communication procedures promoted in STEP are clearly designed to value children's worth and dignity, the natural and logical consequences result in limits that do not allow children to have full democratic rights and power within the family. It is thus easy to see why this program would have considerable appeal to modern-day parents. Nevertheless, practitioners should be aware that the program is not designed or promoted as a solution to clinically significant behavior problems.

ACTIVE PARENTING

The Active Parenting program is essentially a six-session, video-based version of the Adlerian STEP program (Popkin, 1983). The basic program is designed for parents of children ages 5 to 12 years and includes the same skills as those described in the STEP program. A standard program kit is available online and includes the parent's guide (Popkin, 2002a), promotional flyers, overhead transparencies, videotapes, and the leader's guide (Popkin, 2002b), which has instructions about when to use the video and how to lead discussions. Leader training is also available, although the program relies on videotaped presentations as the primary mode of instruction.

In the Active Parenting program, parents attend 2-hour sessions, watch videos, and then discuss, practice, and receive feedback about the skills they are learning. Materials are also available in Spanish. Although no published, peer-reviewed, controlled outcome data are available on the efficacy of this program, it is possible that its outcomes would be similar to those of the original STEP research studies, given that the content is the same. Research needs to be conducted, however, to evaluate this. It remains unknown how the video-based format might influence these outcomes, but results from controlled evaluations of other video-based parent training programs have suggested that video may not be a necessary component of effective parent training (e.g., see Webster-Stratton, Kolpacoff, & Hollingsworth, 1988).

LOVE AND LOGIC

The Love and Logic program was developed by Jim Fay, Charles Fay, and Foster Cline as a 12- to 15-hour program that relies heavily on the parental use of consequences to change and manage behavior in children, from infants through teens (http://www.loveandlogic.com). Materials include instructional videos, audiocassettes, parent handbooks, program transparencies, and a facilitator manual.

The Love and Logic philosophy centers on the notion that, rather than protect a child from consequences or trying to direct and control a child, an effective parent will use love (i.e., empathy) to affirm a child's worth and then logic to establish choices. The program's developers believe this allows children to explore alternatives and make decisions. Much like the egalitarian aspects of the PET program, Love and Logic purports to emphasize "shared control"; however, this program clearly directs parents to limit the options children have available and to choose for them if they are too slow in deciding. Seminars and classes are available for those who wish to become a parent instructor, although promotional materials suggest that no additional training is required if the available, step-by-step facilitator guide is used. Anecdotal testimonials are available, but we could find no controlled outcome data in peer-reviewed journals regarding the effectiveness of this program. Thus, Love and Logic does not meet the minimum criteria used when evaluating the quality of empirical support for a parent training program, and it should be used with caution, if at all, in an evidence-based practice.

PUTTING KIDS FIRST

Putting Kids First is one of a growing number of online parenting programs designed to increase access to parenting information (http://www.puttingkidsfirst.org). This program is specifically designed for those who have been mandated or court ordered to complete a parenting class. Although home study materials are available, the course is intended to be completed online, and a certificate of completion is sent to the participant. The program purports to teach parents better communication and conflict resolution skills, but no other information is available about its content. We found no controlled outcome evaluations describing the efficacy of this program in peer-reviewed publications. Putting Kids First meets none of the criteria used when evaluating the quality of empirical support for a parent training program, and it should be used with caution, if at all, in an evidence-based practice.

NURTURING PARENTING PROGRAMS

Nurturing Parenting is a series of programs developed by Stephen Bavolek, designed for parents of children from infancy to the teenage years. The programs are designed to help parents understand childhood development and to teach them how to use praise, nonviolent discipline, communication, problem solving, and negotiation to improve child self-esteem (http://www. nurturingparenting.com). There are also culturally specific, school-based, and scripture-based programs, as well as programs for foster parents, adoptive parents, and parents of children with special needs.

The programs emphasize empathy as the critical variable in healthy family relationships. Programs range from 7 to 40 sessions depending on the age of the child and whether the program is a home- or group-based training format. Group sessions last 2 to 3 hours and include activities for children. Materials include an assessment instrument for evaluating critical parenting skills and a program manual with planned lessons to assist professionals interested in teaching one of these programs. The Web site has a "Research and Validation" link where the articles and reports are self-published descriptions of program philosophy and program components, rather than scientific studies. No controlled outcome evaluations of relevant variables have been found in peer-reviewed publications describing the efficacy of the program. Nurturing Parenting meets none of the criteria used when evaluating the quality of empirical support for a parent training program, and it should be used with caution, if at all, in an evidence-based practice.

COMMON SENSE PARENTING

The Common Sense Parenting program was developed at the Girls and Boys Town, which is a residential treatment center for abused, neglected, and abandoned youth (http://www.parenting.org). The program is summarized in Table 3.4. It is intended for children 3 to 16 years of age and is typically presented in a group format in weekly 2-hour sessions across 6 weeks. The program

TABLE 3.4
Program Features of Common Sense Parenting

Program domain	Program features
Ages	3–16
Problems	Common nonclinical problems
Materials	Parent book: *Common Sense Parenting Training* (Burke, Herron, & Schuchmann, 2004)
	Manual: Guidebook available at training
	Training workshops: Required to get manual
Format	Group or self-directed
Length	Six sessions, 2 hours each
What to teach	Use of praise, effective commands, and time-out; use of corrective teaching
How to teach	Behavioral skills training, parent workbook, DVD
Unique features	Corrective teaching
Empirical support	Peer review: Yes
	Experimental control: Minimal
	Replication: Minimal
	Relevant outcomes: Moderate

is disseminated through the book *Common Sense Parenting* by Burke, Herron, and Schuchmann (2004). The book is actually a parent workbook that includes a DVD. Together with the DVD, which complements the text with explanations and video clips of parenting skills, the book can be used as a self-directed guide.

The program makes use of basic behavioral skills training with parents, teaching core concepts of using effective praise, clear commands, and consequences (e.g., time-out) and of providing preventive and corrective teaching. The program is also disseminated through the Boys Town National Resource and Training Center. Training is available for practitioners through a 3-day workshop that includes a trainer's guidebook and videotaped examples of parent skills.

The Common Sense Parenting program has been subjected to two outcome evaluations that were published in peer-reviewed journals (R. W. Thompson, Ruma, Brewster, Besetsney, & Burke, 1997; R. W. Thompson, Ruma, & Schuchmann, 1996). Both studies found improvements in parent attitudes. More important, they also found improvements in relevant outcomes such as child behavior and parent–child relationships on the basis of parent reports on rating scales. These findings await replication. Only the 1996 study involved a well-controlled comparison with a no-treatment control group. Participants were not randomly assigned to groups. Nevertheless, the presence of relevant outcome measures within a single controlled outcome evaluation published in a peer-reviewed journal does offer minimal empirical support that the Common Sense Parenting program might be used in an evidence-based practice to improve parent competencies and ratings of clinically significant child behavior problems.

TRIPLE P POSITIVE PARENTING PROGRAM

The Triple P Positive Parenting Program is a multilevel, prevention-oriented parenting and family support strategy developed by Matthew Sanders and colleagues at the University of Queensland in Australia (http://www.triplep.net). It is intended for families with children ages 0 to 16. Although the program is largely based on the social learning models of parent–child interaction described by Patterson and colleagues (e.g., Patterson & Fisher, 2002), it also draws on research in applied behavior analysis, social–informational processing models, developmental psychopathology, and public health (Sanders, 1999).

The program (see Table 3.5) has five levels of intervention along a continuum of prevention services, ranging from a broad media-based universal prevention strategy to an intensive, individualized parent training and family support program. The standard parent training program can be delivered in individual, group, or self-directed formats ranging from 8 to 10 sessions that typically last 60 to 90 minutes. An active teaching approach uses modeling, role-play, practice, homework, and feedback. Manuals, videotapes, and a Web site provide support for practitioners interested in implementing Triple P. The Web site describes the availability of "accredited" training courses, but it is not clear by whom the courses are accredited. Most of the courses are

TABLE 3.5
Program Features of the Triple P Positive Parenting Program

Program domain	Program features
Ages	0–16
Problems	Prevention oriented
Materials	Manual: Available online
	Training workshops: Recommended
Format	Individual, group, or self-directed
Length	8–10 sessions, 60–90 minutes each
What to teach	Observing and recording behavior, pinpointing behavior, effective praise, ignoring, time-out; also incidental teaching, planned activities, reasoning, logical consequences
How to teach	Modeling, role-play, practice, feedback, homework
Unique features	Preventive emphasis
Empirical support	Peer review: Yes
	Experimental control: Strong
	Replication: Moderate
	Relevant outcomes: Strong

offered in Australia. The Web site provides an interesting "decision tree" to guide practitioners in deciding which level of training would best suit their needs, because multiple levels of training are offered depending on whether the practitioner serves individuals or groups, offers brief consultation or intensive face-to-face intervention, works with teens or children, and whether the practitioner serves individuals or organizations.

Unfortunately, the actual skills that are taught in the program are not clearly defined. An early published article indicates that parents were taught skills similar to Patterson and colleagues' program (e.g., see Patterson, Reid, Jones, & Conger, 1975), including how to observe and chart behavior, pinpoint problems, and use contingent consequences such as descriptive praise, ignoring, and time-out (Sanders & Glynn, 1981). However, recent descriptions of the program suggest that the skills parents learn have been significantly expanded. Parents now learn a range of behavior change procedures from a core of 17 child management techniques that might include incidental teaching, task analysis, planned activities, reasoning, and use of logical consequences (Sanders, Markie-Dadds, & Turner, 2003).

The Web site and program descriptions tout the program as "empirically supported" (e.g., see Sanders, 1999), and we did find two well-controlled, peer-reviewed investigations showing that the standard parent training program produced greater reductions in disruptive child behavior and high parent satisfaction compared with a control group that did not receive any treatment (Bor, Sanders, & Markie-Dadds, 2002; Sanders, Markie-Dadds, Tully, & Bor, 2000). There are also randomized controlled evaluations of the Triple P program that involve comparisons of "enhanced" versions with the standard Triple P (e.g., see Sanders et al., 2004) rather than comparisons with no-treatment control groups or alternative (non–Triple P) treatments. The Triple P program has not yet been identified as an empirically supported program by other professional organizations, probably because there remains a need for replication of efficacy by independent investigators. Nevertheless, the empirical support for the program meets strong standards of scientific merit, and Triple P may be considered for use in an evidence-based practice to reduce disruptive behavior in children.

SUMMARY

It is not surprising that there are widely varying degrees of support for parent training programs. Only since the 1990s have the parameters of "empirically supported" been defined, and it is certainly not a universally accepted notion that all programs require proof beyond what is available through subjective, intuitive evaluation and anecdotal experience. What can cause concern about some programs is the extent to which they are marketed and promoted as "proven" programs, using Web sites, books, videos, training materials, lectures, seminars, and even endorsements or association with groups that are widely recognized (e.g., United Way, Office of Juvenile Justice).

This is not to say that these alternative programs are not or could not be important sources of support and change for many families. In many cases, however, we simply do not know. Practitioners must remember that efficacy is not correlated with promotional zeal. Indeed, the most efficacious and best researched parenting programs are often, by comparison, hardly promoted at all.

For consumers truly interested in perusing the empirical support for these programs, the picture is clouded by promotional materials that may claim significant supporting research. On closer inspection, the "research" cited or posted on Web sites often comprises either discussion papers about parenting philosophy, reviews of parent surveys, or testimonials regarding attitudes, perceptions, or satisfaction. Of course, it is possible that parents' attitudinal and perceptual changes are associated with meaningful changes in child behavior or psychosocial adjustment. Unfortunately, with the exception of the Common Sense and Triple P programs, the research we were able to find has not typically directly measured child behavior for the approaches described in this chapter. Finally, although some of the alternative programs do include parenting practices that have substantial research support (i.e., use of rewards and punishment to change behavior in children), many include practices that either have little empirical support (e.g., "I" messages, active listening) or are conceptually suspect (e.g., negotiating and problem solving with toddlers).

Should a practitioner be concerned? Of course. Programs that do not meet the minimum criteria on the continuum of scientific merit constitute a risk for those interested in evidence-based practice. Parents and practitioners may be wasting valuable time and missing opportunities to truly make a difference with their children. This is particularly egregious given the numerous programs available that do meet the standards of good science. What is a practitioner to do? First, evaluate Web-based treatment programs with skepticism. Be equally skeptical of books by self-proclaimed experts. Promotional zeal, slick materials, impressive technology, and personal testimonials should not replace sound data. Programs that are disseminated exclusively through self-published materials, workshops, and advertising rather than peer-reviewed journals should be suspect. Keep in mind that there are no constraints on who may develop Web sites, and there are no standards or regulations regarding the validity or veracity of material posted on the Internet.

Second, be particularly suspicious of programs that are promoted as easy, quick, and broadly effective. Parenting is not easy, and learning new behavior is never quick. If parenting could truly be made easy, the solution would have been discovered long ago, and there would not be such a vast array of programs and resources competing so aggressively for our attention today.

Third, follow the data. The good news is that conceptually sound programs, supported by repeated examples of well-controlled research published in respected peer-reviewed journals, are available, and these programs offer step-by-step guides regarding what and how to teach. They are, admittedly, more difficult to find, and unfortunately, not all of them appear on popular Internet searches. In addition, they are not "easy," and they take time for both practitioners and parents to learn and master. As with anything, however, we reap what we sow. Nevertheless, developers of empirically supported parent training programs would do well to follow the lead of alternative program developers regarding how to market and disseminate their programs. Until then, practitioners need only a healthy dose of skepticism and a small amount of motivation to find meaningful direction amid the cluttered parent training landscape (see chap. 2).

One might ask whether practitioners must limit their pursuit of a parent training program to one that meets the high standards that professional organizations have set for empirically supported programs. The answer is an unequivocal yes if what practitioners desire is a high level of confidence in the validity of the techniques they use to address childhood problems of noncompliance, oppositional behavior, and disruptive social aggression (e.g., tantrums, hitting, arguing). As of this writing, none of the alternatives discussed in this chapter offer the quantity or quality of research support demonstrated by the parent training programs described in chapter 2. Thus, using one of the empirically supported programs is an important component of competent evidence-based practice.

Although important, using one of the empirically supported parent training programs is not sufficient to constitute an evidence-based practice. Even the developers of the empirically supported programs repeatedly claim that their programs require flexibility and adaptation in response to contextual variables. The clinical expertise to know when and how to adapt and flex comes from a strong theoretical and conceptual understanding of each program, from the skillful application of that program, and from attending to individual, social, and cultural contexts. In other words, to maintain an evidence-based approach to treating disruptive behavior problems in childhood, a practitioner will find it necessary, but not sufficient, to include one of the parent training programs reviewed in chapter 2, but other variables must be considered as well. In the following three chapters, these variables are discussed in detail.

II

DEVELOPING CLINICAL
EXPERTISE

4

CONCEPTUAL FOUNDATIONS OF THE EMPIRICALLY SUPPORTED PARENT TRAINING PROGRAMS

As described in chapters 1 and 2, the empirically supported parent training programs have a common conceptual foundation. Knowledge of this foundation can help practitioners understand why the individual components of empirically supported parent training programs work. Perhaps more important, an understanding of the conceptual foundation and the principles derived from it can be an important part of the clinical expertise needed to translate and apply these programs in everyday practice. Indeed, some have argued that standard procedures may be somewhat limited, that practitioners must be innovative, and that being innovative requires understanding theory and underlying principles (Patterson, Reid, Jones, & Conger, 1975). Likewise, some have suggested that refinements and improvements on empirically supported interventions in practice often depend on a clear understanding of the processes by which change is produced (Follette, 1995). Ultimately, those who understand why these parent training programs work may be in a better position to adapt, adjust, and apply the techniques of empirically supported programs as necessary in an evidenced-based practice.

The basic principles that underlie the empirically supported parent training programs are derived from the scientific study of behavior called the *experimental analysis of behavior*, or *behavior analysis* (e.g., see Skinner, 1953). Early experimental research that delineated the basic principles of behavior analysis came from research with laboratory animals (Skinner, 1938). Efforts to study and apply these principles with humans has been called *applied behavior analysis* (Baer, Wolf, & Risley, 1968, 1987). These principles reflect a conceptual foundation that emphasizes the role of immediate environmental events in understanding why humans do what they do.

Events that precede and affect a behavior are called *antecedents*. In behavior analysis, certain principles describe and predict how antecedents affect behavior. Events that immediately follow and affect the future occurrence of behavior are called *consequences*. Behavior analysis also suggests principles to describe and predict how consequences affect behavior. Both antecedents and consequences are considered to be *controlling variables* in that they can be altered to control or change behavior. Strategies that do so are often called *behavioral interventions*, and behavioral parent training programs make explicit use of these controlling variables.

This chapter provides readers with an overview of the behavioral principles that underlie the empirically supported parent training programs. It offers a primer on the basic principles of behavior and includes numerous examples to help practitioners see these principles at work in the everyday behavior of children and their parents. More important, the chapter describes how these principles are revealed in the empirically supported parent training programs and how practitioners can strengthen or weaken the impact of these principles in everyday parent–child interactions. Finally, the chapter provides specific examples of how these principles can be used to guide practitioners in adapting, adjusting, and applying components of the programs to meet the needs of individual clients.

BEHAVIORAL PRINCIPLES: ANTECEDENTS

Antecedents are events that occur before a particular behavior that influence whether, how often, and when that behavior occurs. Although consequences are generally recognized as the "mainsprings of behavior control" (Brady, 1978, p. v), antecedent events have an important impact on behavior (e.g., see Luiselli & Cameron, 1998). In behavioral parent training, two types of antecedents are particularly important—those that help establish the value of consequences (called *establishing operations*) and those that signal the best time to engage in certain behaviors to gain the valued consequences (called *discriminative stimuli*). Practitioners who understand how antecedents influence behavior can engineer the environment to prevent problem behaviors from occurring. They can also arrange the environment to evoke desirable behaviors in both children and adults.

Establishing Operations

Some antecedent events are called establishing operations because, although they occur before behavior, they can help *establish* the value of consequences that occur after the behavior. For example, when a child goes for a long period without food, this helps establish food as a powerful consequence. Sitting for long periods at a desk in school helps establish getting up and moving as an effective consequence. Being cold helps establish the warmth of a coat as valuable. For a teenager, the presence of peers in the room may help establish parent presence as aversive because the teen is embarrassed to be seen with Mom and Dad. In this last example, getting away from Mom and Dad is established as an effective consequence. Of course, these establishing operations occur for parents as well. For example, having guests in the house may establish typical noise from children as more aversive because it is distracting to the adults. Being around demanding children all day long can also establish being alone as a valuable consequence.

Note that after an antecedent event has established the effectiveness of a consequence, any behavior that has, in the past, produced that consequence is more likely to occur. For example, for a child who has gone a long while without food, any number of behaviors that typically produce food will become more likely to occur. These behaviors might include asking for food, rummaging through the refrigerator, or buying candy from a machine at school. A child who is cold will be more likely to do whatever, in the past, has resulted in a sweater or coat, such as getting up and getting a coat or sweater or whining about the cold until a parent brings something warm to wear. For the parent with guests, a noisy child evokes any number of responses that have quieted the child in the past. These might include the "stop it now" glare, a verbal reprimand, or redirection to a quiet activity.

Overall, one can see that establishing operations can be an important part of parent training because they change how much a child wants something (see Table 4.1). Parents who understand how to use establishing operations may

TABLE 4.1
Types of Antecedents

Type	Function	Examples
Establishing operation (EO)	EOs change how much people want something.	Going without food makes food more valuable. Being cold makes warmth more valuable.
Discriminative stimuli (S^D)	S^{D}s signal when certain responses will be most effective in achieving a desired consequence.	Ask Grandma (S^D) for a cookie, not Mom. Wrestle with your younger sister (S^D) and not your older brother if you want to win.

find that the consequences they use will be effective. Practitioners must help parents understand that even when these establishing operations are not under their control or influence, knowing how they work can help them to make good decisions about what consequences their child is likely to value. For example, a practitioner may find it inappropriate to recommend that a parent withhold a meal to establish food as a reinforcer. However, a parent may benefit from knowing that food is likely to be more effective as a reinforcer just before a meal rather than just after the meal. Thus, children may work harder at cleaning up their toys to earn a small snack in the late afternoon (before dinner) than they would immediately after dinner. In this way, parents can be trained to use establishing operations more effectively to change problem behavior over time.

Discriminative Stimuli

In addition to helping establish the value of consequences, antecedents can signal the best time to engage in certain behaviors to obtain a desired result. These stimuli are called *discriminative* because they help people discriminate when valuable consequences are available (see Table 4.1). For example, a child asks for a cookie when his mother walks in the room but not before, because to do so before she is in the room would be ineffective. Asking for a cookie is much more likely to produce a cookie if one's mother is in the room. Therefore, the mother has become a discriminative stimulus (i.e., signal) for asking for a cookie.

Of course, not all signals are equally valuable all the time; their signaling power may change depending on other conditions, such as the time of day. For example, a child may learn over time that his mother walking in the room is a weak signal for the availability of a cookie right before lunch because asking before lunch will rarely get the desired cookie. Yet his mother walking in the room may be a strong signal for the availability of a cookie right after lunch because asking after lunch often will get the desired cookie.

Discriminative stimuli can also play an important role in the development of problem behaviors. Consider that a child who likes interacting with her mother may make more noise when her mother picks up the phone. In this case, the phone has become a discriminative stimulus for noise making. The phone may have developed discriminative properties over time because the girl has learned that making noise while her mother is on the phone is more likely to produce a reaction. The child has also likely found that making noise while her mother is not on the phone does not reliably produce much reaction. In fact, children learn to respond reliably to this type of signal, and parents have been heard to say, "It's as if that darn phone were a signal to my child to start getting noisy." Indeed.

Paradoxically, a parent's attempt to change this situation may provide another discriminative stimulus that signals the child to be noisy. For example, when the phone rings, a mother may put her finger to her lips just before picking up the phone, an action that she believes will signal the child to be quiet. However, parents often use this signal when the call is particularly important, and thus they are most likely to stop and interact with the child if noise is being made. Thus, children often learn that a parent only uses the finger-to-lips signal when the probability is highest that a parent will attend to them for making noise. In addition, if a child happens actually to be quiet while the parent is on the phone, the parent typically does not stop to attend. Rather, the parent keeps talking on the phone. This helps ensure that the phone and the finger are effective discriminative stimuli for being noisy.

By showing parents how their own behavior can become discriminative for both good and bad behavior, practitioners can help parents learn to use these concepts to change child behavior in important ways. As parents learn which antecedents signal undesirable child behavior, they can often arrange for those signals to occur less often. For example, the father experiencing problems while on the phone can stop putting his fingers to his lips. As parents learn which antecedents signal more desired child behavior, they can arrange for those to occur more often. Although parents often do not have many of these antecedents available, it is possible for them to create discriminative stimuli that signal new, more appropriate ways to respond. Building new discriminative stimuli requires pairing new signals with reinforcing consequences. This requires understanding how consequences work.

BEHAVIORAL PRINCIPLES: CONSEQUENCES

Consequences are events that follow behavior, and they influence behavior in two important ways: They can either increase or decrease the probability that a behavior will occur. Consequences are delivered dependent or *contingent* on what an individual is doing. *Contingent consequences* are known to have a powerful influence on behavior (e.g., see Honig & Staddon, 1977) and human development (e.g., see Schlinger, 1992). Contingent consequences are also a reliable feature of each empirically supported parent training program. Contingent consequences in parent training fall into three categories: reinforcement, extinction, and punishment.

Reinforcement

Consequences influence behavior by changing the probability that it will occur. Some consequences strengthen behavior, making it more likely that it will occur again. In the context of parent training, consequences are considered *positive reinforcers* if, when delivered contingent on a behavior, they increase the likelihood that a child will engage in that behavior again. Common reinforcers include social praise, physical touch, edible treats, tangible objects such as toys or dolls, and access to special privileges such as watching TV or playing video games.

Parents reinforce behavior all the time, for example, by praising children when they play nicely, by giving them treats when they remember to wash their hands, or by hugging them when they remember to do a chore. These seem obvious because the consequences appear desirable. In each case, the child is more likely, in the future, to play, wash, or work, respectively. However, parents may also positively reinforce when they reprimand a child for making noise during a phone call. If a consequence such as a reprimand results in the child being more likely to make noise when the phone rings, the consequence is considered to be a reinforcer even though it may appear to others to be aversive, unpleasant, or undesirable. In addition, these types of consequence are considered to be *positive* reinforcers not because they are pleasant or pleasing but because they are consequences that involve presenting or introducing something rather than withdrawing or taking something away (see Table 4.2).

Parents may also *negatively reinforce* behavior by removing something or preventing something from occurring. The consequence is understood to be a reinforcer if the behavior increases in probability and is considered to be a *negative* reinforcer if the effect was achieved by removing or taking something away. Removing some aversive event is usually called *escape*, whereas preventing an aversive event from occurring is usually called *avoidance*. A parent who nags a child to clean his or her room negatively reinforces the child for cleaning when the parent stops nagging. The child escapes nagging, and

TABLE 4.2
Types of Reinforcers

Type of consequence	Operation	Function	Common examples
Positive reinforcement (S^{R+})	Presented contingent on behavior.	Increases the likelihood that a behavior will occur.	Social praise Physical touch Edible treats Tangible objects (e.g., toys)
Negative reinforcement (S^{R-})	Removed contingent on behavior.	Increases the likelihood that a behavior will occur.	Mom stops nagging (S^{R-}) when room is clean. Child stops tantrum (S^{R-}) when parent gives in.

cleaning behavior is negatively reinforced. Consider a child who complains vociferously to a parent who insists that the child do his or her homework before going outside. The complaining is negatively reinforced if it leads the parent to remove the demand and allow the child to go out and play. The child avoids schoolwork, and the complaining is negatively reinforced. Patterson and his colleagues first described the power of negative reinforcement in reciprocal parent–child interactions with what they called the *coercive family process* (Patterson, 1982).

Coercive Family Process

The coercive family process appears to be set in motion early in the parent–child relationship, when parents quickly learn how to quiet a crying infant. Parents' efforts to stop the child from crying, such as picking up and rocking the infant or changing a diaper, are negatively reinforced when the child stops crying. The quieting of the child is a potent reinforcer for picking up, rocking, or changing the infant, and, as a result, the parents are much more likely to do so again when the child cries. The infant is also negatively reinforced when the parents remove hunger, cold, or wetness. Indeed, infants learn early on to "use coercion to train parents in parenting skills" (Patterson, 2002, p. 27).

The fact that negative reinforcement might play a central role in shaping parent–infant interactions is not surprising because it encourages the development of many behaviors, appropriate as well as inappropriate (Iwata, 1987). In some cases, however, as infants grow and mature and when the environment becomes uncomfortable, they begin to exhibit more inappropriate forms of aversive control. For example, a child may cry, fuss, throw a tantrum, and refuse to obey when a parent requests that toys be put away. As with the infant, the child's negative behaviors are negatively reinforced when the parent removes the unpleasant conditions—in this case, the demand. Likewise, the parent is negatively reinforced for giving in as the child ceases the disruptive behavior.

The coercive process expands when parents, from time to time, do not give in but persist with their demands and even intensify their efforts to get a child to comply with or accept the demand. At least some of the time, the child may give in, negatively reinforcing the parent for becoming louder and more aversive. Over time, each is negatively reinforced intermittently for escalating aversive behavior until the other gives in. As the coercive cycle continues over time, there is an increased likelihood of escalation. Both parent and child are exposed to the same sequence, learning that rapid escalation to more aversive behavior may induce the other to capitulate (Snyder & Stoolmiller, 2002). Although a variety of correlational and experimental investigations have supported the coercive process (Eddy & Chamberlain, 2000; Fisher, Gunnar,

Chamberlain, & Reid, 2000), it alone cannot explain or help to resolve all disruptive noncompliance or negative parent–child interactions. This requires an understanding of other types of consequences as well.

CONSEQUENCES: EXTINCTION

Although reinforcement is an important principle for understanding how behavior is increased, several other behavioral principles describe how behavior is reduced. One way for behavior to be reduced is to remove the reinforcer for a specific behavior so that the behavior no longer results in reinforcing consequences. This is called *extinction*, in that the behavior then stops occurring or is *extinguished*. Parents often use extinction when they ignore a behavior that has been reinforced by their attention (see Table 4.3). For example, some children are reinforced by the attention they receive from a parent following tantrums or when they get out of bed at night. Using extinction would require that the parent no longer pays attention to such behaviors, resulting in their eventual termination.

Note, however, that ignoring is not the same thing as extinction. Ignoring a child only functions as extinction when paying attention to the child is the reinforcer. Thus, a parent who ignores a child who gets out of bed at night will find that the behavior does not stop if the child has been getting out of bed to watch TV rather than to interact with parents. Extinction in this case would require unplugging the TV or the cable service so that the reinforcer is no longer available.

Using the principle of extinction in a behavior change procedure is often difficult because behavior that has been reinforced will tend to increase briefly in frequency or intensity once reinforcement is stopped. For example, imagine a child who receives reinforcement from the attention she receives when she throws tantrums. Ignoring the tantrums may

TABLE 4.3
Extinction

Type of consequence	Operation	Function	Common examples
Extinction	Specific reinforcer that is maintaining a behavior is removed.	Behavior stops occurring; a brief increase in intensity (called an *extinction burst*) may occur before the behavior extinguishes.	Parents stop attending to attention-seeking tantrums. Parents stop buying candy at the store in response to candy-demanding tantrums.

briefly increase their intensity, although the tantrums will eventually decrease and stop if the extinction procedure is continued. This *extinction burst*, or increase in intensity, can be punishing for parents and practitioners, leading them to give up on extinction if they are not aware that a burst may occur.

CONSEQUENCES: PUNISHMENT

Other types of consequences that reduce behavior are called *punishers* (see Table 4.4). Consequences are considered to be *positive punishers* if, when delivered contingent on a behavior, they decrease the likelihood that a child will engage in that behavior again. As with the definition of reinforcement, the reference to a punisher as positive refers only to the fact that the consequence was presented contingent on a behavior. Common punishers involve reprimands, spanks, threats, or added chores. Parents punish child behavior by scolding when a child slouches in a chair, swatting the child's behind when he or she runs into the street, or glaring at the child when he or she uses fingers rather than a spoon to eat. Of course, children also punish parent behavior when a parent makes a request and a tantrum results, leading to a parent making fewer requests of the child.

Parents can also punish when they take things away. Consequences are considered to be *negative punishers* if, when removed contingent on a behavior, they decrease the likelihood that a child will do that behavior again. The reference to a punisher as negative refers only to the fact that the consequence was removed contingent on a behavior. Common negative punishers involve taking things away that are reinforcers, such as privileges, toys, or contact with parents or friends. Parents often do this when they ground a child, restrict TV time, or sit a child in the corner for time-out. The reduction in the frequency of a behavior is the critical feature in determining whether a consequence is indeed a punisher.

TABLE 4.4
Punishment

Type of consequence	Operation	Function	Common examples
Positive punishment (S^{P+})	Presented contingent on behavior.	Decreases the likelihood that a behavior will occur.	Reprimands Spanks Threats Chores
Negative punishment (S^{P-})	Removed contingent on behavior.	Decreases the likelihood that a behavior will occur.	Restricts TV Grounds Sits in corner

Note that the distinction between extinction and negative punishment as consequences can be confusing, especially because they both result in reductions or weakening of behavior. In addition, the procedures themselves can appear the same. For example, the loss of TV privileges is described here both as a possible extinction procedure and as a possible negative punishment procedure. The difference is that extinction involves removing the *specific* reinforcer that is maintaining the behavior. Negative punishment, however, involves removing a positive reinforcer other than the one that is maintaining the behavior. So, for example, removing TV privileges contingent on getting out of bed at night is extinction if access to the TV was reinforcing getting out of bed but is negative punishment if parental attention is what is reinforcing the child's getting out of bed. Note also that although time-out may have some elements of extinction, it is also likely a punisher. That is, sitting a child in the corner for a problem behavior may remove the child's access to the reinforcer that was maintaining that problem behavior (i.e., extinction), but it also removes the child's access to many other reinforcers (i.e., negative punishment).

Notice that all of these consequences, including reinforcement, extinction, and punishment, involve *functional definitions*. The consequences are defined, in large part, by their function or the effect they have on behavior. Reinforcers strengthen or increase behavior, whereas punishers and extinction decrease or weaken behavior. This is important because it emphasizes the fact that behavior change is the ultimate judge of whether a consequence is effective and whether the consequence represents reinforcement, extinction, or punishment. It does not matter whether the consequence seems like it should be reinforcing or seems like it should be punishing. What matters is whether the consequence actually produced a change in how the child behaves.

Unfortunately, some consequences that seem rewarding actually function as punishers, and many that seem aversive actually function as reinforcers. The problem occurs when parents (and practitioners) operate as if their perceptions are the determining factor in whether a consequence will be effective or not. Br'er Rabbit took advantage of this error in thinking when he told Br'er Fox that he would prefer to be burned, drowned, or even skinned rather than flung into the briar patch, a place that seemed aversive to the fox but, in fact, was where Br'er Rabbit had been raised.

Consider other examples from everyday life in which parent perceptions do not match behavioral functions. A parent physically restrains a child during tantrums, thinking this to be punishing, but the tantrums seem to be getting worse. By definition, then, the restraints are reinforcing the tantrums because the tantrums are increasing in frequency and intensity. In another example, a parent might sit a child in the corner each time he or she argues with the parent, and yet the behavior is not improving. By definition, then, the corner serves neither as extinction nor as punishment because the behavior is not changing. Finally, a parent might happily greet a teen in front of the school each afternoon when classes let out and praise the teen in front of numerous peers for getting to the car on time. Yet on subsequent days, the parent notices that the teen has begun to come to the car later and later, long after peers have dispersed. By definition, the praise and greeting were punishing to the teen, resulting in a decrease in promptness after school. In sum, the true value of a consequence and how it will function is determined by how hard a child will work to get it or to avoid it and not by a parent's or practitioner's perception of its value.

PARENTS AS CONDITIONED REINFORCERS AND CONDITIONED PUNISHERS

Some events function as effective reinforcers or punishers without requiring any special learning or training. These are usually consequences that meet basic needs. For example, food, water, and sleep meet basic needs and are typically reinforcing without any special learning required. Likewise, there are some things that are typically punishing (e.g., pain), but not always and not for everyone. Indeed, it is unlikely that a parent could find something that is always reinforcing or punishing. For example, even food, water, and sleep lose their reinforcing value just after someone has eaten, drunk, or slept.

In contrast to these natural reinforcers and punishers, many things in life must acquire reinforcing or punishing value, usually through their association with other things that are reinforcing or punishing. Events, objects, or activities that acquire their value as reinforcers or punishers through their association with other reinforcers or punishers are considered to be *conditioned reinforcers* or *conditioned punishers*. For example, coins may have some naturally reinforcing value for toddlers because they are shiny and fun to suck. For most children, however, money only acquires value over time, as they learn that money is associated with other reinforcing things, such as candy and toys. In these latter cases, coins are conditioned reinforcers.

People, too, can become conditioned reinforcers or conditioned punishers if they are repeatedly associated with reinforcers or punishers, respectively. For example, a grandmother who reliably pulls out a piece of candy when her grandson kisses her upon her arrival has established a contingency in which kissing is reinforced with candy. Eventually, the grandmother will become a strong signal or discriminative stimulus for kissing. In addition, the grandmother herself will become valuable because of her continued association with candy. Eventually, her grandson will work to engage in behaviors that produce contact with his grandmother, such as calling her on the phone and inviting her over or asking repeatedly to go to grandmother's house. He will do this because the grandmother has become a conditioned reinforcer, and she will, perhaps unwittingly, reinforce any behavior that brings the boy into contact with her.

Likewise, a father who is critical about his son's hair, clothes, grades, and athletic performance when his son approaches him to talk about how things are going has established a contingency in which talking is punished with criticism. Eventually, the father will become a strong signal or discriminative stimulus for the son to keep quiet. In addition, the father will become aversive because of his continued association with criticism. Eventually, his son will work to engage in behaviors that escape or avoid the father, such as spending more time at friends' homes or talking on the phone in his room. He will do this because the father has become a conditioned punisher, and the father will, perhaps unwittingly, punish any behavior that brings the boy into contact with him.

Thus, over time, not only do individuals deliver and remove consequences that are reinforcing and punishing, but also, as they pair themselves with the delivery of reinforcers and punishers, they acquire two functions. They eventually become conditioned reinforcers or punishers (or both), and they also become signals that reinforcers and punishers are available (see Table 4.5). Parents who deliver numerous reinforcers eventually become valuable to children because they signal that reinforcers are available but also because they are reinforcers themselves. These parents are in a good position to have a considerable influence on behavior because their children want to be around them. This ultimately will make parent training easier.

Conversely, parents who reliably punish behavior signal that punishers are available and also become punishers themselves. These parents are in a more tenuous position and may have more difficulty changing child behavior because their children will not want to be around them. This ultimately

TABLE 4.5
Parents as Conditioned Reinforcers or Conditioned Punishers

Parent action	What child learns	Function	Results
Frequent delivery of positive reinforcers for appropriate behavior	Parent is valuable. Parent signals reinforcement is available.	Conditioned reinforcer Discriminative stimulus	Child works hard to increase contact with parent. Child works hard to exhibit appropriate behavior when parent is near.
Frequent delivery of positive punishers for inappropriate behavior	Parent is aversive. Parent signals punishment is available.	Conditioned punisher Discriminative stimulus	Child works hard to avoid parent. Child works hard to avoid inappropriate behavior when parent is near.

makes parent training more challenging. This should help the reader understand at least one reason why each of the empirically supported programs emphasizes the delivery of reinforcing consequences rather than punishing consequences. Both change behavior; however, the delivery of reinforcing consequences results in parents who themselves become conditioned reinforcers. This increases the probability that a child will want to be around the parent, creating more opportunities for parents to teach, influence, and shape behaviors in a positive direction.

CONDITIONS AFFECTING CONSEQUENCES

Although consequences have powerful influence on behavior, they do not always work the same way. The effects of consequences are strongly influenced by a number of variables. Antecedent events can help establish a consequence as a reinforcer, and the importance of establishing operations was discussed earlier. Yet even if a consequence has already been established as effective through antecedent events, several other variables influence its effectiveness (see Table 4.6). These include the immediacy and frequency of delivery of the consequence, its magnitude and quality, and the effort and choices associated with it.

TABLE 4.6
Conditions Affecting Consequences

Condition	Effect	Recommendation
Immediacy	Reinforcers delivered immediately following behavior are more effective than those that are delayed.	Deliver reinforcers immediately whenever possible.
Magnitude	More is better, to a point.	Give enough to make it worthwhile for the child.
Quality	Highly preferred reinforcers will be more effective than less preferred reinforcers.	Consider individual preferences.
Frequency	The strength of a behavior will increase relative to the frequency with which it is reinforced.	Begin with frequent reinforcement, and then use it more intermittently.
Effort	The value of a reinforcer varies relative to the amount of effort a child must exert to "earn" the reinforcer.	Make sure the task, at least initially, is not too difficult.
Choice	The value of a reinforcer varies relative to the value of other available reinforcers.	Consider competing reinforcers and adjust the other five conditions accordingly.

Immediacy

Consequences that occur immediately after a behavior are more effective than those that are more delayed. Immediate consequences produce faster acquisition during learning. This is not to say that delayed consequences have no impact, but the longer the delay between the behavior and the consequence, the greater the likelihood that intervening behaviors will obscure their relationship.

Many consider this a particularly important variable with younger children and those with developmental disabilities. The thought seems to be that as children mature and develop more advanced cognitive skills, they are more responsive to delays in reinforcement. Yet one needs only to spend a short amount of time observing adolescents and young adults to see that delayed consequences such as grades, health, and adult approval often have significantly less influence over behavior compared with more immediate consequences such as peer approval or risk-taking excitement (Rolison & Scherman, 2002). Immediacy is ultimately an important variable for individuals of any age.

Magnitude

Consequences that come in greater amounts will generate more frequent behavior, to a point. Although it is generally true that "more is better," there are limits. This is particularly true for natural reinforcers such as food, sleep, and drink, for which excessive amounts can result in loss of their value, and they may even become aversive. In fact, it is probably best to use reinforcers such as food and drink in relatively small amounts, especially when developing a new behavior, because (a) a child must spend some time consuming them, leaving less time for practicing the new behavior, and (b) the greater the magnitude, the more quickly the reinforcer will lose its value. That is, the individual becomes "full" or satiated and loses his or her desire. The problem of satiation is less of a concern with conditioned reinforcers such as money, which can be saved and used at a later time.

Quality

The quality of a consequence is tied directly to a child's preferences. For example, for most children, praise delivered with flat affect in a monotone voice would be considered relatively poor quality compared with enthusiastic praise. Likewise, a sucker might be preferred over gum, a cookie over a brownie, being pushed on a swing over playing on a merry-go-round. Discerning a child's preferences can occur in a number of ways. Asking parents what the child prefers is certainly one valuable approach. It can also be valuable simply to ask children what they prefer and to recruit their assistance in making lists of potential reinforcers. A more reliable approach, however, is to simply watch what children do in their free time and the choices they make, especially when choosing between a variety of items or activities (Miltenberger, 2001). In addition, because preferences can change over time, it is important for practitioners to understand that the process of evaluating preferences must be ongoing.

Frequency

Behaviors that are reinforced more frequently are more likely to occur again. When developing new behaviors or training new skills, reinforcing every occurrence of the desired behavior is important. After behaviors have become well established, reinforcement can be delivered less frequently, and this will help make the behavior more durable. That is, behaviors that result in reinforcing consequences some, but not all, of the time are better maintained in a world in which reinforcement is usually intermittent, not continuous.

Effort

The amount of effort a child must exert to "earn" the reinforcer can be an important variable in determining its effectiveness. This variable is often overlooked (Friman & Poling, 1995). Children will work hard for some reinforcers, but there is a limit to what they will do. A child might put a single toy on a shelf for praise and a hug but refuse to put all of the toys away for the same consequence. A youth might agree to shovel 1 inch of light snow from the sidewalk when promised some cookies and cocoa but refuse those same treats if the snow is 6 inches deep and wet. Although we noted earlier that not all reinforcers are equally effective because of differences in quality, what we learn here is that the same reinforcer does not always have the same effectiveness; it depends on what the child is being asked to do. Again, this is particularly important when training or developing new skills for which response effort may be high because the tasks are not yet mastered. Ultimately, reducing response effort can be an important way to enhance reinforcer effectiveness.

Choice

At any given moment, children have a large number of possible behaviors in which they can engage. Each has its own consequences. Generally speaking, the probability that children will engage in a certain behavior is determined by the reinforcement they receive for acting that way, relative to the reinforcement they receive for acting other ways (Herrnstein, 1970). That is, an individual acts on the basis of the relative value of each available response. Although this is often called *choice responding*, the choice is not necessarily a conscious decision because this phenomenon is observed in infants and in nonhumans as well.

There is an important emphasis here on the relative value of the different reinforcers that are available for various behavioral choices. This is important because children are always making choices about how to respond based on the relative reinforcement that has typically been available for each of their responses in the past. For example, praise might, in some cases, function as a potent reinforcer for a child who comes inside when called, but this does not mean the child will always come when called. This is especially true if staying outside on a beautiful evening means more time in the sand, on a bike, and around other children, all of which may, at that moment, be more reinforcing than praise. If a parent offers praise but adds a treat for coming when called, and this works, the parent has simply altered the value of staying outside relative to coming in when called. Altering the relative value of reinforcers often requires increasing the magnitude, frequency, immediacy, or quality of the consequences or reducing the response effort required to get them.

CONCERNS ABOUT THE EFFECTS OF REINFORCEMENT

Although there is widespread acknowledgment that reinforcement can effectively increase the frequency of behavior, since the late 1970s there have been concerns that the use of reinforcement may, in some way, damage children, sabotage their natural desire, and have general detrimental effects on behavior (e.g., see Condry, 1977; Kohn, 2001; Lepper & Greene, 1978). Although numerous authors have rejected these concerns on the basis of disconfirming empirical evidence (e.g., Dickinson, 1989; Pierce, Cameron, Banko, & So, 2003; Strain & Joseph, 2004), concerns persist and the issue continues to be debated (e.g., see Cameron & Pierce, 2002; Urdan, 2003). Indeed, some "experts" continue to advise against the use of any program that involves reinforcing child behavior (Kohn, 2005).

The debate is fueled, in part, by differing assumptions about the importance of the environment in shaping behavior, but concerns about how reinforcement affects intrinsic motivation also come into play. Intrinsic motivation is typically described as motivation to act without needing external rewards. Some claim that there is empirical evidence that reinforcement can undermine natural or intrinsic motivation (e.g., see Lepper & Henderlong, 2000). However, continued research on this subject has revealed that detrimental effects of reinforcement are largely a function of the research methods used to study it (Reiss, 2005). In other words, broad assertions that reinforcement has adverse side effects and that the systematic use of reinforcement in applied settings should be abandoned are unsupported and unwarranted.

CONCERNS ABOUT THE EFFECTS OF PUNISHMENT

Perhaps more compelling is the debate regarding the clinical use of punishment, which might include teaching parents to use time-out, to spank, or to assign chores in response to misbehavior. In general, there is little debate about the effectiveness of punishment as a consequence; punishment can produce a rapid decrease in the frequency of behavior and, in some cases, may lead to complete suppression (for a review, see Lerman & Vorndran, 2002). However, there is not widespread agreement about the extent to which punishment should be used. This issue has been particularly controversial in regard to the use of punishment as a parenting practice; for example, there appears to be no clear consensus regarding the advisability of spanking as a potential form of punishment (e.g., see Benjet & Kazdin, 2003). On the one hand, punishment may be critical when behavior must be suppressed immediately to prevent serious harm or when reinforcement-based treatments are ineffective. On the other hand, punishment can sometimes produce unpredictable side effects, including aggression, escape, and emotional behavior, and some have argued that restrictions should be imposed on the clinical use of punishment (e.g., see Sidman, 1989).

Although some may wish to reject the use of punishment on moral grounds alone, scientific evidence suggests that punishment has advantages as well as disadvantages. In addition, a procedure such as time-out, which in many cases is technically a punishment procedure, is widely regarded as both effective and acceptable. Still, more research is needed to develop empirically sound recommendations for how punishment might be used in treatment (Lerman & Vorndran, 2002). In the meantime, perhaps a reasonable approach to the use of punishment in applied settings is to use it only in combination with positive reinforcement techniques (Kazdin, 2001).

Altogether, these concerns about reinforcement and punishment highlight a second reason why it makes sense for the empirically supported programs to emphasize reinforcing consequences over punishing ones. Punishment can reduce or eliminate problem behaviors, but punishment has side effects, is controversial, and cannot strengthen desirable, appropriate alternative behaviors we wish to see. In contrast, reinforcement can be used to teach new, appropriate alternative behaviors; has few side effects; and is significantly less controversial. It is not surprising, then, that the empirically supported parent training programs begin by teaching parents how to reinforce the behaviors they want and then emphasize reinforcement by setting specific goals for parents regarding their demonstrated competence with these skills. Punishment is relegated to a secondary role, albeit an important one, as evidenced by the fact that all four empirically supported programs recommend the use of both reinforcing and punishing contingencies.

APPLICATION OF BEHAVIORAL PRINCIPLES IN EMPIRICALLY SUPPORTED PARENT TRAINING PROGRAMS

Taken together, these behavioral principles help us understand why children and parents do what they do. Children and parents alike respond to the world around them and learn from consequences, some of which reinforce and strengthen behaviors and some of which punish and weaken behaviors. Some things in the environment signal when to behave in certain ways, and other events change or alter the effectiveness of the consequences children experience, but it is the consequences of their behavior that are the mainsprings of their actions. We see that parents control a child's access to a good deal of these consequences and that parents are similarly influenced by the consequences of their own actions. It is not surprising, then, that each of the empirically supported parent training programs are focused on helping parents to understand basic principles of behavior and, more important, to understand how to use techniques derived from these principles to bring about positive change in child behavior. Because the programs embrace a common behavioral conceptualization of how to change behavior, they are remarkably similar in what they teach parents to do. These similarities can be viewed conceptually as outlined in the sections that follow.

1. Increase Reinforcement for Desired Behaviors

Each of the empirically supported programs emphasize, early in the program, teaching parents to become more reinforcing and to make reinforcement more potent by addressing each of the conditions that have an impact on its effectiveness. This means addressing reinforcer immediacy, frequency, magnitude, and quality, as well as response effort and choice. The programs begin by having parents increase the immediacy and frequency of reinforcement for "good" behavior. Parents are asked to attend to and to catch the child being good. For example, they are asked to look for daily opportunities to praise children immediately for following directions, cooperative play, or completing chores.

The programs emphasize improving the quality of reinforcers, for example, by asking parents to use descriptive praise. Descriptive praise specifically labels the desired behavior the child has exhibited and has been found to be more effective than general praise. In addition, quality is also enhanced through reinforcer variety by, for example, using touch or treats as well as praise. Parents are encouraged to increase the magnitude of the reinforcers by using enthusiastic praise. Targeted behaviors include things such as sharing, using imaginative or pretend play, demonstrating cooperation, practicing turn taking, and especially following directions and following family rules.

Although parents are asked to look more often for naturally occurring opportunities to reinforce desired behavior, these programs also typically take particular pains to involve into the daily routine of all parents some way to ensure that they are reinforcing good behavior in general and compliance in particular. That is, the programs do not leave it to chance that parents will remember to catch their child being good. Thus, parents are taught to schedule daily opportunities to interact with their child. Three of the programs (i.e., Parent–Child Interaction Therapy, Helping the Noncompliant Child, and The Incredible Years) teach parents to schedule a daily play activity in which they engage their child in nondirective play, characterized by verbal descriptions, touch, and praise. In addition, each of these programs asks that parents dramatically reduce the demands that are commonplace in many parent–child play interactions, such as asking questions, directing play, and giving commands. This reduces the response effort required of the child, thereby increasing the relative effectiveness of the reinforcement parents are trying to make available for appropriate behavior. The Living With Children program takes a somewhat different approach, requiring parents to monitor good behavior on a chart and then requiring the parent to review the chart with the child each day, leading to more frequent delivery of reinforcers for good behavior.

Three of the programs also ask parents to schedule compliance training sessions in which compliance is specifically reinforced using praise and touch. Reinforcement for compliance might also involve a program in which parents monitor on a chart and reinforce compliance each day with points that are later exchanged for predetermined reinforcers. In other words, each of these programs is designed to increase the availability and effectiveness of reinforcement for positive, desirable, appropriate behaviors in general and for compliance with directions in particular.

The programs, by virtue of arranging for parents to deliver more reinforcers for good behavior, indirectly increase the value of the parent both as a signal that reinforcement is available and as a conditioned reinforcer. In addition, the low-demand, child-directed play activities can help diminish parents as conditioned punishers by eliminating their association with commands, criticisms, and questions that a child may find aversive and punishing. Thus, parents who previously may have been critical, demanding, and rarely reinforcing become associated with no demands, few questions, and frequent and immediate reinforcement for behavior that requires relatively little effort. Subsequently, children are more likely to exhibit good behaviors in the presence of their parent, because the parent signals that reinforcement is available for being good. In addition, the children are more likely to want to be around their parents simply because the parents have become more valued.

2. Use Extinction With Minor Disruptive Behaviors

In contrast to the increased positive reinforcement for appropriate behavior and especially compliance, the empirically supported programs teach parents to remove the possibility of social reinforcement for minor disruptive behavior. This usually means ignoring minor behaviors by turning away or making no verbal comments or nonverbal responses to these behaviors. It is important to note that the removal of social reinforcement for these minor problem behaviors is always used in combination with the increased social attention for other behavior. This process of combining attention as a reinforcer for good behavior with its removal for minor disruptive behaviors is called *differential attention.*

The combining of attention and ignoring in differential attention is important because ignoring alone can present problems. If social attention is effective as a reinforcer, then after it is removed, children will try to get it back. In doing so, they may try any behavior that has, in the past, recruited social reinforcement from the parent. Of course, they will choose the easiest behaviors and the ones that have been most effective in recruiting immediate and frequent attention. Unfortunately, disruptive behaviors are commonly the most effective in recruiting immediate social responses from parents. Many children simply do not have much experience with cooperative, calm, compliant, independent behavior producing immediate and frequent attention from parents—or frankly, from anyone else. As a result, ignoring alone almost always produces more behaviors that parents will find difficult to ignore. One solution is to make sure the child has other ways to access social attention. Differential attention teaches the child not that social attention is no longer available but that it is unavailable at certain times. It is not surprising, then, that the four empirically supported programs all teach parents to ignore minor disruptive behaviors in combination with increased social reinforcement for other more desirable behaviors.

3. Use Antecedents Effectively

The emphasis on parents' use of reinforcing consequences will likely produce positive changes in child behavior; however, antecedent strategies can significantly affect behavior as well. The empirically supported parent training programs have tended to emphasize improving stimulus control of parental commands. Each of the programs specifically teaches parents how to deliver commands in effective ways. Commands have the potential to signal to children that reinforcement is available for compliance with the command. However, children sometimes may have trouble identifying whether a parent's statement is indeed a command. This might occur when the command is phrased as a question or request or when the command is vague. It is not surprising that compliance is poorer under these conditions because the command does not provide a clear signal of what behavior is expected or that reinforcement is available. As a result, the empirically supported programs teach parents to use a firm, slightly louder voice when giving a command, to use statements rather than questions or requests, and to be specific rather than vague.

Parents are also taught, at least initially, to limit their commands to simple, one-step instructions, thereby reducing the response effort and increasing the likelihood that the child will do what he or she was told. Recall that the amount of effort required to comply with a demand will have an impact on the effectiveness of the reinforcer; if the effort is too great because the command is too hard to understand or there are too many steps, the child may choose to respond with something other than compliance. Parents are also taught to reduce response effort for the child by, at least initially, limiting commands to those that tell a child what to do rather than what not to do. To stop a behavior in response to a "don't" instruction without any behavior to replace it is a much more difficult task than to initiate a new behavior in response to a "do" instruction (e.g., see Vigilante & Wahler, 2005).

Not only do these strategies make conceptual sense, but also research has repeatedly demonstrated that parents' changes in command-giving behaviors indeed bring about improved rates of compliance in children (e.g., see Roberts, McMahon, Forehand, & Humphreys, 1978). It is important to note, however, that it does not matter whether a parent makes firm, specific, simple statements of what is expected if the child has never experienced reinforcement for compliance with commands. In other words, commands must already be established as discriminative stimuli, signaling that reinforcement is available for compliance. In a parent–child relationship in which commands do not signal that reinforcement is available, simply delivering better commands will not make a difference. This is one of the reasons that the parent training programs place such an emphasis on parents delivering reinforcement when compliance does occur. Although parents may complain that their child never does what he or she is told, those who monitor closely and try to catch their child following directions will likely find something to reinforce.

4. Use Punishment When Necessary

Time-out is, in effect, a punishment procedure that involves removing children from an environment in which they are accessing reinforcement to one in which they are not. Access to social reinforcement, such as attention from adults and peers, or tangible reinforcement, such as toys and activities, is terminated. This is usually accomplished by removing the child from a situation in which these are available and involves not only terminating access to reinforcement that was available but also restricting access to reinforcement that might be available. This typically involves moving the child to a chair or room that is away from others and placing him or her in a boring location. However, a time-out from reinforcement could also involve the parent leaving the child where they are and taking the reinforcing environment with them.

Notice that the effectiveness of the procedure depends on the fact that the child is moved from a reinforcing to a less or nonreinforcing environment. Indeed, the effectiveness of the punishment contingency is related to the amount of stimulus change or to the amount of positive and negative reinforcement in time-out relative to that outside of time-out (e.g., see Shriver & Allen, 1996).

Each of the empirically supported parent programs includes time-out. Time-out makes conceptual sense, and there are independent data to support its inclusion in parent training programs. The emphasis is on the removal of reinforcement rather than the introduction of something aversive. Of course, one could argue that the removal of reinforcement is the same as the introduction of something aversive, but many parents believe it to be a qualitatively different punishment procedure and one that is more acceptable than a clearly aversive event, such as spanking (D. L. Miller & Kelley, 1992). Furthermore, time-out has gained widespread acceptance as a punishment procedure of choice in many schools and day-care centers, and it carries with it few pejorative connotations characteristic of other aversive control procedures.

Although none of the programs emphasize punishment, they each offer practitioners specific recommendations for how parents should implement this contingency. Parents are reinforced for adherence to specific guidelines about when to use time-out, how to determine a good location for it, how long to leave a child in time-out, how to decide when to release them, and how to enforce the procedure should a child be uncooperative. These guidelines serve to enhance the effectiveness of time-out as a consequence by ensuring that it is delivered with sufficient quality, magnitude, frequency, and immediacy.

Each of the programs also guides what is to happen immediately after the time-out consequence has been delivered. This is done in an effort to address the fact that sitting in time-out for noncompliance, although potentially punishing, also allows the child to avoid compliance with the demand. That is, time-out may negatively reinforce noncompliance in some children. As a result, parents are asked to bring the child out of time-out and to reissue the original demand. That is, the child is not permitted to escape or avoid the original demand.

We have been unable to find research supporting the requirement that a child comply with the original demand. However, it does fit conceptually with attempts to alter the coercive family process. Children who are subsequently noncompliant are returned to time-out, and upon dismissal, the command is issued again. This process continues until the child is eventually compliant with the original request, at which time the parents are expected to deliver appropriate reinforcers for compliance. Thus, requiring that parents use time-out as a consequence for noncompliance serves to interrupt the escalating cycle of negative reinforcement described by the coercive family process. Rather than capitulate to and thereby reinforce the child's escalating noncompliance, the parent is asked to rely on time-out. Likewise, rather than respond with escalating behavior themselves until the child capitulates, thereby reinforcing the esca-

TABLE 4.7
Principles, Goals, and Strategies of the Empirically
Supported Parent Training Programs

Behavioral principle	Goal	Practical strategy
Reinforcement	Increase desired behaviors.	Catch them being good. Use praise, touch, points. Schedule nondirective play.
Extinction	Decrease disruptive behaviors.	Use ignoring whenever possible.
Stimulus control	Increase command following.	Use direct, simple commands.
Punishment	Decrease disruptive behavior.	Use time-out. Use response cost.

lating parent behavior, the parent relies on time-out. In effect, time-out allows the practitioner to instruct the parent in what to do (i.e., time-out) rather than only what not to do (e.g., yell, scream, threaten, give in).

SUMMARY

Behavior research and theory has identified environment as the primary source of learning in children. Environment includes antecedents that signal or cue individuals as to when to act in certain ways, and it includes consequences that are ultimately responsible for choices children make. Empirically supported parent training programs have taken advantage of this understanding about the impact of environment on child behavior and have developed interventions that use parents as the primary means of changing the child's environment.

These programs emphasize positive reinforcement as a means of increasing desirable behaviors but recognize that a plan for consequences that reduce problem behaviors is necessary as well. The skills taught rely on four basic principles (see Table 4.7) and the techniques that are derived from them. Parents who use these strategies rely on these principles, whether consciously or not. Empirical support provides confidence that the use of these strategies produces meaningful changes in child behavior. However, the parent–child relationship is not unidirectional; it is reciprocal. Child behavior affects parent behavior in the same way that parent behavior affects the child's. These programs do not ignore these influences of the child on the parent per se, but the emphasis is clearly on mediating changes in the parent–child relationship through changes in parent behavior. How, then, does one bring about changes in parent behavior? Through the practitioner, of course. The practitioner must have a good grasp of not only what to teach but also how to teach these skills to bring about desired behavioral changes in the parents. These issues are considered next.

5

HOW TO TEACH PARENTS

The preceding chapters have demonstrated that the empirically supported parent training programs offer robust empirical and conceptual support for their inclusion in everyday practice. Using the step-by-step manuals and protocols that are included with these programs can help ensure that practitioners deliver critical features of the programs as prescribed (e.g., Nezu & Nezu, 2005).

Manuals typically assist the practitioner by providing specific guidance about which behaviors (i.e., skills) to teach and in which order to teach them. Yet success is dependent on more than this alone. The success of any parent training intervention is dependent on at least two critical practitioner teaching components: (a) whether the practitioner knows how to teach the critical skills and (b) whether the practitioner can motivate parents to use the skills that have been taught. Fortunately, the general concepts of how to teach have received considerable attention in the literature, and effective approaches to skill teaching are relatively well established.

Getting parents actually to use the skills they have been taught, however, is more problematic. Whether skills learned are used is typically referred to as treatment adherence (or nonadherence), and it has not received nearly the same attention as treatment effectiveness (Allen & Warzak, 2000). Of course, parent behavior, like any behavior, is subject to the environmental influences discussed in chapter 4 of this volume (e.g., antecedents, consequences). Antecedents help establish what will function as a reinforcer for adherence and also help signal when reinforcement is available. Consequences serve sometimes to reinforce and sometimes to punish parents for their use of the skills they have been taught, and a variety of conditions serve to enhance or diminish the impact of those consequences. Ultimately, parents who do not do what they have been taught to do are often called "unmotivated" or "resistant," but these labels are not particularly useful for the practitioner because the poor motivation and resistance themselves must be explained. Close inspection of the environment provides that explanation (Allen & Warzak, 2000): We can look at the influences of antecedents and consequences as barriers to success when they discourage adherence. More important, understanding how antecedents and consequences affect a parent's motivation to act and willingness to adhere provides the practitioner with tools for strengthening motivation and reducing resistance. In this chapter, we address both—how to teach the behavioral skills that parents will need to be successful and how to overcome some of the motivational barriers to parents using those skills in the home.

COMPONENTS OF BEHAVIORAL SKILLS TRAINING

Teaching parents the skills they need to be effective parents typically requires four components: instruction, modeling, rehearsal, and feedback (e.g., Miltenberger, 2001). This has commonly been called behavioral skills training (BST), and researchers have demonstrated that this approach is superior to education and discussion alone when teaching new behaviors to children and parents (e.g., Bromberg & Johnson, 1997; Crane, 1995). In addition, parents complete more homework and achieve better outcomes when BST is used compared with, for example, problem-solving skills (e.g., Magen & Rose, 1994).

Instruction

BST begins with instruction (see Table 5.1). Instruction commonly involves a description of the specific skill that is to be taught and includes a rationale for why that skill is important to teach (see Developing Rationales later in this chapter). Of course, complex skills are much more difficult to learn and teach than simple skills. Effective skills training commonly requires breaking complex or multicomponent skills into smaller, more manageable, easy-to-learn steps. For example, when teaching parents to attend to their children, skills such as describing, reflecting, touching, and praising are often taught separately before combining them. Praise can be further simplified into unlabeled and labeled praise.

TABLE 5.1
How to Teach Parents—Behavioral Skills Training

Teaching technique	Description
Instruction	Analyze components.
	Start with simple skills.
	Describe skill to be taught.
	Use written description (i.e., protocol) as aid.
Modeling	Match the model to the parent(s).
	Demonstrate each skill.
	Model correct and incorrect.
	Model learning as you go.
Rehearsal	Practice easy skills first.
	Do whole-task practice.
	Practice outside the clinic (i.e., homework).
Feedback	Use encouragement more than critique.
	Be descriptive more than general.
	Be immediate with feedback.
	Use prompting if necessary.

In some instances, the component skills must be used in a specific sequence. The practitioner can initially teach the skills separately, later "chaining" the skills back together in sequence. Compliance training, for example, involves first teaching how to give effective instructions and then providing opportunities to practice giving instruction. Only then are parents taught how to use time-out for noncompliance. Learning to use time-out also involves learning a sequence of skills such as selecting and setting up an appropriate time-out location, giving well-worded warnings, and escorting the child to time-out. Instruction in each of these skills should be provided separately before combining them into a sequence.

Certainly the extent to which skills need to be simplified into easier components depends, in part, on the skills parents bring with them to the clinic and the ease with which they are observed to learn new skills. Nevertheless, decades of research from the medical and the behavioral literature have demonstrated that the complexity of a skill is one of the most consistent predictors of follow-through with implementation (Meichenbaum & Turk, 1987).

Some experts have promoted written prescriptions (e.g., Cox, Tisdelle, & Culbert, 1988) or brief protocols to assist practitioners with instructing parents who are learning new behavioral techniques (e.g., Danforth, 1998; McMahon & Forehand, 2003). These protocols list, in simple language, step-by-step instructions for completing an intervention and may help support verbal instructions that have been provided (e.g., clear instruction → child does not comply → warning → child does not comply → time-out). Nevertheless, although instructions and protocols may improve parents' knowledge of what to do, knowledge does not reliably translate well into practice. That is, practitioners who assume a high correspondence between what parents know and what they actually can do are likely to be disappointed (e.g., Myers & Midence, 1998; Parrish, 1986). More is required, and the modeling of skills that have been described enhances learning.

Modeling

After parents have received instruction regarding the skill they are to learn, modeling or demonstrating it allows them to see the skill in action, ask questions, and clarify how it is to be implemented. In many cases, the practitioner performs this modeling. If the practitioner plans to model a skill in interaction with the child, he or she may wish to advise the parent of the plan and ask permission, especially if the skill requires physical contact with the child, such as providing a positive touch, physical prompting, or guiding a child to time-out. However, skills can also be modeled initially with the parent posing as the child or, in some cases, using a doll. The practitioner should plan, however, eventually to model the skills directly with the child to demonstrate how the parent is to respond to unique instances that arise.

In general, the effects of modeling have been found to be enhanced when the model (a) resembles the people who are observing, (b) shows coping or learning from experience, (c) demonstrates simple rather than complex behavior, (d) demonstrates the behavior in context (i.e., a "real" situation), and (e) points out for the observer the specific behaviors of importance. For example, individuals have generally been found to be more likely to imitate a model of the same gender than a model of the opposite gender (e.g., Begin, 1978) and are more likely to benefit from modeling when the modeled skills are perceived as easy and relevant (e.g., Bruch, 1978). More specifically, modeling has long been used to train parents (e.g., Johnson & Brown, 1969), who have been found to benefit more from modeling when models are observed to be learning parenting skills rather than to have already mastered them (e.g., Cunningham, Davis, Bremner, Dunn, & Rzasa, 1993). In addition, some have found that videotapes provide a particularly effective way to enhance the effects of modeling by showing other parents modeling both mastered and incorrect examples of relevant skills in real-life situations (Webster-Stratton & Hancock, 1998). Of course, for modeling to be beneficial, observers must be able to imitate what they have seen. This can be confirmed by asking parents to demonstrate or rehearse the skill themselves.

Rehearsal

Following instruction and modeling, behavioral rehearsal provides the opportunity for parents to practice the parenting skills just reviewed and, in fact, rehearsal has been found to enhance the retention of modeled behaviors (e.g., Sims & Manz, 1982). This component is critical because, as with any behavior, practice is necessary before a parent can master each skill. In addition, if the skill instruction has been arranged so that the easiest skills have been taught first or so that the first in a sequence is practiced before the others are added, parents will be able to experience initial success, increasing their motivation to continue with training. However, evidence suggests that ultimately, whole-task rehearsal is important for long-term retention of a skill (e.g., Naylor & Briggs, 1963). That is, it is not adequate to practice the various components of a complex or sequenced skill without eventually putting it all together.

It is also important to understand that the skills rehearsed in clinic will not necessarily generalize to the home setting (Stokes & Osnes, 1989). Indeed, the more different the clinic is from the home, the less likely the skills will transfer. However, the more the practice situation resembles the actual situation in which the skills will be used, the more likely parents will be able to carry those skills out of the clinic and into the home. In fact, actual rehearsal of parenting skills in the home has been found to be the most potent means of ensuring generalization of parenting skills into the home (e.g., Bakken, Miltenberger, & Schauss, 1993).

Unfortunately, it is typically impractical for the practitioner to accompany the parent to the home to supervise rehearsal. Alternatives include rehearsal in as many settings as possible, such in the waiting room, the hallway, and various rooms in the clinic. It may also prove valuable to rehearse parenting skills in the presence of those who reside in the home even if the practice itself does not take place in the home. In addition, using written protocols to prompt parents during rehearsal in the clinic can help with the transfer of learning between settings if those protocols are then taken home. Ultimately, however, the parents need to practice in the home, whether supervised or not, and homework is an important component of a good skills training program. Sending protocols home and requiring parents to record the frequency and quality of home practice can help increase the probability that parents will rehearse the skills on their own. However, it is supervised rehearsal that allows the practitioner to assess what the parent has learned and to shape and strengthen those skills through feedback.

Feedback

After parents have begun to demonstrate the skills that have been described and modeled, the practitioner can begin to provide feedback to help them achieve mastery of those skills. Providing feedback allows the practitioner to shape the required parenting skills. Effective feedback allows parents to encounter learning as a positive experience and contains the following elements:

1. Feedback should initially focus on reinforcing rather than correcting. Just as parents are taught to "catch 'em being good," practitioners must do the same with parents, offering initial feedback that reinforces even the smallest successes. As the parent improves, the practitioner can gradually expect more and more elements to be correct before reinforcement is offered.
2. Feedback should emphasize specific, descriptive praise of the desired skills.
3. Feedback should be delivered immediately after the behavior is exhibited, whether that feedback is positive or corrective.
4. Feedback should ask the parent to correct or change one behavior at a time.
5. Feedback should include prompts (i.e., guidance) if necessary during practice to help parents know when or where to change specific behavior.

Many practitioners have found bug-in-the-ear devices (see chap. 2, this volume) to be extremely valuable in providing feedback to a parent from behind a two-way mirror as the parent rehearses the skills that have been described and modeled (e.g., Packard, Robinson, & Grove, 1983). Modern two-way radios can serve this function, are inexpensive and widely available, and require nothing more than parents wearing a small earphone. With these devices, practitioners can provide immediate feedback directly to parents without disrupting the rehearsal or distracting the child.

It is not critical, however, that one have access to remote feedback devices. A practitioner can provide direct verbal feedback to parents as they rehearse, praising correct demonstrations and offering corrective feedback for others. For example, a parent who is just learning how to give descriptive praise might, on a first attempt, offer several unlabeled praise statements (e.g., "Wow, that's neat!") to a child who is engaged in creative play with blocks. The practitioner might choose initially to offer immediate, labeled praise of that behavior (e.g., "That was a very good praise statement") to encourage the parent and to begin the shaping process. However, the practitioner's next feedback statement might be "OK, that was good, unlabeled praise. This next time, let's use labeled praise and be very specific about what it is you like." Thus, the practitioner has offered another labeled praise statement to the parent and only then offered a corrective request. The practitioner might also provide several verbal prompts for the parent by telling him or her exactly what to say (e.g., "Try saying, 'It is neat to see you using your imagination and creating your own design!'") but also by verbally signaling to the parent the exact moment when the practitioner wants the parent to say it (e.g., "Say it now!").

In group-based parent training, learning can be enhanced by having parents train other parents in the skills they have already mastered. For example, one parent or caregiver learns the desired skills through instruction, modeling, rehearsal, and feedback provided by the practitioner. At a subsequent session, the trained parent uses instruction, modeling, rehearsal, and feedback to train another caregiver while the practitioner observes. Results of studies that included parents or teachers as intervention agents in a pyramidal training paradigm have generally found that serving as a trainer enhanced the training parent's own skills (F. H. Jones, Fremouw, & Carples, 1977; Neef, 1995).

One benefit of having parents train other parents in the clinic is that it provides the practitioner with considerable latitude in developing practice scenarios. These scenarios can incorporate obstacles that parents may not anticipate and provide practice in overcoming them. In addition to parents training other parents in the clinic, they can be encouraged to train relatives (e.g., grandparents) and other caregivers in specific skills. Asking that a parent train multiple caregivers may help ensure more consistency in responding to the child and also provide the parent with additional opportunities for practice.

ENHANCING PARENT MOTIVATION

Although instruction, modeling, rehearsal, and feedback are well-established methods of training parents, motivating parents to participate enthusiastically in the clinic and then use what they have learned in the home can be a significant challenge. Developing convincing rationales for practicing skills may require using language skillfully before and during the training process to enhance parent motivation. Practitioners must also pay careful attention to what is reinforcing for parents and to how contingencies are managed, both in the clinic, where parents need to learn the skills, and in the home, where parents need to use the skills.

Developing Rationales

Practitioners do not typically need to spend much time developing rationales for why a child's behavior needs to be modified. The fact that a parent has come to the clinic with his or her child is usually evidence that the parent recognizes something needs to be done. However, the process of developing rationales to explain why the parent is the focus of the treatment can be critical to a parent's motivation to learn and use the skills that are being offered. A rationale can function as a type of establishing operation (see chap. 4) that practitioners can use to enhance a parent's motivation to participate in training. Parents often assume their child will be the focus of one-on-one counseling.

When parents learn that parent training will be the means of intervention, they may become defensive or be offended that treatment focuses on them—as though they were the cause of the problems. This issue must be addressed from the start. Consider the following example:

> I would like to point out that just because we consider you, the parent, to be part of the solution, does not mean that you are the cause of the problem. In fact, the *solution* to a problem is rarely the *cause* of the problem, and there are many examples in which this is quite clear. The doctor who repairs a broken arm is an important part of the solution but certainly not the cause of the problem. Likewise, aspirin can successfully treat a headache, but no one would conclude that the cause of a headache is the lack of aspirin in the head. Aspirin is the solution but not the cause of the problem. Finally, you came to our clinic today looking for help for your child not because you believe we caused the problem but because you recognize we may be part of the solution. In the same way, we now turn to you because we recognize that you, too, can be part of the solution.

In addition, an effectively delivered rationale will help parents see that they are the logical choice to implement treatment because they have the greatest amount of contact with the child and control over the home environment (McMahon & Forehand, 2003). The role of the home environment can be emphasized given that the home is where most of the daily life learning experiences occur. Some parents may also be particularly pleased and motivated to participate in parent training knowing that the skills they will be taught have been validated as effective in scientific studies.

In addition to developing rationales for parent training as the method of choice for treating a child's problem, the practitioner must also be prepared to develop rationales for each of the skills parents will be required to learn. For example, consider a parent who is motivated to address a child's noncompliance but does not see how participating in child-directed play will address the problem. The practitioner must convince the parent of the necessity of this activity, or the parent may not implement the activity at home.

The practitioner might explain to the parents how child-directed play helps their child learn what constitutes acceptable behavior (e.g., turn taking, sharing) before addressing what constitutes unacceptable behavior (e.g., McMahon & Forehand, 2003). Likewise, one could explain that these play activities can help improve the parent–child relationship and child frustration tolerance (e.g., Hembree-Kigin & McNeil, 1995), both conditions that may make discipline more effective. Together, these rationales should help establish child-directed play as reinforcing and motivate parents to participate effectively with their child in this skill-building activity.

Finally, arranging time for home practice of newly learned skills can require considerable effort. Practice can also be disruptive to typical routines in the home. As a result, practitioners need to develop strong rationales for taking the skills that have been learned at the clinic and practicing them in the home setting. For example, a practitioner might say,

> You have done a nice job of practicing these new skills here in clinic, and I can see that you are really getting the hang of it. Now I need to ask you to take these skills and practice them at home. I am not asking for a lot of practice, but I do ask that you practice a little bit each day. I ask that you practice at home for two important reasons. First, if we really want Anna to learn to make changes in her behavior, then she needs practice every day, and she will only practice if you do. Just like at school, where we give children practice every day with reading, writing, and math, they need practice at home every day using good play skills, sharing, and following directions. Second, the more you practice these skills at home, the more natural they will become and the less you will need to concentrate to use them effectively.

Most parent training manuals provide some assistance with developing effective rationales, and Webster-Stratton has an entire chapter describing rationales designed to help parents understand and be motivated to adhere to parent training recommendations (Webster-Stratton & Herbert, 1994, pp. 169–197). However, when developing rationales, practitioners can be most effective when they appeal to the unique perspectives and expectations of the individual parent. Information about parental expectations can be acquired most easily simply by asking parents what they expect, but observing how parents talk about problem behaviors and the solutions they have pursued in the past is also useful. The language they use can not only reveal information about parents' expectations but also provide the practitioner with information about how to modify his or her own language, choosing to use similar language when describing rationales or strategies to use.

Choosing Language Carefully

There is some evidence that descriptions of behavioral interventions for children are viewed as more acceptable when nontechnical terms are used (e.g., Witt, Moe, Gutkin, & Andrews, 1984; Woolfolk & Woolfolk, 1979). Recent research has also demonstrated that more conversational language and colloquial descriptions of behavioral procedures produce better understanding among the public about what is to be done, as well as more favorable emotional reactions to it (Rolider, Axelrod, & Van Houten, 1998). Clinical language may also need to highlight aspects of behavioral technology that are consistent with highly valued cultural constructs such as freedom, self-confidence, individual responsibility, and independence (Bailey, 1991). For example, a token reinforcement program for compliance with a response cost component for noncompliance might be presented something like this:

> We are going to be asking Tim to make some very difficult behavior changes. These are important changes, because his noncompliance is unacceptable and because he should want to be more compliant; it is the right thing for him to do. However, these will be difficult changes for Tim because they require him to learn independence and responsibility. Children make changes toward independence and responsibility most easily when they are helped with three things: (a) they receive reminders each day of skills and choices they are working on, (b) they receive positive encouragement and acknowledgment so that they can feel positive about the good choices they make, and (c) they encounter natural consequences each time they choose not to work on changing their behavior. The daily reminders can be handled nicely by placing a chart on the wall or refrigerator that lists the behavior(s) on which Tim is working. The encouragement can come from points or tokens that Tim can earn each time he independently makes responsible choices. Because children appreciate attention and encouragement in concrete ways, Tim can then trade his points for a special privilege, activity, or treat. You and Tim can make a list of things he can work to earn. However, each time Tim makes a poor choice, he will lose one of the points or tokens he has earned. Of course, our goal is to have Tim do as you ask because it feels good when he does so and because he has learned it is the right way to behave. This program will help Tim to be more compliant, help him feel good about his success, and build self-control so that we can slowly withdraw the program and have Tim following rules without daily reminders.

Notice that in this example, the practitioner is true to the conceptual underpinnings of empirically supported behavioral parent training but has couched the concepts in ways that are consistent with culturally valued constructs (Allen & Warzak, 2000).

One alternative to behavioral language is to use language that is not only valued but also simple. For example, the practitioner's use of simple, jargon-free language should improve parents' comprehension of the intervention and increase its acceptability as a problem-solving tool. In addition, the use of analogies help make language more experiential because they often draw on direct experience. Analogies allow the practitioner to take issues or concepts that may be complex and ground them in common sense. Finally, because analogies often function like pictures, they can be more easily remembered. For example, the following analogy has been found helpful to parents who have expressed concern about the need to use rewards to motivate children to do things they should be doing anyway.

When a child has a broken leg, we use a cast because doctors know a cast is necessary to allow the leg to heal properly. The cast is uncomfortable, itchy, and sometimes gets in the way of normal activities, but we know that without it, the leg might not correctly heal. In addition, we know that the cast is temporary, so we are more tolerant. A reward program functions in much the same way. Your child is having trouble learning to be a good listener, and we have plenty of evidence, as with a cast, that a reward program can help the learning process. Using a reward program can be cumbersome and sometimes disruptive to normal everyday activities, but we know that without it, your child is having a hard time learning to behave. In addition, we know that the program is temporary, so we can be more tolerant.

In many ways, the practitioner is an interpreter who must translate concepts and principles into words and behaviors that parents can easily understand and apply. Analogies can help this translation process, although finding real-life experiences and situations to which the parents can relate may change depending on the parent's culture, class, age, and education.

Finally, no matter how good we are at translation, pictures still speak the most universally understood language. It is not surprising, then, that all of the empirically supported parent training programs use pictures to help practitioners translate concepts and principles to parents. The Incredible Years relies heavily on videotaped depictions of parents demonstrating both correct and incorrect use of skills, in large part because video modeling has been demonstrated to be an important learning tool for parents. The Helping the Noncompliant Child program also asks practitioners to draw pictures (i.e., bar graphs) to help parents visualize the importance of teaching children "OK behaviors" (which we want more of) as well as "not OK behaviors" (which we want less of). In addition, the manuals for the Parent–Child Interaction Therapy and Living With Children programs both include sample charts for use with reward and discipline programs. Still others (e.g., Jensen, Rhode, & Reavis, 1994) have dedicated entire books to providing visual aids and pictorial resources to help parents understand and implement behavioral programming.

OVERCOMING BARRIERS TO TREATMENT ADHERENCE

Although carefully selected rationales and language can help develop parent motivation to learn and practice the procedures suggested by the practitioner, at times they are not enough. Fortunately, there are other strategies that can help parents stay dedicated (see Table 5.2). These include predicting outcomes, using reminders, developing rapport, providing tangible incentives,

TABLE 5.2
Overcoming Barriers to Treatment Adherence

Strategy	Description
Rationale for BST	Parent(s) are part of the solution.
	It is important to learn new skills.
	Practice is important to success.
Language in session	Use nontechnical terms.
	Value child responsibility and independence.
	Translate principles into pictures.
Predict outcomes	Predict extinction bursts.
	Predict social disapproval.
Provide reminders	Engage in frequent contact with practitioner.
	Use partners and relatives.
	Post checklists of skills.
	Train in different settings.
	Teach general principles of behavior.
Build rapport	Use reflection and empathy.
	Schedule practices to avoid likely conflicts.
	Use self-disclosure and humor.
	Balance expert versus collaborative model.
Use incentives	Reimburse parents for adherence.
Use technology	Consider use of electronic monitors.
Use resources	Offer group format as support group.
	Add sessions on communication training.
	Refer for marital or drug counseling.
	Teach problem solving and self-management.
Incorporate flexibility	Adjust performance criteria.
	Modify skills and sequences as needed.

Note. BST = behavorial skills training.

using technology, addressing parental resource barriers, and using program guidelines flexibly.

Predicting Outcomes

One of the first barriers to treatment adherence is parental expectations that if they follow the practitioners advice, change will occur quickly. In part this derives from the many years of experience parents have had with medical professionals who provide recommendations that generally produce relatively quick improvements in health (e.g., antibiotic treatment of bacterial infections). After years of associating health care recommendations with rapid improvements in health, parents often expect similar success from mental health practitioners and their recommendations.

Unfortunately, behavior often does not change fast, and many times there are negative bumps in the road along the way. In this way, parents' efforts to adhere to recommendations are punished. However, the practitioner may be able to say things in a way that establishes slow behavior change, even temporary negative changes, as reinforcing. Consider, as an example, a parent who has participated in an empirically supported parent training program and is expecting immediate improvement in child compliance but instead encounters tantrums by the child when time-out or ignoring is used. A practitioner may be able to establish these behavior changes as reinforcing rather than punishing, by predicting these changes, and by describing them as a sign of progress (e.g., Hobbs, Walle, & Hammersly, 1990). For example, a practitioner might say,

> It is not uncommon to see a brief increase in tantrums when you begin to ignore them. This reassures us that your attention is valuable and that your child experiences being ignored as unpleasant. So an increase in tantrums is an early indication of success.

The practitioner may be particularly effective in this regard if these changes are identified before their occurrence so that he or she is predicting rather than explaining observed changes.

Practitioners can also predict ahead of time that there will likely be negative reactions from others when they use the recommended behavior change procedures, thus preparing and supporting the parent when and if these reactions occur. For example, a parent may have been taught to ignore whining but is punished by disapproving glares and comments from family members, relatives, and people in public who disapprove of the child's behavior. Alternatively, social approval establishes a child's silence as a powerful reinforcer, and any parental behavior that quickly brings about silence is reinforced. Unfortunately, parent techniques that bring silence quickly are often either aversive control procedures (e.g., spanking) or giving in to the demand that produced the whining in the first place.

Although there are probably few strategies a practitioner can use that will alter the responses of the social community, the practitioner who can predict these reactions from others may be able to frame them in a way that disestablishes their influence. For example, the practitioner might suggest the following to parents:

> People around you may not understand the strategies that you will be using to solve this problem. This is much like someone who is wearing braces on their teeth and must endure teasing by others, knowing that the end results, although not immediately visible, will be pleasing to everyone involved. You will have adults who will disapprove of allowing your child to whine, and it may be tempting to give in to your child's demands, or perhaps even to spank your child, but you must remember that your child's whining in these situations is simply an understandable, although unacceptable, attempt to communicate his or her desires. Our goal is to teach your child that this behavior will no longer work while teaching an alternative adaptive behavior that does.

Finally, a parent's attempts at implementation of positive reinforcement may initially be punished by unpleasant and aversive child behaviors that occur when the parent delivers the reinforcer. This is why parents are so often reluctant to interrupt a child who is playing nicely, despite practitioner appeals to "catch 'em being good." Parents have often experienced that praising and acknowledging good behavior can, at times, result in disruptive acting out. This *response induction* (Balsam & Bondy, 1983) occurs when the process of attending to one behavior induces other behaviors to emerge that have, in the past, produced attention. Unfortunately, for many children who are seen in clinic, the behaviors that have most reliably recruited parental attention are often the very behaviors the parent is hoping to eliminate (e.g., whining, interrupting, throwing toys, hitting a sibling). One would expect this effect to diminish rapidly if a parent persists with implementation of differential attention, but the immediate effect is punitive for parents, and they may not, as a result, persist. Anticipating and predicting this reaction from a child may help diminish some of the punitive aspects of the child's behavior. In addition, the practitioner may be able to reassure parents that the reaction from their child helps confirm the power of their attention.

Using Reminders

Although using effective rationales, language, and predictions may help increase parent motivation to learn and use the skills necessary for child behavior change, there simply are not many cues in the natural environment that signal a parent when to use these skills. Sadly, the transfer or generalization of skills from one setting (e.g., a clinic) to another (e.g., a home) does not happen automatically (e.g., Stokes & Osnes, 1989). Indeed, when left to chance, it does not happen often or well. Rather, it requires the presence of signals or cues (i.e., discriminative stimuli) that remind parents when to use the skills they have learned. Arranging for reminders can be accomplished in a number of ways. First, frequency of contact with the practitioner can serve as one type of reminder. Frequent visits to the clinic allow parents to review, rehearse, and receive feedback on a regular basis and allow the practitioner not only to reinforce successes but also to emphasize (i.e., cue) how and when to use skills in the home. In addition, phone calls allow greater frequency of contacts and serve as regular reminders to enhance consistency of implementation. Phone calls to the home were a regular feature of the Living With Children program during its development and an important source of ensuring program integrity and parent adherence.

A second means of arranging reminders involves training parents to place cues or reminders in every situation in which problems are likely to occur. This might involve rehearsing new parent behaviors in a variety of settings (e.g., clinic, school, home), with a variety of people present, under a variety of everyday conditions (e.g., Lundquist & Hansen, 1998). This, of course, could be extremely labor intensive and expensive. An alternative would be to include cues and reminders in training that can be transported to new situations. For example, it may involve arranging for a spouse or relatives from multiple settings to be present during training (Hansen & MacMillan, 1990), and, as the next chapter of this volume indicates, this may have cultural benefits as well. Others have suggested presenting and reviewing a simple list of intervention steps during training and then posting the list on the wall at home or carrying it in a pocket and reviewing it from time to time. The protocols (see Instruction section earlier in this chapter) as well as the graphs and charts (see Choosing Language Carefully) described earlier can serve these functions. The homework self-monitoring forms (see Rehearsal) that parents use to track their rehearsal of skills they are learning can also serve as reminders to use the skills learned in clinic. In addition, some researchers have evaluated teaching parents to create their own reminders (Sanders, 1982). The parents in this study created a checklist of how to respond to child behavior. They reviewed with the child their expectations and how they would respond to misbehavior; they then self-recorded their performance and arranged for cues (e.g., charts on walls, notes on mirrors) to be present across settings to remind themselves to use the parenting skills they had learned. Results showed marked improvement in adherence in a number of settings where training did not originally occur.

Third, consider that a child's behavior itself can serve as one form of cue or signal. A parent who has been taught a skill in clinic may not use it in the home because the child's behavior does not signal that it is time to use the particular skill. This may be because the child's behavior is slightly different from behavior seen during training. For example, a parent may learn to use a time-out routine effectively to deal with a child who pinches a sibling but is confused and does not respond when confronted with the same child who chases a sibling with a stick. This suggests that the practitioner may need to include a greater variety of behavior examples during training. This effort to train diversely might involve arranging for parents to receive training with a wide range of potential problem behaviors. In fact, when parents of young infants were taught to recognize multiple problem behaviors as cues or reminders about when to use new parenting skills, the parents were found to be much better at recognizing when to act (Lowry & Whitman, 1989).

Finally, parents may need fewer reminders to use their parenting skills if they have been taught general principles of behavior management rather than or in addition to learning specific techniques for changing child behavior (Forehand & Atkeson, 1977). In this way, parents can learn that all behaviors, not just specific ones, are changeable, increasing the likelihood that many problem behaviors will remind parents to use the general principles they have learned. Indeed, some laboratory data suggest that teaching parents general principles of behavior modification can enhance generalization of skills to untrained behaviors and settings (Glogower & Sloop, 1976).

Developing Rapport

Although positive child behavior change is sometimes too delayed to reinforce immediately parents' adherence, developing good rapport can serve as an important source of motivation. A relationship in which the practitioner's approval is reinforcing for the parent is one in which rapport is said to have been established. This may require the practitioner to use words and actions that reflect interest and concern (e.g., eye contact, reflective comments) and that are supportive and positive (e.g., praising past parenting efforts). Indeed, practitioners who engage in these empathetic and nonjudgmental behaviors are thought to be effective parent trainers (Bernal, 1984) and may produce higher levels of satisfaction and skill acquisition in parents. Parents may also find it reinforcing to hear practitioners reveal their own struggles or lessons they have learned from work with other families—or even their own families. Consistent with theories of modeling, observers are more likely to imitate models who have experienced some of the same problems but have learned to cope with or overcome them.

Practitioners can also develop rapport with parents by openly acknowledging the need for parents to enjoy activities that do not involve their child. For example, parents also have TV shows they like to watch, e-mails to exchange, other children to feed and tuck in at night, and sleep to accrue. Indeed, a parent may find that these activities provide more immediate, potent, and easily and frequently accessed enjoyment than activities involving the parenting skills learned in clinic. Practitioners can show empathy and increase rapport by asking parents about their own needs. Although parents will ultimately need to use skills such as differential attention, time-out, or effective commands throughout the day, it may be valuable initially to ask parents to schedule and practice these skills only during times that they will be least likely to interfere with preferred parent activities.

Humor can also be a rapport-building technique, rendering social exchanges more reinforcing. Some have suggested, for example, including opportunities for parents to participate in role-plays in which they try to do everything wrong, an activity that can be entertaining and humorous (Webster-Stratton & Herbert, 1994). In addition, demonstrating incorrect responses has also been found to help individuals become more aware of and recognize their own undesirable behaviors. In fact, awareness training is now recognized as an important part of other empirically supported behavior change programs, such as habit reversal (e.g., Woods & Miltenberger, 2001). Humor can also be added to sessions by incorporating entertaining anecdotes from past experiences. For example, we have found that during parent training, using the following real anecdotes from experiences with our own children can allow parents both to laugh and to learn about the limits of using logic and reason with young children, who are so concrete in their thinking:

When driving into Manhattan one time, I commented to my young daughter that the cab we were in was about to go under the Hudson River, and she wondered out loud if we should roll up the windows.

After my young son went out the front door and stepped on a plate of muffins, left for us in celebration of May Day, he brought them to me, crying as he showed me his footprint on several of the smashed muffins. When I asked where he had found the muffins, he explained that he had found them under his foot!

Rapport may also be influenced by the style with which the practitioner engages the parent. Some have suggested that the *expert model,* in which a practitioner is directive and prescriptive, may result in less reinforcing interactions and generate more resistance from the parent. Indeed, some research has found that directive techniques that teach and confront can result in increased parental resistance and nondirective behaviors that facilitate and support lead to less resistance (Patterson & Forgatch, 1985).

An alternative to the expert approach is a *collaborative approach* in which parents actively participate in setting goals and even setting the individual session agenda. In this model, the practitioner is not an expert who dispenses advice or lectures but is instead a collaborator who asks parents to problem solve and to help write the specific treatment protocol. The thought is that this approach will build better rapport, make the session more reinforcing, and lead to improved adherence (Webster Stratton & Herbert, 1994).

Note, however, that there have been no direct comparisons of these models with regard to the adherence they produce. In addition, three of the four empirically supported parent training treatment programs use primarily expert models of treatment delivery. Nevertheless, it is easy to imagine that a style that allows parents to participate in some aspects of decision making could improve rapport and enhance adherence. For example, BST might begin with the parents reviewing a menu of behaviors that can be taught first, allowing them to choose which skills to learn first on the basis of which would be easiest to incorporate into the home environment. In this way, the practitioner can, if desired, both direct, by limiting choices, and collaborate, by allowing choices.

Ultimately, we think the relation between "expert" and "collaborator" may be better described as a continuum rather than a dichotomy, because "teaching" and "confronting" are not mutually exclusive from "facilitating" and "supporting." Even practitioners who adopt a collaborative model will, at times, be called on to teach, lecture, and give advice, especially if the practitioner is also using a BST approach that includes instruction, modeling, rehearsal, and feedback. Perhaps it is more important for practitioners to remember that whether they consider themselves experts, collaborators, or both, those who reinforce frequently and who acknowledge parents' unique strengths and perspectives in a nonblaming relationship are likely to have better rapport and encounter less resistance.

Using Tangible Incentives

Practitioners may also be able to add additional sources of reinforcement for adherence to treatment recommendations by adding tangible sources of reinforcement. For example, the practitioner might have parents deposit money (e.g., $50–$100) that would be refunded contingent upon attendance at training sessions, assignment completion, or even demonstration of meeting training criteria (e.g., Eyberg & Johnson, 1974). Others have promoted the idea of parent "salaries" in which payments are delivered contingent on compliance with treatment (e.g., Bernal, Klinnert, & Schultz, 1980; Fleischman, 1979). These systems may produce significant improvements in attendance, participation, and homework completion; however, there are practical problems with interventions that require parents to make large monetary deposits or that require practitioners to access funding sources for salaries. A more practical solution may be to recruit a spouse or family member to deliver rewards contingent on completing homework assignments or using those skills daily in the home. Rewards could be decided in advance in consultation with the parent and might include activities such as going out to dinner, going to a spa for a massage, or going out to a movie.

Using Technology to Reduce Effort

Electronic technology is playing an increasingly important role in everyday life, in large part because of the extent to which it can significantly reduce the effort required to complete many tasks. As we saw in chapter 4, individuals are more likely to engage in behavior that requires less effort, and response effort is understood to have an important impact on both parent and child behavior. Using electronic technology to reduce response effort for parents has an attractive appeal, but it requires product development, a process in which behavioral practitioners have not generally engaged (Bailey, 1991). This is somewhat surprising given that behavioral scientists were widely involved in the early development of electronic technology for use in modifying behavior, including for training relaxation (e.g., Budzynski & Stoyva, 1969), developing teaching machines (e.g., Cleary & Packham, 1968), and controlling activity level (e.g., Schulman, Stevens, Suran, Kupst, & Naughton, 1978). Yet although some recent efforts have explored adaptations of technology from the medical community (e.g., Costa, Rapoff, Lemanek, & Goldstein, 1997; Rapp, Miltenberger, & Long, 1998), efforts at product development have not kept pace with the promise afforded by available electronic technology, especially for facilitating parent training. There are, however, some exceptions.

Jason (1985) developed a token-actuated electronic timer for use with a token-exchange system to control TV access. The electronically controlled device was actually developed as a means to check the accuracy of parent-reported data, but it had remarkable potential as a means of enhancing parental adherence. For example, an electronic token-activated timer could reduce the response requirements for parents who are implementing reinforcement programs in which access to TV is to be delivered contingent on desired changes in child behavior. Indeed, there are now Web sites where electronic devices of this type that are designed specifically to help parents implement and follow through with contingencies designed to control children's access to reinforcers are available (e.g., http://familysafemedia.com/index.html). These include devices that monitor and control TV, phone, computer, and video-game use without requiring constant parental supervision. Of course, access to these types of devices is limited to those parents who have sufficient resources to own electronics and to purchase the monitoring devices.

Enhancing Parent Resources

Parents not only bring their child and differing expectations about how treatment will progress to clinic, they also bring vastly different resources to aid them in the process. Family resources can be influenced by poverty, mental health, physical health, cognitive functioning, and marital status. For example, intellectual impairment can make parenting skills difficult to learn and significantly increase the amount of time a practitioner will need to spend with a family teaching even basic skills (e.g., Bakken, Miltenberger, & Schauss, 2002). Cognitive impairments in children can also significantly increase stress in the family (e.g., Innocenti, Huh, & Boyce, 1992). Parents with affective disorders may find that memory, concentration, and sensory–perceptual skill impairments make parenting difficult (Herwig, Wirtz, & Bengel, 2004), and maternal depression, in particular, has been identified as a negative factor in child outcomes following parent training (Conley, Caldwell, Flynn, Dupre, & Rudolph, 2004). Restricted economic resources can limit access to and benefits from interventions that require time and materials beyond the means of the family (e.g., Chin & Phillips, 2004). Physical health impairments in either a child or an adult can place significant stress on family functioning (e.g., Streisand, Kazak, & Tercyak, 2003), and social isolation can place immense burdens on single or divorced parents who may have fewer supportive relationships than those found in traditional two-parent households (e.g., Utting & Pugh, 2004).

Various types of family resources are important for the practitioner to assess and address because they affect not only personal well-being but also the extent to which parents will do what they are asked to do (Dunst, Lee, & Trivette, 1988). As a result, clinical researchers have explored how best to meet the unique needs of families with limited resources. For the most part, the emphasis has been on adding supplemental components to the basic skills training that has already been found effective. For example, several parent training programs developed specifically for divorced mothers begin by training mothers in the same basic child management techniques common to the empirically supported parent training programs. However, the programs have also focused on using group-based formats to reduce isolation and allow participants opportunities for peer support and problem solving. They have also added sessions that include communication training and managing emotions (e.g., Forgatch & DeGarmo, 2002; Martinez & Forgatch, 2001; Weiss & Wolchik, 1998).

Some family resource barriers are probably best addressed before attempting parenting training. Parents with significant mental health problems or drug addictions may present barriers too difficult to address in session. Even marital distress can prove to be a significant barrier to successful outcome in parent training and may require referral for additional services before parent training can begin. Indeed, one of the empirically supported programs recommends against beginning parent training before marital issues are resolved (Hembree-Kigin & McNeil, 1995). However, Patterson's (1976) *Living With Children* book includes a chapter on addressing marital conflict in session, and Webster-Stratton has developed a supplemental component to The Incredible Years that is a 14-session, group-based treatment called ADVANCE to address parental risk factors such as marital distress. Finally, parent training can be supplemented by teaching problem solving and self-management skills to help parents deal with everyday interpersonal, vocational, and family stress (e.g., McMahon & Forehand, 2003; Sanders, 1996; Sanders & Dadds, 1993).

Treatment Program Flexibility

Although some family resource barriers can be overcome by supplementing the basic parent training skills with additional components, other barriers may require modifying the parent training program itself; rigid adherence to a parent training protocol or manual may not always be in the best interest of a child or family. Indeed, Patterson and colleagues have described the need for flexibility since the inception of their parent training program (Patterson, Reid, Jones, & Conger, 1975), and each of the other empirically supported parent training programs emphasizes the importance of flexibility when considering the unique needs of individual families (Hembree-Kigin & McNeil, 1995; McMahon & Forehand, 2003; Webster-Stratton & Herbert, 1994).

None of the programs specify exactly how their programs might be modified, but this is not surprising; just as a *flexible standard* is nearly an oxymoron, so, too, is a *standard flex*. It is difficult to describe a standard way in which to flex parent training. Competency criteria may be lowered, the order in which skills are taught may be altered, the format might be changed from individual to group, or the number of sessions spent on a particular skill might be extended—all in the name of adjusting a program to meet unique family needs. Unfortunately, there is almost no evidence to guide practitioners regarding the extent to which a program can be modified without substantially negating the empirically demonstrated benefits. So should it be done?

Yes, and modifications to the empirically supported programs can be done successfully if practitioners are guided by sound principles of evidence-based practice. Evidence-based practice integrates clinical expertise (American Psychological Association, 2005). Clinical expertise is what results from scientific training, conceptual understanding, and experience. Indeed, in a study of practitioners conducting parent training, those with more scientific training, conceptual understanding, and years of experience obtained better parent and child outcomes relative to less experienced, less trained, and less knowledgeable parent trainers (Moore & Patterson, 2003).

A practitioner dedicated to evidence-based practice can reasonably combine knowledge of empirically supported treatments with a conceptual understanding of why those treatments work to modify parent training programs to meet the unique needs of any individual family. Rigid adherence to specific performance criteria, session sequence, attendance requirements, and even specific behaviors taught are not as critical when practitioners understand that their goal is to increase reinforcement for desired behavior, reduce reinforcement for minor problem behaviors, use antecedent control strategies when possible, and use time-out from reinforcement when necessary. For example, a token program can function in much the same way as child-directed interactions and is a better alternative if the parent will be more likely to deliver a contingent token than to use descriptions and reflections during play. Likewise, parents removing themselves from a situation can function in much the same way as putting children in the corner if parents are the critical source of reinforcement and are more willing to "put themselves in time-out" than the child. Finally, none of the empirically supported programs encourage teaching punishment techniques before reinforcement techniques, but punishment has been found to be as effective in reducing noncompliance (Eisenstadt, Eyberg, McNeil, Newcomb, & Funderburk, 1993) and may be critical in responding to unique parent needs for immediate intervention with high-risk behavior. Together these examples demonstrate how knowledge of research and concepts can help practitioners flex programs within the context of evidence-based practice.

SUMMARY

Practitioners need to look beyond the contingencies that control the behavior of the child and also to look at those that control the behavior of the parent. It is these contingencies that determine whether parents will learn what practitioners teach and then do what they have learned. BST provides the foundation for skill development, but getting parents to use these skills requires overcoming barriers to adherence. Practitioners who develop rapport and craft effective rationales, who adjust their language and talk of outcomes, and who use reminders, incentives, and technology will find more successful outcomes because parents will be more likely to do what they have been asked to do. Note, however, that even when attending fully to the contingencies that affect parent behavior and directly supervising implementation outside the clinic, generating 100% adherence to practitioner recommendations is difficult (e.g., Volmink, Matchaba, & Garner, 2000).

Practitioners must also broaden their perspective and consider the contingencies that govern their own behavior. Practitioners, like parents, must work to catch parents "being good," use differential attention with parents, and incorporate effective commands. Yet practitioners may struggle to remember to do these things for the same reasons that parents do (e.g., they forget!). In addition, practitioners, like parents, want solutions to problems that do not require them to expend considerable effort or to alter their clinical routines to any great degree. It would be preferable to think that a child's welfare would come first and that issues related to the practitioner's effort and motivation were not relevant factors, but they are relevant. As a result, practitioners need to acknowledge their influence, as well as program-specific sources of support, for adherence. For example, practitioners may need to incorporate reminders into their own clinic, including protocols that prompt each component of BST. Practitioners may need to program their own sources of reinforcement, such as including students or interns who are there to learn the mechanics of parent training. Or practitioners may need to ask a colleague to observe and provide feedback regarding a parent training session. In these ways, practitioners can increase the likelihood of their own adherence to empirically and conceptually sound aspects of parent training.

Although the focus in this chapter has been on the immediate environment and the impact on adherence, there are broader influences to consider. In particular, culture provides a context in which all parenting is conducted and all treatment is provided. Culture describes the beliefs, values, and behaviors that are shared by a racial, ethnic, religious, or social group, and it is not difficult to imagine that culture profoundly affects the antecedents and consequences of everyday life as both a parent and a practitioner. Cultural competence as a practitioner comes from an understanding of shared cultural beliefs, values, and behaviors and the manner in which these can affect parent training. Chapter 6 provides an overview of major cultural influences on parenting in the United States and suggests how these influences may affect parent training. It also considers how this information might be used to enhance treatment outcome.

6

CULTURAL ISSUES IN PARENT TRAINING

Parents encourage behaviors viewed as culturally acceptable and discourage those viewed as culturally unacceptable. Culture heavily influences the specific parenting practices used to encourage and discourage child behavior. In addition, it influences which child behaviors are considered troublesome, the meaning that parents give to those troubles, the stigma associated with seeking help, the people parents go to first for help, and the trust they have in providers. Finally, culture influences the very recommendations that a practitioner provides about how to raise children properly and can be expected to influence parents' acceptance of and adherence to those recommendations.

As a result of these cultural influences, practitioners must use a so-called cultural lens as a central focus of professional behavior. That is, practitioners must recognize that all individuals, including themselves, are influenced by historical, ecological, sociopolitical, and disciplinary aspects of culture (American Psychological Association, 2003; http://www.apa.org/pi/multiculturalguidelines.pdf). A step toward ensuring that ethnically different children and families receive quality services is the adoption of culturally sensitive parent training practices. Although there are only limited data regarding empirically supported decision making in this regard, this chapter attempts to provide information and recommendations that are grounded in religious, social, educational, familial, and legal contexts that shape the experiences and beliefs of Asian American, African American, Native American, European American, and Latino American individuals and the practitioners who serve them.

It is important to note from the outset that cultural bias and stereotypic thinking influence us all. Across cultures, there is a tendency for individuals to exaggerate the differences between groups and the similarities within groups and then favor their group versus others (Fiske, 1998). At the heart of this bias lies an attribution error: a tendency for individuals to attribute positive behaviors to the similarities with their group but negative behaviors to the similarities of the other group. As a result, those within the same group tend to be more valued and more trusted, engendering more cooperation within groups and competition between groups. In addition, those with the strongest in-group affiliation show the strongest prejudice (Fiske, 1998).

Stereotypic thinking can cloud many evaluation and intervention efforts (Stuart, 2004). Bias can also lead to miscommunication because normative behavior in one culture may not necessarily be understood or valued by another. For example, addressing an individual by his or her first name may be a sign of disrespect in cultures that highly value authority and respect. These biases may also result in those in the out-group not seeking services, or they may seek services but not be well understood because cultural values may influence how they present their symptoms.

One strategy to overcoming these biases in parent training is to promote a color-blind approach in which racial, ethnic, and cultural differences are minimized. However, ignoring differences has been found to result in the perpetuation of out-group inequalities (Sue, 2004). Instead, practitioners must avoid being trapped in their own cultural worldview, which may prevent them from seeing the world from alternative perspectives. This requires awareness from all practitioners that we bring our own culture into the clinic or classroom and commonly operate from a predominantly ethnocentric perspective.

Unfortunately for practitioners doing parent training, awareness of one's own cultural assumptions is often elusive because views shared by the predominant culture are likely to seem "natural" rather than cultural and thus seem universal (Gone, 2004). Improving awareness requires understanding that one's own worldview about how parents should be trained or what they should be taught may be only partially accurate. Improving awareness also requires entertaining the notion that one's worldview may represent a false impression of what is normal or natural.

It is ironic that the very process of trying to increase awareness of one's own as well as other cultures serves as much to strengthen cultural stereotypes as it does to expand cultural sensitivity. That is, descriptions of a specific culture tend to list unique behavior, values, and lifestyles shared by a group of people (Tseng, 2003) but say nothing about any within-group differences that may, in fact, be substantial. For example, descriptions of African American culture imply commonalities among 40 million people in the United States because of ties with some 800 million people in Africa who represent 50 countries and speak 1,000 languages. Descriptions of Asian American culture ignore within-group differences between people from China, Japan, India, or Korea who embrace doctrines as diverse as Islam, Hinduism, Shinto, Christianity, and Buddhism. Similarly, efforts to generalize conclusions about Native Americans, who represent some 500 tribes, or Latino Americans, who represent numerous countries, territories, and islands across three different continents, assume a homogeneity that does not exist (Stuart, 2004).

Given such within-group diversity, it is misleading to draw broad conclusions about all members of any group. To ascribe naïvely to individuals the average properties of large groups is to perpetuate a "myth of uniformity" or an "ecological fallacy" (Lawson, 2001). Thus, efforts to increase cultural sensitivity and awareness may provide information about what some groups may believe but offer little information about a given individual. Nevertheless, practitioners must make some effort to identify areas of culture that are potentially relevant to their clients. Perhaps the best way to do this is to develop sensitivity to cultural differences without overemphasizing them (Stuart, 2004). Toward this end, this chapter reviews and discusses five major cultural influences on parenting practices in the United States today.

EUROPEAN AMERICAN CULTURE AND PARENTING

European American is a label used to describe individuals who are Caucasian and who can trace their ethnic heritage largely to European countries. The culture is often described as individualistic, in that the focus tends to be on the individual. That is, children and youth are encouraged to be "their own person." Children are often encouraged to allow their own interests to take precedence over the interests and welfare of the group. In this way, the self is seen as separate from rather than interconnected with all others within the social realm (Romero, 2000).

In the European American culture, social groups, social connectedness, and family ties are important; however, the needs, goals, and desires of the individual are encouraged to take priority. In contrast to many other cultures, children are encouraged, for example, to make decisions about which college to attend, which career to pursue, which job to take, and whom to marry, with little or no interference from parents. This emphasis on individualism appears to be tied to the American values of freedom, individual rights, and free choice (Hall & Hall, 1990). The result is a culture that values, encourages, and reinforces behaviors that are considered to be independent, self-directed, and autonomous (Markus & Kitayama, 1991). For example, European American parents have been found to socialize children for independence and to view dependent behavior as "clingy" and worrisome in that it suggests the child may be experiencing some sort of problem (Harkness & Super, 2002). This emphasis on the value of independence is also clear from early on when parents put infants to bed by themselves, a practice some cultures consider tantamount to child neglect (Morelli, Rogoff, Oppenheim, & Goldsmith, 1992). Indeed, much of the European American focus on developing children's independence is unappreciated in other cultures because it seems contrary to meeting a child's basic needs and wishes.

In European American culture, great value is placed on independence, and there is an equally strong focus on achieving success and pursuing personal goals (American Psychological Association, 2003). Those who work hard, are action oriented, achieve success, and accumulate goods tend to be valued individuals. It is not surprising that parents, too, are driven to achieve success in raising their children. Vast numbers of books, tapes, seminars, and workshops are available to assist parents with doing it "right," reminding them of the consequences if they fail or do it "wrong." Indeed, even the recent emergence of and relative importance placed on evidence-based parenting training programs might be considered the result of European American cultural values and priorities. Furthermore, pursuing personal goals with a direct and assertive way of communicating is encouraged in European American culture (Althen, Doran, & Szmania, 2002), and as a result, behavioral parenting programs often tell rather than suggest to parents what they should and should not do. Thus, both the existence and the content of behavioral parent training programs have been strongly shaped by European American cultural influences.

The European American culture also tends to be monochronic, emphasizing punctuality in all things. Schedules and time commitments are commonly taken very seriously. A culture that places an emphasis on punctuality might encourage someone to take on one job at a time, concentrate on that job, take deadlines seriously, and adhere strictly to job plans. This stands in contrast to cultures that place more emphasis on patience and human relationships in which an individual might take on many jobs, be less focused on any one of them, be committed to relationships more than the job, and change plans easily and often (Hall & Hall, 1990).

The impact of these cultural values on empirically supported parent training programs is evident and should not be surprising given that each was developed in the United States, where the dominant culture is European American influenced. Consider, for example, the following European American assumptions, values, and expectations in each empirically supported parent training program:

- Success depends on individual parent effort.
- Achievement is measured through performance requirements.

- Parents are expected to attend sessions alone or with the target child only.
- Practitioners are viewed as experts, and trust is expected.
- Practitioners' communication is directive and assertive.
- Effective command giving requires that parents be directive.
- Homework is expected to be done in a timely fashion and with integrity.
- The practitioner is to follow detailed lesson plans.
- The Child's Game (see Helping the Noncompliant Child, chap. 2, this volume) assumes that allowing a child's interests to direct the parent is acceptable.
- Reward elements assume rewarding children for expected behavior is acceptable.
- When given a command, children are expected to comply immediately.
- Parents must implement consequences immediately.
- Time-out assumes placing the child alone, and making the parent unavailable is acceptable.

The fact that European American culture places value on certain ways of parenting is not, by itself, a reason for concern. Likewise, it is not particularly problematic that parent training programs have been derived largely out of and reflect the values of European American cultural practices. The problem comes when parenting practices of other cultural, ethnic, or minority groups are compared against "standard" Euro-American practices (Garcia-Coll & Pachter, 2002). Differences between groups are then often described in terms of deficits. This approach assumes that there is a universal way to parent. To reject this approach is not to reject the need for scientific data to inform practitioners about the effectiveness or value of some child-rearing practices over others. Instead, it merely acknowledges that culture influences parenting and that this influence generally reflects adaptive strategies responsive to unique environmental and historical demands (Forehand & Kotchick, 1996). In this regard, practitioners should recognize that there is no cultural parenting standard.

AFRICAN AMERICAN CULTURE AND PARENTING

In many ways, enslavement, segregation, legal subjugation and their aftermath have shaped and continue to shape the culture and parenting of African Americans (Raajpoot, 2000). In contrast to other immigrant and cultural groups, who came to the United States to escape oppression or to seek new freedoms and economic possibilities, Africans arrived in the United States oppressed and without freedom or opportunity (McAdoo, 2002). The legacy of slavery and the racial caste system also left African Americans disproportionately in the lower class and at an economic disadvantage. As a result, the cultural experience of African Americans is a result of the overlapping influences of racism and oppression, minority status, economic disadvantage, and African heritage (Hill, 1999).

Adaptation to these influences has shaped a culture that often values communal family traditions and a matriarchal family system (Prince, 1997). For example, there is a strong communal aspect of child rearing in West African cultures, in which children are taught to regard parents and other relatives equally as caregivers (Caldwell, 1996). Similarly, many in the African American community view child care as a communal task. Considerable emphasis is often placed on the caring role for women, including sisters, aunts, and grandmothers. Parents may even take particular pride in infants being held and cuddled by an array of people without fussing or crying (Hill, 1999). In addition, extended family networks and church members may function as parents. In fact, informal adoption practices in which adults take in and parent children of family or friends in times of adversity continue to be an important part of the culture (McAdoo, 2002). It is not difficult to imagine that this "child sharing" has its origins both in African traditions and in response to early experiences with oppression, poverty, and disadvantage in this country. Regardless, it may be important for practitioners to explore the parenting roles played by siblings, grandparents, family friends, and church members and to explore whether they will or should be involved in parent training (Canales, 2000).

Both African and American influences have shaped a culture that encourages early self-care and self-reliance in children. African American parents may strive to have children weaned and toilet trained at an early age. In addition, the affection and attention directed to infants and toddlers may be less available to older children, who are expected to be more self-reliant. African American child-rearing practices have also been perceived as harsh and authoritarian, relying on emotional withdrawal or physical discipline (or both) to develop obedience.

In fact, there is some evidence that African American parents are actually more likely than European American parents to have and enforce strict rules and limitations (Bartz & Levine, 1978). In addition, African American parents have been found to be significantly more likely than Caucasian parents to define themselves as disciplinarians and to describe spanking as a frequently used method of discipline (Hill, 1999). This may be more a reflection of socioeconomic than cultural influences; there is considerable evidence that individuals with lower socioeconomic status are more restrictive and use more corporal punishment, regardless of cultural background (Hoff, Laursen, & Tardif, 2002). However, controlling for social class diminishes but does not eliminate these differences. Still, spanking is not the first choice in discipline for a vast majority of African American parents. In addition, it is important to remember that interpretations of any parenting practices as harsh or restrictive are culturally influenced. Other cultures may view these same practices as responsible and protective (Hill, 1999).

In many African American communities, spirituality is a valued communal tradition, and religion is an important source of guidance and support for child rearing. Although the African American emphasis on religion had its origins in ancient Africa, this emphasis was subsequently influenced by slavery and oppression such that religion and spirituality now play a central role in the lives of a majority of African Americans (Carter, 2002). Church membership is often an essential element in the family, and, as we have already seen, fellow church members and ministers are often considered part of the extended family (Paniagua, 1994).

Finally, culture may negatively influence the likelihood that many African Americans will seek assistance with parenting. For many African Americans, the need to seek treatment is associated with weakness and diminished pride, particularly in women, who are considered to be the anchor and source of strength in the family (V. L. Thompson, Bazile, & Akbar, 2004). There is also a general tendency for many African Americans to be cautious and skeptical, reflecting what many consider to be a healthy suspicion as a way of coping with a biased environment (Carter, 2002). Slavery and racism have shaped the cultural development of African Americans, and the development of a "healthy cultural paranoia" (M. K. Ho, 1992) may result in a highly suspicious reaction to mental health practitioners and the recommendations that they make. Indeed, professional degrees earned in and under the auspices of institutions marked by the presence of the dominant culture may be a poor basis for trust in individuals who consider that dominant culture to have been insensitive to their needs (Garcia, 1992). It is not surprising that practitioners who are described as older White men (perhaps perceived as more strongly reflecting the dominant culture) are more likely to be seen as unsympathetic, uncaring, and unavailable (V. L. Thompson et al., 2004).

Some evidence exists that African American culture tends to embrace environmental causes to problems and concrete, solution-oriented approaches to those problems—that is, approaches that are directive, active, and structured may be favored because they offer specifics about what the problem is, what role parents will play in the process, and what exactly the practitioner is recommending to solve the problem (Paniagua, 1994; Sue & Sue, 1990). As a result, many African Americans may be comfortable with the overall approach of empirically supported parenting programs.

LATINO AMERICAN CULTURE AND PARENTING

Latino is a label used to describe people who have their origins in Mexico, Central or South America, and the Spanish-speaking Caribbean (Cauce & Domenech-Rodriguez, 2002). The largest percentage of Latinos in the

United States claim Mexican heritage, but Latinos are a diverse group represented by countries from Central and South America as well as Europe, and they are projected to comprise one fourth of the U.S. population by 2050. Much has been made of Latinos being at risk for receiving poor education, having trouble finding employment, and living in poverty, yet the majority of Latinos in this country are here legally, complete high school, obtain employment, and live above the poverty line (Markus & Kitayama, 2001). Although Latinos are a heterogeneous group and there are wide variations with respect to individual and family cultural preservation, there are some common cultural beliefs and practices regarding child rearing and parenting that might be expected to influence the process and success of parent training.

There is substantial evidence that Latinos, when compared with European Americans, tend to adhere to child-rearing beliefs and values that are consistent with a more sociocentric perspective (Cauce & Domenech-Rodriguez, 2002). That is, individuals are encouraged to consider the thoughts, feelings, and actions of others in the group when making decisions. This stands in contrast to the European American culture, which encourages and reinforces behaviors that are considered to be independent and autonomous from the group when making decisions. The Latino emphasis on interdependence strongly affects parents' interactions with their children. For example, Latino American parents may tend to be less strict in their discipline and more permissive and placating as they consider and value a child's thoughts and feelings about their parenting. Furthermore, the emphasis on interpersonal connectedness means Latino Americans might be less likely to pursue parent training, independent of a spouse or partner. Indeed, research on parent training with Latinos has found that mothers consider husbands' involvement and encouragement in parent training to be extremely important (Armenta, 1993).

The Latino culture also values a strong family orientation. The family often reflects traditional male–female roles, and loyalty and solidarity of family members are considered critically important (Cortes, 1995). Men are often the dominant authority, and *machismo* (i.e., physical strength, masculinity, sexual attractiveness, and aggressiveness), *rispeto* (i.e., respect for authorities, especially men), and *marianismo* (i.e., women who are obedient, dependent, gentle, and spiritual) are valued (Paniagua, 1994). Women commonly care for children and do activities that benefit children and husbands. The extended family, primarily relatives, is also important to the cohesive family network, and parent training may benefit from inclusion of these extended family members (Paniagua, 1994).

In general, Latino culture also places emphasis on proper demeanor and respectfulness (R. L. Harwood, Leyendecker, Carlson, Ascencio, & Miller, 2002)—that is, the culture strongly encourages appropriate courtesy and decorum in relation to others, especially parents. For example, Latino American adolescents have been found to place more importance on respect for parental authority than individual autonomy (Fuligni, 1998). Indeed, Latino American youth describe strong feelings of respect for their parents and are more likely to assist parents rather than openly disagree (Fuligni, Tseng, & Lam, 1999).

There also tends to be a greater emphasis in Latino American culture on full participation in household chores and everyday tasks. Perhaps it is this emphasis on participation in family life that leads to Latino American children being expected to participate in and be self-reliant with household responsibilities at an earlier age than European American children. This seems consistent with the Latino cultural emphasis on social and family interdependence (Cortes, 1995). Family networks are vital, and participation in family life is not just encouraged but expected.

Latino mothers observed during parent–child play have been found to be more didactic, to spend more time directing, and to spend less time watching their children play than European American mothers (R. L. Harwood, Scholmerich, Schulze, & Gonzalez, 1999). Indeed, studies have also suggested that Latino parents do not spend much time talking about their children's emotions. Again, these observations seem consistent with a cultural emphasis on the child's obligations to the family and the larger group, with less emphasis on interactions that center on the child's actions, wishes, thoughts, and desires (R. L. Harwood et al., 2002). As a result, Latino Americans may find some aspects of the child-directed interactions (see Parent–Child Interaction Therapy, chap. 2, this volume) to be particularly difficult to accept or perform.

In studies comparing European American and Latino American families, Latinos have also been found to discourage competition and confrontation (Flannagan, 1996; Knight, Cota, & Bernal, 1993). For example, Latino American children have been found to be more likely to choose cooperative rather than competitive solutions to problems. In addition, Latino parents have been found to rely on appeals for cooperation rather than on confrontation to influence their children's behavior. Although many parents from all cultures would choose cooperation over confrontation, for Latino parents, cooperation is a deeply held cultural value in all relationships.

These cultural attitudes may have important implications for delivery of empirically supported parenting practices that encourage parents to use direct commands, to confront noncompliance, and to leave children alone in time-out when being disciplined. Thus, activities in parent training that rely on confrontation may be more difficult for Latino parents than for other parents to accept.

Empirically supported parent training, of course, involves much more than confrontation of child noncompliance. It involves relationship building and efforts to nurture parent–child interactions through play and cooperation. In fact, many aspects of parent training actually emphasize behaviors that reflect strong consideration of the thoughts, feelings, and actions of others—

behaviors that are very consistent with a sociocentric perspective characteristic of the Latino American culture. In addition, the empirically supported parent training programs do emphasize the interdependence in family relationships, and the group-based programs offer the possibility of including a community of families together in training.

ASIAN AMERICAN CULTURE AND PARENTING

The term *Asian* can refer to individuals from East, South, and Southeast Asia with extensive regional, ethnic, linguistic, and religious differences within regions. Yet even with this diversity, there are important parenting commonalities or themes across Asian societies (Chao & Tseng, 2002).

The most prominent theme found in Asian culture is that of family and family interdependence. This interdependence stresses the relation of a person to others, in contrast to the European American emphasis on independence and the person as separate or unique from others. Although the concept of interdependence emphasizes the importance of harmonious relationships in general, Asian cultures view the family as the prototype for all relationships (D. Y. E. Ho, 1996). This results in prioritizing of family goals over personal ones.

As a result, the interactions of Asian American parents with their young children tend to be characterized by more social–relational and "empathy" training than would typically be observed in European American parents (Clancy, 1986). Asian American parents have been found to spend more time appealing to social norms, directing their children's attention to fulfilling the wishes of others, and attempting to improve the ability of children to anticipate the needs of others. This has interesting implications for parents asked to participate in the child-directed interactions portion of the Parent–Child Interaction Therapy program (see chap. 2, this volume), which emphasizes a warm parent–child relationship but does so by allowing a child to pursue personal rather than relational goals. In addition, Asian Americans tend to pursue the social–relational goals through directive rather than nondirective interaction.

The value placed on family interdependence also involves a strong emphasis on respect for and obedience to parents and elders. Great importance is placed on parental authority in general, but the father often assumes the role of disciplinarian, teaching children to behave and orient themselves toward parents and others, often with little tolerance for emotional indulgence (Jankowiak, 1992). However, this approach does not typically begin until children are school-age. Before that time, parents may be rather indulgent, with minimal demands or expectations (Chao & Tseng, 2002).

Once children reach school-age, they are traditionally thought to be more responsible for their actions. There is then a general shift to more strict discipline, which is thought necessary to bring about proper development of character, emotional maturity, self-control, and social courtesy. It would not be unusual for a parent to select a child's interests and ambitions, and any attempt by the child to self-direct might be seen as a threat to the parents' authority (Paniagua, 1994).

Parental advice and guidance is expected to be sought even after a child becomes an adult. Although European American interpretations often view Asian parenting as controlling, Asian cultural frameworks suggest that parental authority reflects caring within an interdependent system. Parental authority and firm control are thought to reflect love, sacrifice, and concern that are critical for harmonious relationships. Parenting in this way is thought to bring pride, honor, and harmony. Indeed, parents who do not exert authority or control with their children would be viewed as negligent and uncaring.

In this context, compliance training and activities such as parent-directed interactions (e.g., see Parent–Child Interaction Therapy, chap. 2, this volume) might be expected to fit comfortably within an Asian American cultural framework. However, evidence-based parenting programs that encourage parents to be expressive, enthusiastic, and praising may offend those who have been exposed to Asian cultural sanctions against expressing strong emotions. Instead, silence, passive expression, and lack of eye contact are considered to be signs of respect and politeness, and significant self-worth is often derived from the ability to restrain expression of individual feelings and wishes (Okazaki, 2000).

Finally, family interdependence includes a strong expectation of family obligation. This begins in early childhood, when young children often are expected to take on day-to-day chores. Financial and caregiving obligations to family continue into adulthood and are one source of motivation behind a cultural emphasis on educational achievement. Schooling is considered to be a primary parental responsibility, and the quality of parents is often judged by how well their child does in school (Chao & Tseng, 2002). As a result, Asian American parents tend to have higher expectations for educational attainment, the grades they consider acceptable, and the amount of effort they believe their child can apply to educational activities. Academic success is considered important for self-improvement, social mobility, and economic betterment, all of which are understood to benefit the interdependent family system. It is not surprising that Asian American parents of young children tend to be more heavily involved in school activities and programs, to arrange supplemental learning opportunities, and offer significant home structure that supports learning (e.g., rules about homework; Chao & Tseng, 2002).

Perhaps the most significant cultural barrier between Asian Americans and access to empirically supported parent programs involves the stigma associated with seeking treatment. Public admission of mental health problems is not generally acceptable (Sue & Sue, 1990). Typically, family problems are shared only with family members, just as all successes are shared by family members. Public exposure of a family seeking services might be expected to engender significant shame and guilt. In addition, mental health practitioners in general, and Western psychological approaches in particular, have relatively low ascribed credibility, further reducing the probability of many Asian Americans seeking treatment. However, there is some evidence that increased credibility is often assigned to those who are older, male, or authority figures and that using official titles during introductions and displaying degrees may improve credibility (Okazaki, 2000). At least initially, maintaining formality and distance may also prove important.

NATIVE AMERICAN CULTURE AND PARENTING

Native Americans today represent considerable diversity because they practice numerous religious traditions, speak dozens of languages, and live in hundreds of communities, both rural and urban. Their cultural history has been strongly influenced by disease, racism, and discrimination brought on by European immigrants pursuing the expansion associated with Manifest Destiny. Most Native Americans were eventually forced onto reservations or into assimilation with European culture (Paniagua, 1994). Despite these events, cultural traditions have survived. Although descriptions of the culture cannot accurately reflect the diversity described by the term *Native American* (Gone, 2004), there do appear to be some cultural commonalities that influence parenting.

Perhaps the strongest cultural commonality among Native Americans is the emphasis placed on the inviolability of person: One person ultimately cannot speak for or control another. Every individual is self-responsible and self-accountable from the time of early childhood. As such, individuals make their own decisions, and no one person is responsible for anyone else's behavior (Brink, 1982). This applies even to parent–child relationships, in which parents can influence, but are generally not responsible for, the way a child turns out.

This is not to say that parents take no interest in guiding their children, but too much adult interference in the form of disciplining, lecturing, and controlling is thought to insulate a child from important experiential learning (Dillard & Manson, 2000). In fact, parents do not consider it critical to prevent children from making mistakes (Sprott, 1994). Furthermore, young children who have not yet developed the ability to reason are expected to behave badly from time to time. Thus, the child-rearing practices of many Native Americans often involve minimal discipline and might likely be considered permissive according to other cultural standards.

Although isolation from others (e.g., use of time-out) would be considered a severe punishment that might be used in some situations, Native

American parents have been found to be less likely than other parents to structure or intervene in children's activities. Instead, they are more likely to rely on indirect parenting strategies such as persuasion, shame, and nonverbal redirection (Seideman, Williams, & Burns, 1994). Given the cultural view that it is unacceptable to force someone to do something he or she does not wish to do, attempts by outsiders to discipline or correct a child might not be viewed kindly, even if others viewed it to be in the best interest of the child.

Consistent with many cultures worldwide, Native American traditions tend to place an emphasis on family first with the self as secondary. The family, rather than any individual, works to solve problems, and working together is emphasized. The extended family is important and often includes tribal elders and traditional medicine men (Paniagua, 1994). Mutual respect between all family members is rewarded and valued. Cultural expressions of interpersonal respect often involve nonverbal behaviors such as downcast eyes and a composed demeanor.

In many Native American communities, much authority is placed on tribal elders, yet there is also a strong sense of independence for children; they are rarely told directly what to do and are encouraged to make their own decisions (M. K. Ho, 1992). There may be few household rules, and those that do exist are likely to be flexible. There is also likely to be a de-emphasis on household routines and schedules. This may arise out of not only the cultural emphasis on child independence but also the cultural view that time is a natural event. When viewed this way, time does not control life, nor is it a measuring tool (M. K. Ho, 1992). Time would also not take precedence over a task or event. Instead, the cultural emphasis tends to be on living patiently in the here and now, and time, like goods, would be something to be shared with others. In this context, the European American cultural emphasis on rules, structure, control, schedules, and discipline that are clearly seen in the empirically supported parenting programs might be resisted by Native American parents. A practitioner might reasonably expect that cultural influences could make it less likely that Native Americans would seek treatment in the first place, show up in a timely fashion for sessions, or adhere to many of the controlling aspects of behavioral parent training programs.

TRANSLATING SENSITIVITY INTO PRACTICE

Table 6.1 summarizes some of the values from the five cultural groups discussed in this chapter and describes their possible implications for behavioral parent training. Clearly, culture does influence a wide range of values, customs, and traditions that may affect parent training. Reviewing these values and implications may help improve one's sensitivity to the ways that culture can influence a family's perception of parent training and the specific skills that are taught.

TABLE 6.1
Cultural Values and Parent Training Implications

Culture	Cultural values	Parent training implications
European American	Independence Self-directed Autonomy Achievement Punctuality	Empirically supported behavioral parent training programs are likely to be valued.
African American	Matriarchal Communal parenting Self-reliance Obedience Healthy suspicion Spirituality	Many aspects of empirically supported parent training are likely to be valued but may need to include extended family. Consider sibling in parent role. Match client–practitioner race.
Asian American	Self control Emotional maturity Family privacy Respect Social courtesy	Less likely to seek treatment. Formality may be expected. Praise may be discouraged and enthusiasm muted.
Latino American	Family loyalty Respect Interconnectedness Communal parenting Traditional gender roles Cooperation	Include extended family. Emphasize group rather than individual effort. Formal and direct approach. Compliance training may need to be reframed to emphasize teaching cooperation.
Native American	Centrality of family Self-responsible Independence of child Time as natural event	Empirically supported treatments may not be valued because of reliance on rules and control in a highly structured, directive format.

Armed with specific knowledge about how culture might influence perspectives on parent training, practitioners should be able to incorporate specific questions into the initial assessment to tap those influences. Table 6.2 includes some examples of questions that might be used during an initial assessment with a family to acquire important information about how behavioral parent training might be received (see Pedersen, 1997, for a comprehensive culture-centered interview guide). Rather than assume any individual has adopted "typical" cultural beliefs and practices, a sensitive practitioner can use knowledge of common practices to guide the questions asked during the initial assessment. This might begin with an open-ended question such as, "Are there any particular cultural identities or traditions that are important to you that I should be aware of as we get to know each other?" Note, however, that many individuals may not be aware of the ways in which their values and parenting practices reflect cultural influence. As a result, the practitioner must

TABLE 6.2
Culture-Relevant Assessment Questions

Cultural domain	Interview questions
Social customs	Is it acceptable to show affection in public (e.g., hugs, kisses)?
	Is it acceptable to praise and acknowledge accomplishments?
	How does one show respect (e.g., bow, lower eyes, hats off)?
	What behaviors are considered rude (e.g., showing soles of feet)?
	What is considered proper personal space?
	What is the family attitude toward punctuality?
Family life	What are the duties of men and women in the family?
	Who functions as caregivers or parents in the family?
	Who makes decisions about upbringing of the children?
	How is good behavior encouraged?
	How is bad behavior discouraged?
	What encounters between boys and girls are acceptable before marriage?
Clothing and food	What types of clothing are taboo?
	What parts of the body must be covered?
	Are there foods your family eats that are unique?
	How many meals a day are customary?
	What are your family's views on snacking?
Religion and folk beliefs	Are there any religious beliefs that influence daily life?
	What objects or places have sacred value?
	What religious traditions are taught?
Value systems	What is more valued: competition or cooperation?
	What is more valued: politeness or honesty?
	What types of activities are considered chores?
	What types of activities are considered play?
	What views are held regarding children earning allowances?

be careful in assuming there are no such influences simply because a parent reports none. In fact, many of the suggested assessment questions are appropriate to ask regardless of the response to the initial query.

The answers to these questions will help practitioners know how a client may perceive or accept parent training and determine whether it is an appropriate service delivery model. Of course, the assessment process can also help build rapport and allow the practitioner to select appropriate language, reframe important concepts, and develop appealing rationales that fit relevant cultural values. Ultimately, the practitioner may also need to adjust which skills are taught and how to teach them to overcome potential cultural barriers. In the overview of cultural values and their possible implications for parent training practices (see Table 6.1), note that, in some cases, there may be such a poor match between the client's cultural values and those embedded in the empirically supported treatments that the practitioner may not have the clinical expertise or the cultural competence to address the incongruity adequately. It is unlikely that this will be a common situation because individuals whose cultural values are so critically different from the dominant culture are not apt to seek the services of a practitioner associated with it. However, when this situation does rise, a referral may be necessary. In other cases, modifications may be necessary to ensure a match. In all cases, given that both parent values and behavioral parent training are culturally derived, some effort to assess and match values and training is required.

SUMMARY

The United States is a nation with many cultural influences, each with its own views on the nature of childhood, the importance and structure of families, and the roles and functions of ideal parents. Although there is no evidence that one particular style of child rearing or parenting is better than any other (Sprott, 1994), members of each culture have a tendency to view their own practices as good and desirable. This, by itself, is not a concern, but it can become problematic when one culture is dominant. Dominant cultures enjoy greater status, power, and privilege and commonly represent the majority of the professionals in health care programs and services. In the United States, although the mix of cultural diversity is increasing and will, by 2050, represent half of the population, the dominant culture is, and will probably continue to be, European American for some time.

With the growing diversity among families and children in the United States, it is particularly important for health care professionals to acknowledge and incorporate culturally sensitive practices into parent training. Ideally, cultural sensitivity means understanding that culture influences all parenting practices, including those of the dominant culture and the science that informs those practices. As a result, parents and children from nondominant cultures may find some or all aspects of dominant culture parenting practices to be objectionable. This is important because effective treatment requires not only practices that can change behavior but also those that parents are willing to use.

Unfortunately, predicting which individuals will find which practices objectionable is difficult, even for culturally sensitive practitioners. Stereotyped generalizations about cultural influences provide some information about what some groups may believe but provide little information about the beliefs of a given individual. The solution is for practitioners to make few assumptions about probable cultural influences. Indeed, the only reasonable assumption is that there are likely to be cultural influences and that the practitioner must assess them. The information in this chapter provides some guidance for practitioners about where to look for possible influences and their likely impact on parent training, but none of the information can take the place of a competent assessment. Although there have not been adequate empirical studies of the effect of cultural sensitivity on parent training outcomes, it is reasonable to suggest that the practitioner's ability to "package" the parent training program and to reframe the rationale for specific interventions in a culturally congruent way may have a positive impact. Such strategies (e.g., Forehand & Kotchick, 1996) can be an important means of enhancing treatment acceptability and encouraging parents to try alternative parenting strategies.

III

INTEGRATING AND TRANSLATING RESEARCH INTO EVERYDAY PRACTICE

7

BEYOND NONCOMPLIANCE: DEVELOPING EVIDENCE-BASED PARENT TRAINING INTERVENTIONS

Every day, practitioners are faced with a wide range of child problems including inattention and hyperactivity, sleep problems, feeding problems, toileting problems, academic problems, adolescent–parent conflict, internalizing problems, and a host of other potential concerns. In this chapter, we discuss how parent training can be used to address child problems beyond noncompliance. Historically, child noncompliance has received most of the attention in the parent training literature because it is one of the most common problems that practitioners will face regardless of whether they work in mental health outpatient clinics, primary care, or schools (e.g., Arndorfer, Allen, & Aljazireh, 1999; Bear, 1998; Schroeder, Gordon, Kanoy, & Routh, 1983). In addition, noncompliance is a predictor of poor developmental outcomes and is considered a keystone behavior in the development of other childhood problems (McMahon & Forehand, 2003; Nelson & Hayes, 1986). For example, bedtime problems often include noncompliance with bedtime routines. Toilet training struggles may include noncompliance with sitting on the toilet when requested. Mealtime problems often include children's noncompliance with attempting to eat new foods. Academic problems may include or be exacerbated by children's refusal to complete homework. Even children's adherence to medical treatments may be negatively affected by noncompliance,

159

such as refusal to take medicine, monitor blood glucose, or wear splints. Thus, the empirically supported parent training programs described in chapter 2 of this volume can be helpful to address noncompliance associated with other common child problems (e.g., Barkley, 1997; Wells, 2003; Wells et al., 1996).

Unfortunately, there are to date no parent training programs that meet previously defined criteria as empirically supported (e.g., Chambless & Hollon, 1998; Kumpfer, 1999) in the treatment of child problems other than noncompliance. This includes the four empirically supported parent training programs. For example, although the Parent–Child Interaction Therapy (PCIT) manual suggests that the program is appropriate for treating childhood problems as wide ranging as stealing, hyperactivity, self-injurious behavior, perfectionism, and separation anxiety (e.g., Hembree-Kigin & McNeil, 1995), there are no empirical data offered to support these claims. In addition, the manual provides no guidance regarding how a parent trainer might adapt the PCIT protocol to address these other types of behavior problems.

McMahon and Forehand (2003), in their book *Helping the Noncompliant Child* (see also chap. 2, this volume), discuss adaptation of their parent training program to other populations of children, such as children with attention-deficit/hyperactivity disorder (ADHD), children with developmental disabilities, in-patient populations, children who have been abused and neglected, and children with elimination disorders such as enuresis and encopresis (Wells, 2003). However, the Helping the Noncompliant Child program is typically applied for the purpose of reducing the noncompliance that often accompanies these populations of children. McMahon and Forehand do not suggest that the program would actually treat ADHD, encopresis, or developmental disability.

In their clinician manual and parent books, Patterson and colleagues discuss how parents may address other types of child problems, such as stealing, bed-wetting, toilet training, sleep problems, whining, and temper tantrums (Patterson, 1975; Patterson, 1976; Patterson, Reid, Jones, & Conger, 1975). Webster-Stratton also discusses how parents can solve other child problems such as dawdling, bedtime resistance, television addiction, stealing, mealtime problems, and hyperactivity in her parent book (Webster-Stratton, 1992). In both of these programs, parents are taught to apply basic scientific principles and intervention techniques to address these other child problem behaviors. In both programs, the emphasis is on describing what to teach parents to do, but there is relatively less emphasis on how to teach parents to do it.

Numerous individual research studies have demonstrated that parents can be trained to solve child problems other than noncompliance (e.g., Briesmeister & Schaefer, 1998; Dangel & Polster, 1984). For example, online literature reviews reveal published research showing that parents have been used to treat bedtime problems (e.g., Mindell, 1999), enuresis (e.g., Azrin, Sneed, & Foxx, 1974), academic problems (Valleley, Evans, & Allen, 2002), and stealing (e.g, Luiselli & Pine, 1999). Unfortunately, most research is not explicit or detailed in describing how to train parents to implement interventions that address these other child problems. Researchers may write in their intervention procedures that parents were trained to deliver an intervention, but they often do not provide details about how they were trained. This is not a small obstacle because getting parents to do what is necessary is at least as important as knowing what it is necessary for them to do (Allen & Warzak, 2000).

A FRAMEWORK FOR DEVELOPING INTERVENTIONS

As part of an evidence-based practice, practitioners need to review the research literature on interventions for particular child problems of interest. However, given that most treatment research does not provide clear information about how to conduct parent training, practitioners may benefit from a structured approach to gleaning the most relevant information from the research for purposes of developing parent training interventions. We now describe a framework that can assist the practitioner in organizing information and procedures from research to determine specific steps in the parent training process. This framework is based on the behavioral principles and training process inherent in the empirically supported parent training programs (see chaps. 4 and 5). The framework helps the practitioner decipher and organize the research literature on interventions for other child problems to identify what and how to teach parents.

Exhibit 7.1 presents this organizing framework, derived from knowledge of the empirically supported parent training programs described in this book. Practitioners can use the framework as a clinical tool when reviewing research on effective interventions for child problems beyond noncompliance.

The information for column 1, "What to teach," will come from a review of the research on the specific child problem. Column 2, "Why it works," integrates the practitioner's understanding of the behavioral principles underlying parent training (i.e., reinforcement, extinction, stimulus control, and punishment) with the steps toward the goals for the intervention. Column 3, "How to teach: parent training," outlines the four behavioral parent training methods (i.e., instruction, modeling, rehearsal, and feedback) for each component listed in column 1. Practitioners can complete each of these cells as they become familiar with the research on a particular child problem area. Table 7.1 shows how these cells would be completed after reviewing the four empirically supported parent training programs described in chapter 2.

The empirically supported parent training programs summarized in Table 7.1 all have manuals and a voluminous amount of research support, making the use of the table in daily practice unnecessary. Nevertheless, it is presented here because it helps to summarize visually the common key aspects of these programs. This organizing framework can be beneficial for the

EXHIBIT 7.1
Organizing Framework for Research and Parent Training

What to teach	Why it works	How to teach: parent training
	Reinforcement	Instruction Modeling Rehearsal Feedback
	Extinction	Instruction Modeling Rehearsal Feedback
	Stimulus control	Instruction Modeling Rehearsal Feedback
	Punishment	Instruction Modeling Rehearsal Feedback

practitioner who is reviewing treatment research related to other child problems for which there is not much research or no treatment manuals. In many cases, not all cells in the framework will be completed because, for example, the research may not support use of punishment in some situations, or the intervention may not include each of the elements represented in the "Why it works" column. Clinical expertise is needed in these instances to determine whether these are cells that need to be completed before the intervention and parent training can reasonably be expected to be effective. It is recommended, however, that practitioners attempt to complete all cells to increase the probability of intervention and parent training success.

To summarize, practitioners should begin with a review of the literature to formulate a plan of what to teach. At the same time, consideration of why it works should help practitioners identify whether intervention components derived from the research literature are designed to increase a desired behavior through reinforcement, decrease behavior through extinction, prompt a behavior through stimulus control, or decrease a problem behavior through punishment. Parent training is then sequenced in the framework so that reinforcement is considered first when implementing treatment, then extinction and stimulus control techniques before consideration of punishment techniques. This is consistent with the approach of each of the empirically supported parent training programs for child noncompliance. Note that this preference for implementation of reinforcement procedures over punishment is also consistent with some

TABLE 7.1
Parent Training for Child Noncompliance

What to teach	Why it works	How to teach: parent training
Teach parents social attention skills such as praise and positive touch, descriptions, and reflections contingent on compliant and appropriate behavior.	Reinforcement: Social attention delivered contingent on compliance or other desired child behaviors increases the probability of the behavior recurring.	Instruction: Describe and provide rationale for using social attention. Present information orally and provide handouts. Modeling: Demonstrate with the child or parent how to provide praise, descriptions, and reflections. Rehearsal: Have the parent practice providing praise, descriptions, and reflections with the child. Have parents practice social attention skills daily at home during the child-directed interaction or Child's Game activity. Feedback: Provide positive and corrective feedback during rehearsal to shape parents' behavior toward the desired goal.
Teach parents to ignore minor misbehavior.	Extinction: Removal of social attention contingent on noncompliance or other defined misbehavior reduces probability of the behavior recurring.	Instruction: Describe and provide rationale for ignoring minor misbehavior, particularly in relation to the use of social attention for compliance (i.e., differential social attention). Modeling: Demonstrate use of ignoring during the Child's Game activity with the child. Rehearsal: Have the parent practice ignoring with the child during the Child's Game activity. Have parent use ignoring at home daily during the Child's Game practice. Feedback: Provide immediate positive and corrective feedback to the parent during rehearsal.

(continues)

TABLE 7.1
Parent Training for Child Noncompliance *(Continued)*

What to teach	Why it works	How to teach: parent training
Teach parents how to provide direct, one-step, developmentally appropriate commands.	Stimulus control: A parent command that signals reinforcement is available for compliance (a discriminative stimulus).	Instruction: Describe and provide rationale for giving effective commands. Modeling: Demonstrate giving effective commands with the parent or child. Rehearsal: Have the parent practice giving effective commands with the practitioner or child. Have the parent practice using effective commands at home daily and track practices and/or child responses. Feedback: Provide immediate positive and corrective feedback to shape parents' commands.
Teach parents how to apply time-out contingent on noncompliance or other target misbehavior.	Punishment: The child is removed to a less reinforcing environment contingent on noncompliance decreasing the probability of noncompliance recurring.	Instruction: Describe and provide rationale for using time-out. Provide step-by-step protocol or procedure. Modeling: Model with the child how to implement time-out. Rehearsal: Have the parent practice time-out in the clinic with the child. Have the parent begin using time-out at home, collecting data on the procedure and the child's response. Feedback: Provide immediate positive and corrective feedback to parent to shape effective implementation of time-out.

ethical guidelines for intervention (Behavior Analyst Certification Board, 2004). Although clinical expertise would suggest that the most potent intervention is likely to include aspects of all four concepts, we do not suggest that an intervention should include all four, only that doing so may enhance the probability of a desired outcome.

On the basis of the information in the "What to teach" and "Why it works" columns, practitioners can then develop a plan for parent training that will be completed in the "How to teach: parent training" column. In each step listed under "How to teach: parent training" in Exhibit 7.1, parents are taught using a sequence of behavioral skills training including instruction, modeling, rehearsal, and feedback. Practitioners can complete these cells as they become familiar with research in a particular topic area with consideration of the basic scientific principles that support why the intervention works.

CASE EXAMPLES FOR COMPLETING THE ORGANIZING FRAMEWORK FOR PARENT TRAINING

In the remainder of this chapter, we illustrate how research material can be organized for six common child problems often encountered in schools, clinics, and other community agencies. These examples[1] include sleep problems, bed-wetting, picky eating, classroom behavior problems, academic problems (e.g., reading fluency), and problems common in adolescence (e.g., breaking curfew). The information presented throughout the chapter presents elements of good evidence-based practice. The interventions are derived from the best available treatment research for each child problem, integrated with knowledge about why the interventions work, coupled with practitioner expertise in the application of a behavioral skills training model.

The reader will note in reviewing these examples that elements of teaching children to be more compliant are often included as a component of effective interventions for these other child problems, particularly teaching parents to provide effective commands. In addition, the dependent variable, or problem behavior, is often operationally defined in research, and careful monitoring or repeated measurement of the problem behavior is inherent in research. Similarly, the empirically supported parent training programs for noncompliance include parent training for defining and monitoring both problematic and desirable child behaviors. More discussion of this step is provided in chapter 8, but the reader will note in the following examples that teaching parents to define and monitor child behavior is one of the first skills taught.

---

[1]The cases presented in this chapter are provided for illustrative purposes only and do not represent a single actual case. Rather, they represent composites of actual cases presenting to our clinic.

A thorough review of the research for each problem presented here is beyond the scope of this chapter. Readers should also note that the examples provided may not pertain to individual children and families that they see with similar problems. The intervention strategies actually used by an individual practitioner must be carefully selected on the basis of an initial assessment of the unique needs of the child and family. So, for example, although attending to all four basic concepts in developing an intervention may help ensure a high probability of success, it may prove to be overkill for a child who presents with a fairly circumscribed problem of mild intensity. In addition, including unnecessary components may increase the response effort required of parents, reducing their adherence to recommendations and also the probability of a successful outcome.

Thus, the following examples are not meant to be used as treatment protocols for every child presenting with the same problem but as examples for how practitioners may use the framework to plan parent training interventions for children they see. These multiple, prototypical examples provide information about how to use the framework to organize information. Chapter 8 provides additional information about how to use the framework as a component of a comprehensive model of parent training service delivery that is tailored to the needs of individual children and families.

Sleep Problems

Problems with sleep are relatively common in young children. More than 30% of children will exhibit sleep problems sometime during their first 3 to 4 years (Wolfson, 1998), although sleep problems may also occur in later childhood, adolescence, and adulthood. Poor sleep habits contribute to poor developmental and educational outcomes (Fallone, Owens, & Deane, 2002; Wolfson & Carskadon, 2003). Interventions for sleep may consist of establishing a bedtime routine, changing the expected sleep schedule, fading a parent's presence, systematically ignoring awakenings, rewarding staying in bed, or some combination of these strategies (Kuhn & Elliott, 2003; Kuhn & Weidinger, 2000; Wolfson, 1998). Each of these approaches or techniques involves manipulating environmental contingencies to establish good sleep habits in children.

In Table 7.2, information is presented regarding an intervention and parent training protocol developed for a 7-year-old boy, Daniel, brought to an outpatient psychology clinic by his mother because of concerns regarding poor sleep. Information gathered from his mother revealed that Daniel refused to go to bed. He had access to TV and a computer in his room. A light was left on in his room at bedtime. There was no clear routine before bedtime, such as changing clothes, brushing teeth, or voiding, nor was there time with his mother before bed in which Daniel was engaged in a calm activity such as reading. Typically, Daniel watched TV until he fell asleep, sometimes in his

TABLE 7.2
Parent Training for Child Resisting Bedtime

What to teach	Why it works	How to teach: parent training
Teach parents to define goal behavior and monitor bedtime routine. Teach parents to implement token reinforcement system for bedtime routine and remaining in bed. Tokens are cashed in for rewards in the morning. Teach parents to develop list of rewards child may earn daily.	Reinforcement: Tokens and praise increase the probability of compliance with bedtime routine and the child remaining in bed.	Instruction: Describe and provide rationale for using a token reinforcement system and rewards. Modeling: Demonstrate how to provide tokens and exchange them for a reward. Rehearsal: Have parents role-play with child providing tokens and reward. They may also role-play the bedtime routine. Feedback: Provide positive and corrective feedback during rehearsal to shape parents' use of the token system and bedtime routine.
Teach parents to ignore minor misbehavior that may occur when the child is in bed and reduce verbal interaction when the child arises from bed for drinks, bathroom, and so on	Extinction: Removal of social attention contingent on minor misbehavior in bed or arising from bed reduces the probability of the behavior recurring. It may also briefly increase problem behavior through extinction burst.	Instruction: Provide description and rationale for ignoring minor misbehavior and reducing verbal interaction. Predict temporary increases in behavior. Modeling: Demonstrate the use of ignoring during role-play with parent or child. Rehearsal: Have the parent practice ignoring during a role-play with the child. Feedback: Shape effective ignoring during role-play.
Teach parents to establish a bedtime routine, including a consistent time schedule and activities such as changing clothes, brushing teeth, toileting, drinking, and reading.	Stimulus control: Chart functions as discriminative stimulus.	Instruction: Describe and provide rationale for the bedtime routine, chart, structuring of the bedroom environment, and changing bedtime.

(continues)

TABLE 7.2
Parent Training for Child Resisting Bedtime *(Continued)*

What to teach	Why it works	How to teach: parent training
Teach parents to provide direct commands and clear expectations for following the routine.	Commands are discriminative for compliance.	Modeling: Demonstrate how to make a bedtime routine chart with the parent or child.
Teach parents to set up the bedroom environment to encourage sleep such as lights off, TV off, and no toys in bed.	Environment is discriminative for sleep onset.	Rehearsal: Have the parent role-play with the practitioner or child how to give effective commands and monitor completion using the chart.
Teach parents to start with a later bedtime that increases probability of falling asleep faster. Gradually return to desired bedtime as child demonstrates success with falling asleep.	Later bedtime strengthens sleep as a reinforcer (establishing operation).	Feedback: Shape the parent's use of the bedtime routine chart and effective commands for bedtime.
Teach parents to implement a "bedtime pass." The child gets several free tokens at bedtime but loses one each time he or she rises from bed and leaves the room.	Punishment: The loss of a token decreases the probability of child getting out of bed.	Instruction: Describe and provide rationale for the response cost procedure. Modeling: Model how to implement response cost procedure. Rehearsal: Have the parent role-play in the clinic with the child. Feedback: Shape effective implementation of the response cost procedure.

clothes. If he fell asleep in bed, he would frequently get up at night and move to the couch in the living room. He was expected to go to bed at 8 p.m. but often did not fall asleep until close to 11 p.m. He was awakened at 6 a.m. to prepare for school. Additional information was provided during the initial intake session regarding family structure, dynamics, and daily routine. It appeared that Daniel was generally compliant throughout much of the rest of the day. His mother appeared to be inconsistent with providing punitive consequences for noncompliance when it did occur, however. Although sleepy, he was still doing well academically and behaviorally at school. His mother noted no other concerns with behavior.

For a young child refusing to go to bed, treatment begins with efforts to reinforce going to and remaining in bed, or at least in the room. Tokens or stickers can be effective with young children and have been used in the treatment of bedtime problems in previous research. It is important, however, that tokens or stickers be exchanged for rewards because tokens or stickers alone may not increase behavior. Next, treatment involves removal of social attention from the parents for minor misbehavior or for arising from bed without permission. The environment is also made conducive to sleep by reducing distractions in the bedroom, and bedtime may be moved to later to ensure the child is tired. Finally, if the child is persistent in getting out of bed, a punishment procedure may be implemented in which the child loses a token for this behavior.

Teaching each of the strategies included in this framework involves a behavior skills training approach. Preplanning for parent training using the framework will reveal, however, that some strategies may require more careful explanation and supportive rationale before modeling and rehearsal can begin. For example, ignoring often seems like an obvious, although perhaps impossible, strategy to many parents, and the need for a later bedtime is often less than apparent. In addition, rehearsal of skills is almost always limited to role-playing because it is difficult to recreate bedtime outside the home, but the practice can be important nonetheless. Asking the parent and child to walk through the steps can assist in identifying aspects of the intervention that were not communicated effectively during instruction. The practitioner may also consider ranking the skills to be taught in terms of difficulty so that the easiest are taught before the more difficult ones. In this case example, it may be that the reinforcement program will be easier to implement relative to ignoring the child or implementing punishment. Punishment strategies may at times be much easier to implement than reinforcement strategies. Nevertheless, reinforcement strategies remain the focus of almost all child interventions for the numerous conceptual, practical, and ethical reasons described in chapter 4.

Toileting Problems

Bed-wetting, or enuresis, affects at least 10% of children ages 5 to 16 years (Mellon & Houts, 1998). Although enuresis may co-occur with other problems of childhood, it is not typically indicative of other behavior problems (Friman & Jones, 1998). Rather, enuresis is problematic for children because of the negative effect it may have on parent–child interaction that comes with unmet parental expectations as well as the need to waken at night and clean sheets and nightwear. Bed-wetting is also problematic for socialization with peers, particularly when children reach an age when sleeping over at friends' homes or participation in campouts becomes more common. Enuresis is typically nocturnal, although children may exhibit diurnal enuresis as well, which can also lead to additional difficulties related to socialization and school adjustment.

A review of the best available research indicates that there are several effective methods to treat enuresis (Christophersen & Mortweet, 2001). Medication can be effective but does not appear to have the long-term positive outcomes that behavioral techniques demonstrate. Nevertheless, medications can provide a valuable short-term adjunctive treatment option, and thus it is important that the practitioner communicate with the child's physician. The standard behavioral treatment involves a urine alarm, which has consistently been shown to be the single most effective treatment (Friman & Jones, 1998). With the urine alarm, small sensors are snapped to the child's pajamas or underwear. When the child begins to urinate, the sensors trigger an alarm. The intent is that the alarm awakens the child, and the child stops urinating and finishes voiding in the toilet. The alarm has been shown to be effective compared with numerous other treatments and typically requires from 8 to 12 weeks of intervention (e.g., Doleys, Ciminero, Tollison, Williams, & Wells, 1977; McKendry, Stewart, Khanna, & Netley, 1975). The urine alarm can be used alone but has also been found to be effective when combined with other treatment components, such as positive reinforcement for successes (van Londen, van Londen-Barentsen, van Son, & Mulder, 1993), cleanup routines, retention training, overlearning (e.g., Houts, Liebert, & Padawer, 1983), and positive practice (Azrin & Foxx, 1974).

Table 7.3 provides an example of how research on treating enuresis was used to develop an intervention and parent training strategy for a 9-year-old child with enuresis. The 9-year-old boy, Adam, was brought to a primary care physician's office because of concerns regarding bed-wetting. The psychologist working in the office interviewed the parents and gathered information indicating that Adam had never consistently had a dry night in bed. There were no concerns with toileting during the day. He was described as a generally compliant child who was doing well at school, had friends, and participated in extracurricular activities. His parents had primarily attempted punishment procedures in the past, including removal of privileges and having Adam assist with cleanup of the bedsheets and laundry. He was described as generally compliant with loss of privileges but resistant to cleanup activities, occasionally leading to arguments with his parents.

On the basis of a review of research, an intervention using a urine alarm was used in this case. Contrary to the other examples in this chapter, this intervention is probably best conceptualized as being based on the behavioral principle of punishment. The application of the alarm decreases voiding. There may well also be a negative reinforcement component because the probability of the child's awakening when his or her bladder is full may be negatively reinforced by the avoidance or termination of the alarm. Understanding the behavioral principles underlying the interventions we use is important because not all research-based interventions necessarily emphasize positive reinforce-

TABLE 7.3
Parent Training for Nocturnal Enuresis (Bed-Wetting)

What to teach	Why it works	How to teach: parent training
Teach parents to monitor and collect data on bed-wetting incidents. Teach parents to develop list of rewards. Teach parents and child to use the alarm. Each night the alarm is worn to bed. The child is prompted to get up immediately when alarm sounds and finish voiding in toilet. Alarm is worn to bed again.	Reinforcement: Avoidance of alarm sounding functions as negative reinforcement of awakening when bladder is full and compliance with other treatment components.	Instruction: Describe and provide rationale for alarm and for using praise and reward system. Modeling: Demonstrate how the alarm works and how to praise and deliver tokens. Demonstrate token exchange. Rehearsal: Role-play praise, delivery of tokens, and exchanges.
Parents provide praise and stickers or tokens for compliance with alarm routine (i.e., up within 3 minutes of alarm going off and finish voiding in toilet)	Tokens and praise increase probability of alarm use.	Feedback: Provide positive and corrective feedback during rehearsal to shape implementation of the reward system and proper wearing of the urine alarm.
Parents may also provide praise and stickers or tokens for retention training and/or compliance with cleanliness training.	Tokens and praise increase retention training practices and wait time before voiding and compliance with cleaning.	
Reduce reprimands and lecturing contingent on accidents or poor adherence to routine.	Extinction: Removal of attention may reduce the probability of inadvertently reinforcing accidents or resistance (i.e., arguing).	Instruction: Provide description and rationale for reducing reprimands and lectures. Modeling: Demonstrate the use of ignoring in role-play. Rehearsal: The parent practices ignoring during a role-play. Feedback: Provide positive and corrective feedback to the parent to shape effective ignoring.

(continues)

TABLE 7.3
Parent Training for Nocturnal Enuresis (Bed-Wetting)   *(Continued)*

What to teach	Why it works	How to teach: parent training
Teach parents and child retention training. Child is encouraged to drink fluids during the day and then delay urination as long as possible after the first urge to void.	Stimulus control: The mechanism may involve classical conditioning so that urine in the bladder does not elicit the urge so quickly. Practice may also result in the urge becoming discriminative for waiting longer, even when asleep.	Instruction: Describe and provide rationale for retention training. Determine appropriate fluid intake for the child. Describe and provide rationale for clear commands and expectations throughout the intervention procedure.
Teach parents to provide clear commands and expectations regarding intervention components.	Commands are discriminative for compliance.	Modeling: Demonstrate how to encourage waiting with the child. Demonstrate how to provide clear commands.
		Rehearsal: Have the parent and child increase fluids before session and practice waiting in session. Practice clear commands.
		Feedback: Provide immediate positive and corrective feedback to shape parent skills in implementing toileting expectations.
Teach parents to have child clean self, clothes, and bedding materials, as well as remake the bed with clean bedding after accident.	Punishment: Alarm functions to decrease voiding. Cleanup decreases frequency of accidents.	Instruction: Describe and provide rationale for having child participate or independently clean bedding and clothes.
		Modeling: Model with child and parent how to implement cleaning expectations.
		Rehearsal: Have parent and child role-play cleaning expectations.
		Feedback: Shape parent's skills in instructing child to implement cleaning expectations.

ment as the mechanism of behavioral change. It is important for purposes of planning parent training that the practitioner acknowledge the potentially aversive aspects of the intervention. Of course, one way for a child to avoid the alarm is to refuse to wear it. Noncompliance with the treatment regimen is a common problem. Certainly a practitioner could use standard treatments for noncompliance if this problem were to arise, but it is probably more judicious simply to add a positive reinforcement program for compliance to complement the negative reinforcement and punishment features of treatment.

Notice that extinction procedures specific to enuresis have not been researched and probably have received little attention because enuresis is not considered to be a problem maintained by the attention the behavior receives. Nevertheless, minimizing parental reactions to noncompliance and bed-wetting accidents can reduce the probability of adventitious reinforcement of related behaviors, such as resistance to treatment procedures. Finally, positive practice and cleanliness training components are often cited in the literature because they have been included as a part of enuresis treatment packages. These are also most accurately described as punishment procedures, and their independent effects are unknown. This is not to suggest that these strategies should not be used; a balance of strategies from the various conceptual domains can be valuable. In this particular case, a cleanliness training component was included. Note again that an understanding of the behavioral principles involved in the intervention components allows the practitioner to plan for adding reinforcement into the program to help facilitate child compliance with procedures as well as parental adherence. Adding reinforcement to the program may also help reduce any negative side effects that arise from use of punishment procedures.

Teaching these strategies to parents will require not only good behavioral skills training but also creativity. The practitioner will not be able to observe bed-wetting in clinic. For this reason, one may need to pay particular attention to teaching parents to monitor dry and wet nights, as well as to specific times when accidents are likely to occur and even the amount of urine released (e.g., measure the size of the urine spot to see if the child is awaking earlier or releasing less urine as the alarm sounds). Modeling and role-playing will not be a central aspect of treatment in the clinic, but a walk-through of each of the intervention steps can be important to help ensure that the parents and child understand each of the steps involved in the intervention and their roles, particularly in regard to first awakening (i.e., Will child be expected to awake independently, or will parents assist with wakening child?) and follow-up cleaning (i.e., Where are extra sheets kept, where will wet sheets be placed, and who will make up the bed?). In addition, it may be helpful for the parents and child to walk through the steps at home so that they all know what their roles in the intervention will be.

Feeding Problems

Problems with feeding may include restrictive food preferences (e.g., "picky eaters"), overeating, spitting up, rumination, chronic food refusal, or pica. Prevalence estimates for feeding problems range from 20% to more than 60% for children under 12 years of age (Budd, Chugh, & Berry, 1998). Poor eating habits may lead to developmental and physical concerns, such as failure to thrive. Educational concerns may also co-occur. For example, children who regularly eat breakfast tend to perform better academically in the classroom (Mahoney, Taylor, Kanarek, & Samuel, 2005; Wesnes, Pincock, Richardson, Helm, & Hails, 2003). Eating problems, such as overeating, may lead to socialization problems, particularly teasing by peers or lack of opportunity for active play participation because of the physical limitations of obesity. In childhood, parents are often the primary source of food and can assist with establishing and maintaining appropriate eating patterns. Parent training is typically a component of effective treatment for childhood feeding problems (Linscheid, 1998; M. M. Mueller et al., 2003).

A common feeding problem in childhood is picky eating. Picky eating in young children typically involves intake of a limited variety of food. The child will only eat certain foods, and this may be detrimental to his or her physical health. Foods the child will eat are often referred to as *high preferred foods* and those he or she will not eat as *low* or *nonpreferred foods*. Here the research provides important information about how to reinforce a child's intake of nonpreferred food. Generally, there is some research support for interventions that intersperse high preferred with low preferred food as a means to reinforce eating the latter (Piazza et al., 2002). In addition, food intake may be limited between meals to increase hunger, creating an establishing operation that increases the reinforcing value of all food, even low or nonpreferred foods.

In Table 7.4, parent training procedures culled from intervention research to address picky eating are presented. In this particular case, a single mother brought in her 3-year-old daughter, Madeline, who was refusing to eat much of what was presented to her. Madeline was the youngest of four children. No concerns with the other children's eating habits were noted. Madeline would only eat jelly sandwiches and potato chips. She drank juice but refused milk and water. She would eat snacks throughout the day when provided, typically consisting of cakes or other sugary foods. She would eat applesauce and yogurt on occasion. No medical or developmental concerns were noted. Her pediatrician reported that she was growing adequately.

In this example, particular attention to how to teach parents to implement the intervention is needed because providing preferred food and social attention or reward contingent on eating low or nonpreferred food can be difficult to master. The practitioner should consider which decisions par-

TABLE 7.4
Parent Training for Picky Eating

What to teach	Why it works	How to teach: parent training
Teach parents to identify preferred foods and nonpreferred foods. Teach parents to monitor food intake with a food diary. Teach parents to intersperse high preferred food with low preferred food.	Reinforcement: Interspersing high preferred foods increases the rate of eating less preferred foods.	Instruction: Describe and provide rationale for identifying high and low preferred foods and monitoring food intake. Describe and provide for using interspersal, social attention, and rewards.
Teach parents to provide social attention contingent on compliant behavior and food intake. Teach parents to provide reward contingent on food intake.	Social attention and reward also increase the likelihood of nonpreferred food intake.	Modeling: Demonstrate how to intersperse food and provide contingent social attention and reward with the child or parent. Rehearsal: Have parents practice with the child during role-play or actual meal. Feedback: Shape parents' skills in the feeding intervention.
Teach parents to ignore minor misbehavior during mealtime. Teach parents to delay delivery of preferred food in response to minor misbehavior.	Extinction: Removal of reinforcement (both social and food) reduces the probability of the behavior recurring. May also briefly increase problem behavior via an extinction burst.	Instruction: Describe and provide rationale for ignoring minor misbehavior as part of differential attention. Predict possible temporary increase in misbehavior. Modeling: Demonstrate use of ignoring during role-play or actual mealtime. Rehearsal: Have parent practice ignoring with child during practice of mealtime in session. Feedback: Shape effective use of ignoring and differential attention during meals.
Teach parents to limit or eliminate food and drink between mealtimes.	Stimulus control: Decreasing access increases the reinforcing value of even nonpreferred food (i.e., establishing operation).	Instruction: Describe and provide rationale for reducing other food intake and for giving effective commands and clear expectations. (*continues*)

TABLE 7.4
Parent Training for Picky Eating *(Continued)*

What to teach	Why it works	How to teach: parent training
Teach parents how to provide direct, one-step, developmentally appropriate commands and expectations during meals.	Clear commands are discriminative for compliance.	Modeling: Demonstrate with parent or child how to give effective commands and set clear expectations. Rehearsal: Have parent practice how to give effective commands during role-play or mealtime with the practitioner or child. Feedback: Shape parents' use of effective commands.
Teach parents how to apply time-out contingent on food refusal or other noncompliance or target misbehavior.	Punishment: Removal from reinforcing environment (food and praise available) to less reinforcing environment decreases food refusal and other problem behavior.	Instruction: Provide description and rationale for using time-out. Provide step-by-step protocol or procedure. Modeling: Model with child how to implement time-out. Rehearsal: Have parent practice time-out in the clinic during role-play or actual meal with the child. Feedback: Shape parent's effective implementation of time-out.

ents need to make as part of mealtime feeding and how this decision making will be taught. For example, some of the decisions that need to be made include determining the ratio of high preferred to low preferred food, how quickly food should be presented, what amounts of food will be provided, and how other rewards will be used. Thus, modeling by the clinician, rehearsal by the parent, and immediate feedback by the practitioner are particularly important in making these types of decisions and helping teach parents to make these decisions outside the clinic setting. Modeling, rehearsal, and feedback will be more effective if parent training can take place during a typical mealtime, with parents bringing preferred and nonpreferred foods to the session. The practitioner also needs to prepare a place for the rehearsal meal to take place.

Behavioral Problems in the Classroom

At least 50% of children seen for noncompliance and oppositional behavior problems in clinical settings also demonstrate school-related problems (McMahon & Forehand, 2003; Webster-Stratton & Reid, 2003). Some previous research has demonstrated generalization of positive child outcomes to school settings following parent training for noncompliance, particularly PCIT (Funderburk et al., 1998), whereas other research has demonstrated that improvement in compliance at home following parent training does not necessarily generalize to improvement in behavior in the classroom (Wahler, Vigilante, & Strand, 2004). As with other common child behavior problems, treating noncompliance at home may be necessary to address behavior problems in the school setting, but it is often not sufficient.

Including parents in the treatment of children with school-related problems has been a component of clinical service delivery since 1896, when Lightner Witmer started the first psychology clinic in the United States (Levine & Levine, 1992). Working with parents to address school-related issues is important because providing services directly in the school setting is difficult for many practitioners who work in clinical or other community settings. Practitioners in clinical settings may not be reimbursed for school-based services and may find the time and travel commitments to be fiscally inefficient.

In school settings, parent involvement has been a recognized feature of children's success in school for years (Christenson & Sheridan, 2001). It is only recently, however, that models have been developed to describe how practitioners may include parents in collaborative consultation with teachers to address school-related concerns (Sheridan, 1997; Sheridan, Kratochwill, & Bergan, 1996). Effectively including parents in collaborative consultation with teachers and intervention with children requires parent training.

Early in the history of behavioral parent training, parents were trained to implement home–school note interventions in collaboration with teachers (Patterson, Reid, Jones, & Conger, 1975). Subsequent research on this form of intervention has found them effective for improving children's behavior in the classroom (Kelley, 1990; McCain & Kelley, 1994). An example of parent training to implement a home–school note that is based on this research is presented in Table 7.5.

In this example, a 10-year-old boy, Roger, was brought to an outpatient psychology clinic by his mother. She reported that he was exhibiting difficulty at school with following directions, completing work, and poor peer interactions. He frequently pushed or touched peers in class and grabbed at their school materials. Roger's mother reported that she had some difficulty with noncompliant and impulsive behavior at home but believed that she was effectively managing this. His behavior at school was contributing to failing

TABLE 7.5
Parent Training to Implement a Home–School Note

What to teach	Why it works	How to teach: parent training
Teach parents to introduce the home–school note procedure to the teacher and collaborate to identify target behaviors. Teach parents to work with the teacher to set criteria for child to earn a reward at home. Teach parents to instruct the teacher in how to provide praise for target behaviors and mark the note accordingly. Teach parents to develop a reward list with the child. Teach parents to provide social attention and a reward to child contingent on positive marks on the home–school note.	Reinforcement: Social attention from the teacher increases the probability of target behavior occurring in school environment. Social attention and rewards from parents increase the probability of the target behavior occurring in school environment.	Instruction: Describe and provide rationale for using social attention and reward for targeted school behavior. Emphasize the critical role of collaboration with the teacher. Modeling: Demonstrate parent–teacher collaboration skills. Also demonstrate how to provide social attention and reward based on home–school note. Rehearsal: The parent practices teacher collaboration skills with the practitioner. Homework will be to discuss the home–school note procedure with teacher. Feedback: Provide positive and corrective feedback during rehearsal to shape parents' reward and collaboration skills.
Teach parents to collaborate with the teacher to minimize verbal responses when child does not earn a positive mark on the note. Teach parents to ignore or eliminate reprimands and lectures for target behaviors on the note for which child did not receive a positive mark. Teach parents to ignore misbehavior that may occur in response to not achieving criteria for reward or if child receives punishment.	Extinction: Reduction of teacher attention for negative child behavior may reduce child misbehavior. Reducing attention and ignoring child misbehavior when reviewing the note or if child resists punishment will decrease child misbehavior. Note in school and home the possibility of increased child misbehavior due to an extinction burst.	Instruction: Describe and provide rationale for ignoring behaviors not marked positively on the note, particularly in relation to use of social attention for compliance (i.e., differential social attention). Also provide instruction to the parent about how to work with the teacher to reduce attention to negative child behavior. Modeling: Demonstrate use of ignoring with parent or child when reviewing a home–school note. Model how to present ignoring to the teacher. Rehearsal: Have the parent practice ignoring with the child during in-session role-play. Have parent role-play a meeting and discussion with the teacher about ignoring.

TABLE 7.5
Parent Training to Implement a Home–School Note

What to teach	Why it works	How to teach: parent training
Teach parents to work with the teacher to have the note posted at the child's desk or work area. Teach parents to provide clear commands and expectations regarding behavior and consequences.	Stimulus control: The note on the desk signals (i.e., reminds) the child of availability of reinforcement. Parent commands and expectations are discriminative for compliance with note procedures.	Feedback: Shape effective ignoring skills and teacher collaboration skills. Instruction: Describe and provide rationale for giving effective commands and posting the note at the child's desk. Modeling: Demonstrate with the parent or child how to give effective commands relative to home–school note procedures. Model collaboration skills for the parent to use with the teacher. Rehearsal: Have the parent practice how to give effective commands relative to home–school note procedures with the practitioner or child. Have parent practice teacher collaboration skills regarding posting note. Feedback: Shape the parent's use of effective commands and continued collaboration with the teacher.
Teach parents how to apply *grounding* (i.e., short-term loss of all privileges for the evening) or loss of specific privileges for failure to meet criteria.	Punishment: Loss of access to preferred activities reduces the probability of behaviors that result in unearned marks.	Instruction: Provide description and rationale for using short-term grounding or loss of privileges. Provide a step-by-step protocol or procedure. Modeling: Model with the child how to implement grounding. Rehearsal: Have parent role-play grounding with the child or practitioner in the clinic. Feedback: Shape effective implementation of the grounding procedure.

grades, and an evaluation for eligibility for special education services and perhaps a self-contained classroom was being considered. Completed work and other school assessments suggested that Roger had the ability to complete the academic work.

When conducting parent training to address school behavior problems, parents are taught not only specifics about implementing the program at home but also specific skills for how to communicate and collaborate with a child's teacher. Skills for collaborating with teachers are not typically found in the research literature on home–school notes, and practitioners need to rely on other research literature regarding effective collaboration (e.g., Sheridan, 1997) to train parents effectively. These skills are important because the critical component of the program that the parent delivers at home is dependent on information provided by notes from the classroom teacher. If the teacher does not agree with the target behaviors or complete the note accurately or on a frequent basis, the consequences the parent delivers may be less effective.

Academic Problems

In addition to behavior problems that may occur in the classroom, children may also demonstrate academic performance problems. This fact was recognized early in the parent training literature, and Patterson and colleagues described a program designed to teach parents to act as reading tutors (Patterson et al., 1975). More recently, additional examples of teaching parents to address academic skills have been published (Erion, 2006; Resetar, Noell, & Pellegrin, 2006; Valleley, Begeney, & Shriver, 2005). Although academic problems may seem to constitute a different type of child problem compared with behavior problems, parents can be trained to implement academic interventions. In the example provided in Table 7.6, research on using a repeated-reading strategy to improve reading fluency is integrated with knowledge about effective parent training to develop a procedure to address reading fluency problems.

Kimberly was an 8-year-old girl in second grade brought to a school psychologist by her father because of concerns with reading. She was receiving extra assistance at school for reading difficulties but had not been identified as eligible for special education services. According to her father, she did not appear to be making progress with reading. Her father indicated that there were no other behavioral, social, medical, emotional, or developmental concerns. Information about family structure, dynamics, and daily routine was gathered. No other family concerns were noted other than a history of reading problems on the father's side of the family. Kimberly's father worked with her daily on reading, but she was resistant to reading with her father, and he did not know what to do to improve her ability or to encourage her to be pos-

TABLE 7.6

Parent Training to Improve Reading Fluency

What to teach	Why it works	How to teach: parent training
Teach parents to provide social attention and reward contingent on participation in the repeated-reading intervention. Teach parents to provide performance feedback and help the child graph progress. Teach parents to provide social attention and reward contingent on child's attainment of reading fluency goals.	Reinforcement: Attention, data on fluency, and rewards all help increase the rate of participation in the repeated-reading procedure and also possibly fluency.	Instruction: Describe and provide rationale for use of social attention, performance feedback, and reward during reading. Provide instruction in counting words correct per minute and number of errors. Modeling: Demonstrate with the child or parent how to provide social attention, performance feedback, and reward. Rehearsal: Have parents practice providing social attention, performance feedback, and reward with the child. Feedback: Provide positive and corrective feedback during rehearsal to shape parents' skills in the use of reward and social attention during reading intervention and performance feedback.
Teach parents to ignore minor misbehavior that may occur during reading activity.	Extinction: Misbehavior typically allows the child to avoid or escape reading. Ignoring decreases the probability of this because escape is no longer available.	Instruction: Describe and provide rationale for ignoring in context of differential attention. Modeling: Demonstrate the use of ignoring during a reading activity with child. Rehearsal: Have the parent practice ignoring with the child during a reading activity. Feedback: Shape effective use of parental ignoring during a reading activity.
Teach parents to implement the repeated-reading procedure with child.	Stimulus control: Repeated reading of the same material plus reinforcement brings fluent reading behavior under control of letters and words.	Instruction: Describe and provide rationale for the repeated-reading intervention. Modeling: Demonstrate with the parent or child how to implement the repeated-reading intervention. *(continues)*

TABLE 7.6

Parent Training to Improve Reading Fluency   *(Continued)*

What to teach	Why it works	How to teach: parent training
Teach parents how to graph and post the child's reading performance.	Public posting of the graph provides a reminder that reinforcement is available for fluent reading.	Rehearsal: Have the parent practice the repeated-reading intervention with the child. Feedback: Shape accurate implementation of the repeated-reading intervention.
If errors are problematic during reading, parents may be taught to point out the error, model the correct form, and have the child accurately repeat the word or sentence three times. Parent may also be taught to chart errors.	Punishment: Error identification and repeating the word correctly decreases the probability of errors recurring.	Instruction: Describe and provide rationale for the error correction procedure to the parent and child and provide rationale. Modeling: Model the procedure with the child. Rehearsal: The parent practices error correction with the child during training. Feedback: Shape effective implementation of the procedure.

itively and actively involved in reading activities at home. Assessment of Kimberly's reading indicated that her primary difficulty was reading fluency.

As an intervention for reading fluency, repeated reading has been demonstrated to be effective for enhancing reading skills in general education students, as well as those with disabilities (e.g., Blum & Koskinen, 1991). Much like compliance training in which a parent requires a child to practice following commands (e.g., parent-directed interactions; Hembree-Kigin & McNeil, 1995), in repeated reading, a parent requires a child to practice reading a short passage two to three times. The child receives immediate reinforcement in the form of improved reading fluency with each repetition, as well as attention from the parent and rewards for participation or increased fluency.

This intervention requires changes in how parents may typically read with their child. When training parents to implement this intervention, special attention may be needed to provide a clear rationale about why to implement this type of reading strategy. Written protocols may be helpful for parents to improve treatment adherence at home. Modeling and feedback by the practitioner and rehearsal by the parent with the child in the presence of the practitioner may also assist in improving treatment adherence at home. Note also that the practitioner should give careful consideration to how the steps in the program are presented. Stimulus control is a particularly important behavioral principle of repeated reading to improve reading fluency. When examining what to teach and how to teach, the steps associated with how to teach that correspond to stimulus control may be most important to present first, followed by reinforcement, punishment, and extinction.

Problems Common in Adolescence

Children, typically considered to be individuals from ages 2 to 10, have traditionally been the focus of parent training programs. This is true for the empirically supported parent training programs reviewed earlier in this book, as well as for other examples of research-based parent training strategies to address other types of child problems (e.g., Briesmeister & Schaefer, 1998). This age range is most frequently targeted for parent training approaches to treatment delivery because it is typically at younger ages that parents have the most control over environmental contingencies that may affect child behavior. As children mature into adolescence, they begin to have more contact with influences over which parents have little control. These influences come from peers, coaches, employers, teachers, and sometimes from a youth's increased interest in self-directed or high-risk behaviors.

If parents establish instructional control (i.e., the child is compliant to parental instruction) and positive parent–child relationships early in childhood, the transition to adolescence and adulthood has a greater likelihood of a positive outcome. Sometimes, however, even a child who is relatively well adjusted in childhood will experience behavioral, social, and emotional difficulties through adolescence. More likely, however, is that a young child who is not under instructional control, is oppositional, and who grows up with coercive parent–child interaction will have an adolescence fraught with difficulties. Negative peer interactions, depression, sexual activity, drug and alcohol experimentation and use, motivation, and conduct problems are all examples of adolescent issues parents may have to address.

The literature on parent training for adolescent problems is limited relative to parent training for childhood noncompliance and other childhood problems. This area of parent training is in clear need of additional research. However, there are examples of applying parent training to address problems common in adolescence. For example, a two-part, parent-oriented series was published by Patterson and Forgatch (1987, 2005; Forgatch & Patterson, 1987, 2005). These books are meant to be read by parents, but practitioners may use them with parents in individual or group parent training contexts. However, there are no empirically supported or research-based protocols or manuals for doing so.

Part 1 (Patterson & Forgatch, 1987, 2005) essentially follows the process of parent training outlined in Patterson's (1976) earlier work with young children (see *Living With Children*, chap. 2, this volume). These first basic steps include developing an understanding of parent–adolescent interaction and the parents' role in establishing contingencies that support positive adolescent compliance and socialization. Parents are provided information on developing clear rules, expectations, and commands; monitoring adolescent behavior specific to rules and expectations; and reinforcing desired behavior using parental attention and reward systems, including point charts and reward menus. Parents are also provided information on implementing punishing consequences such as brief work chores, longer work chores, removing privileges, response cost techniques such as monetary fines, and adaptation of time-out for adolescents or sending them to their room. Homework assignments are provided at the end of each chapter. Case examples appear throughout the text to illustrate implementation of procedures and the difficulties in working with adolescents.

Part 2 of this series (Forgatch & Patterson, 1987, 2005) focuses on teaching parents how to communicate and problem solve effectively with their adolescent. The indirect benefit of this approach may be that the adolescent also learns to communicate and problem solve situations so that positive outcomes occur. Information is provided regarding effective communication, particularly listening skills, as is information on establishing family forums for problem solving, brainstorming solutions, evaluating solutions, and addressing specific topics related to sexual activity, drugs and alcohol, and school problems. Similar to Part 1 of the series, homework assignments are recommended at the end of each chapter so that parents are actively implementing and monitoring both their own and the adolescent's behavior. The authors of these two books highly recommend that parents read and implement the techniques written in Part 1 before attempting those in Part 2.

A practitioner can work with parents to facilitate implementation of the strategies outlined in both books and to answer questions, monitor treatment integrity, and assist parents with making adjustments to the strategies as needed to fit their unique family situation or adolescent problem. Making decisions about how to proceed with parent training to address an adolescent concern may be facilitated by using the organizing framework for research and parent training. In the example that follows (see also Table 7.7), information from these books and research on contingency contracting is integrated to train parents to intervene with an adolescent who is breaking curfew.

A mother and father brought their 16-year-old son, Julio, to an outpatient psychology clinic. Julio was frequently out late at night, throughout the week and on weekends, in violation of his parents' rule that he be at home by 10 p.m. on weeknights and 12 p.m. on weekends (i.e., Friday and Saturday). Julio was described as generally compliant at home and school. His friends were described as "good kids," and there was minimal concern that Julio and his friends were engaged in drugs or alcohol or other illegal activities. Julio believed that he had "earned" the right to be out as

TABLE 7.7
Parent Training for Adolescent Breaking Curfew

What to teach	Why it works	How to teach: parent training
Teach parents how to negotiate a reward list with the adolescent. Teach parents how to negotiate a curfew rule with the adolescent. Teach parents how to develop a behavior contract with the adolescent. Teach parents how to monitor adolescent behavior and curfew compliance.	Reinforcement: Reward increases the probability of compliance with curfew.	Instruction: Describe and provide rationale for negotiating with the adolescent and providing a reward for curfew compliance. Provide instruction for how and when rewards will be provided. Modeling: Role-play with parent how to negotiate the curfew and reward list with adolescent. Rehearsal: Have parents practice with adolescent curfew rule and reward list negotiation. For homework, have parents negotiate rules and rewards at home. Feedback: Provide positive and corrective feedback during rehearsal with the parent and adolescent.
Teach parents to ignore minor misbehavior and eliminate reprimands and lectures contingent on curfew rule violation.	Extinction: Ignoring decreases probability of misbehavior because avoidance of consequences is not available. Parent attention is also not available.	Instruction: Describe and provide rationale for ignoring minor misbehavior in context of differential attention. Also, verbal mediation may reinforce avoidance of punishment, and attention may reinforce complaining. Modeling: Model use of ignoring during role-play with the parent, with the practitioner or parent acting as the adolescent. Rehearsal: Have parent practice ignoring and negotiation with the adolescent during session. As part of homework, have parents practice ignoring during negotiation at home. Feedback: Shape ignoring skills during practices in session. Practitioners may wish to target non-emotional negotiation skills in particular.

(continues)

TABLE 7.7
Parent Training for Adolescent Breaking Curfew *(Continued)*

What to teach	Why it works	How to teach: parent training
Teach parents how to provide direct commands and a clear rule regarding curfew. Post the curfew rule or behavior contract.	Stimulus control: A clearly defined parent command or rule that signals reinforcement is available for compliance. Posting the contract provides a reminder that reinforcement is available for following the rule.	Instruction: Describe and provide rationale for developing a clear rule or expectations, as well as for posting the contract. Modeling: Demonstrate with the parent how to develop a clear curfew rule and give commands regarding consequences for follow-through or violation of curfew. Rehearsal: Have the parent practice providing expectations and commands regarding consequences for follow-through or violation of the rule with the practitioner or adolescent. Feedback: Shape parents' effective use of commands and house rules.
Teach parents how to implement a response cost procedure (e.g., loss of "night out" privilege) contingent on curfew violation. The parent may also need to implement a job-card grounding procedure contingent on more serious infractions of the curfew rule.	Punishment: The loss of privilege or the application of an aversive stimulus (i.e., job) decreases the probability of curfew violation recurring.	Instruction: Describe and provide rationale for using the punishment procedures. Provide step-by-step protocol. Emphasize follow-through. Modeling: Model with parent or adolescent how to implement the procedure. The practitioner or parent may act as the adolescent. Rehearsal: Have the parent practice or role-play the response cost procedure with the adolescent or practitioner in the clinic. Feedback: Shape the parent's use of the response cost or job-card procedure.

late as he wanted because of his history and his parents' general level of trust. His parents were concerned with the risks involved with being out later. The curfew violations were leading to frequent arguments and were beginning to affect other aspects of the parent–adolescent relationship because negative emotional responding was occurring in other previously neutral or positive interactions. Julio was generally silent during sessions and kept his eyes downcast. He would interrupt to correct or dispute his parents' reports of events.

In Table 7.7, note that the process of parent training to address problems in adolescence is essentially the same as that for problems in childhood. One important difference, however, is that there is a greater emphasis on communication and negotiation strategies with adolescents than is found in the literature on childhood problems. Similar to teaching parents to collaborate with teachers when addressing school-related behavior problems, practitioners should consider the literature that provides information on effective communication and negotiation with adolescents (e.g., McIntire & McIntire, 1991).

SUMMARY

The empirical support for parent training to address child noncompliance is substantial, but similar levels of research support are not available to address other child problems. Practitioners can, however, train parents to intervene with other types of child problems. What practitioners must do is review the best available research evidence and integrate this with their expertise regarding the foundational components of effective parent training. That expertise comes from knowledge about why behavior change procedures work and how to teach them effectively. It also comes from knowledge of common behavioral change strategies revealed through examination of the empirically supported parent training programs for child noncompliance. These parent training programs support application of a behavioral skills training model to train parents and of behavioral principles to help identify what to teach parents and why interventions work. These components can be used to create a common organizing framework for parent training. This organizing framework is a tool that practitioners can use to review and apply research in the development of parent training procedures whenever they are presented with a child problem beyond noncompliance.

Although the organizing framework for research and parent training presented in this chapter can help translate research into practice, this is but one, albeit crucial, step in the process. There are still other considerations to which the practitioner must attend. In the next chapter, we discuss additional considerations in translating research into practice and describe all of the steps of a comprehensive approach to evidence-based practice in parent training.

8

DELIVERING EVIDENCE-BASED PARENT TRAINING: FROM RESEARCH TO PRACTICE

The organizing framework found in chapter 7 was offered as a tool to help organize research findings and develop parent training protocols for children presenting with problems beyond noncompliance. This chapter extends the discussion about translating research into practice. In particular, we present issues specific to examining the match between research and practice, which will assist practitioners in making decisions regarding whether and how to adapt interventions to meet the unique needs of children and families. Following this discussion, we present a comprehensive series of steps that compose an evidence-based approach to delivering parent training.

EXAMINING THE MATCH BETWEEN RESEARCH AND PRACTICE

When examining the match between research and practice, it is important to know whether the research was designed to evaluate the efficacy or the effectiveness of the intervention. *Efficacy* refers to research examining whether an intervention works under ideal or laboratory conditions (Kratochwill & Shernoff, 2004). If an intervention is not useful under ideal conditions, it is typically deemed unnecessary to evaluate it under less than ideal or real-world conditions. In the area of parent training, efficacy studies largely compose the foundation for the empirically supported programs.

In contrast, studies that examine whether particular interventions work in actual practice conditions are termed *effectiveness studies* (Kratochwill & Shernoff, 2004). Effectiveness research seeks to evaluate whether an intervention shown to result in positive outcomes in an efficacy study under laboratory conditions will produce positive outcomes in actual practice (Shriver & Watson, 2005). Effectiveness studies are particularly important to the translation of research into practice because they are conducted to demonstrate whether an intervention that works under research conditions also works under practice conditions (Ringeisen, Henderson, & Hoagwood, 2003; Shriver & Watson, 2005). This type of research is important for practitioners because interventions that appear useful under the relatively ideal conditions of controlled research may not be effective under the less than ideal and uncontrolled conditions in which many practitioners work (Weisz, Weiss, & Donenberg, 1992).

Many have called for more attention to and support for conducting effectiveness studies to provide a firmer empirical foundation for evidence-based practice (Kratochwill & Shernoff, 2004; Messer, 2004; Ringeisen et al., 2003; Wampold & Bhati, 2004). Unfortunately, there are barriers to conducting and disseminating effectiveness studies that must be overcome (Shriver & Watson, 2005). In the meantime, it is incumbent on practitioners to consider how the research conditions found in efficacy studies actually match the practice conditions under which the treatment will be implemented (Kazdin, 2004).

Typically in research examining the efficacy of an intervention, many variables are controlled, including characteristics of the sample population, resources available in the setting in which treatment is taking place, and the clinical skills of the practitioner administering the intervention being evaluated. The subject sample is carefully controlled by recruitment procedures that often include specific exclusion criteria. The setting is controlled by ensuring that there are adequate resources and time available to implement the intervention with integrity. The clinical skills of the practitioner are controlled by requiring implementation of specific procedural steps often described in manual form, as well as extensive training of the practitioner in the procedures and frequent supervision and feedback to the practitioner administering the intervention procedures.

Control over these client, setting, and practitioner variables helps provide confidence that it was the treatment that led to positive outcomes for a particular sample of children and not some other undefined variable related to the sample of children, aspects of the setting, or practitioner characteristics. In the real world, however, the population receiving treatment, the setting characteristics, or the provider skills are not controlled but are often determined by a unique history of events. These three variables have substantial effect on the outcomes of any intervention (Messer, 2004; Schoenwald & Hoagwood, 2001; Wampold & Bhati, 2004).

Practitioner Characteristics

Much of the discussion to this point has focused on the quality of research, but evidence-based practice involves integration of the best available research evidence *with clinical expertise*. The quality of a practitioner's training, experience, and expertise plays an important role in evidence-based practice. Practitioners should consider the level of training and experience needed to implement an intervention in parent training successfully relative to their own training and level of expertise (McCabe, 2004). Efficacy studies often provide their practitioners with explicit training in the parent training procedures, including frequent supervision in the application of the treatment protocol. When translating those procedures or interventions into practice, practitioners must consider whether the procedures and interventions have been demonstrated to work when implemented by practitioners in settings where that same level of training and supervision may not be available. A study with this type of demonstration would be considered an effectiveness study (e.g., Irvine, Biglan, Smolkowski, Metzler, & Ary, 1999). To the extent possible, the practitioner should examine the research to determine the level of training and supervision required to implement a specific intervention effectively. Often this information is not readily available for efficacy studies in which the focus is on the concise presentation of treatment procedures, not on practice implementation issues. Review of the manuals of the empirically supported parent training programs for noncompliance may provide guidance for practitioners in determining whether they have the skills to implement the parent training procedures.

A practitioner's clinical skills and expertise are largely determined by training and experience. Training includes formal graduate training such as coursework and practica. Training may also include in-service workshops, participation in professional conferences, and maintaining a mentoring relationship with a senior practitioner for consultation, collaboration, or supervision purposes. Experience also heavily influences practice. All practitioners learn from direct experience with children and families, with colleagues both within and outside of the discipline, and with both successes and mistakes.

Our training and experiences make each of us unique in how we interact with clients and implement interventions. It is the responsibility of practitioners to recognize the limits of their knowledge and skill base when working with children and families and to refrain from offering services that they are not trained to provide. This is an ethical issue, in addition to an evidence-based practice issue (see the American Psychological Association's, 2002, "Ethical Principles of Psychologists and Code of Conduct," Standard 2.01, Boundaries of Competence; http://www.apa.org/ethics/code2002.html). Reading books or manuals can be important aspects of developing expertise about parent training. Likewise, reviewing the research literature is a necessary aspect of providing evidence-based parent training. However, knowledge alone is not sufficient. There are also specific skills in clinical decision making, conducting observations of child and parent interaction, interviewing, data collection, and other areas of clinical practice that require supervised training and experience. If practitioners believe that their skills do not match with those necessary to conduct parent training, they should seek to identify training or supervision opportunities before implementing behavioral parent training in practice or refer to another practitioner with the necessary expertise.

On a more personal level, it is important that practitioners consider the type of skill repertoire required in behavioral parent training and whether this skill set is a good match for their unique personality characteristics and interaction style with children and adults. For example, an effective practitioner must frequently model parenting skills and techniques. The practitioner must be comfortable with the notion that the child and parent may not respond as expected during rehearsal or implementation of the intervention, requiring some impromptu flexibility in modeling and rehearsal strategies, as well as in instruction, rationale, and provision of feedback.

Effective behavioral skills training also often requires that a practitioner be relatively direct, assuming some semblance of an expert role, during parent training. The practitioner is asked to model actively during training sessions and to role-play with the child and parent rather than just sit and talk. In addition, there are collaborative aspects to parent training in terms of working with parents to problem solve difficulties or barriers to implementing interventions. Practitioners need to consider whether their personality and interaction style with clients matches this approach to the delivery of services for children. If not, the practitioner should develop these skills, work around this issue, or reconsider whether parent training is the right match for service delivery.

Setting of Research and Practice

Efficacy research on parent training has taken place largely in university-affiliated clinical settings. Practitioners, however, will typically work in outpatient clinics, primary care settings, school settings, inpatient units, and community agencies that may have limited resources, space, and personnel. These practical realities may constrain how parent training is delivered and the subsequent effectiveness of parent training. Practitioners must examine the degree to which their respective settings match that in which the research took place. This is true whether the practitioner is reading efficacy or effectiveness research. It is expected, however, that effectiveness research would provide more description or discussion about possible influences of setting variables on treatment effectiveness.

In efficacy research, resources can typically be bought or accessed through research grant funds that allow for advantages not available in many practice settings. These advantages may include equipment such as one-way mirrors, bug-in-ear receivers, or video cameras for monitoring, training, and supervision. These advantages may also include extra personnel for providing supervision of practitioners, conducting phone calls to clients, or making home visits. Finally, even the perceived expertise of university faculty by clients may influence adherence to treatment recommendations. Parent training implemented under these conditions may be more likely to be successful compared with training implemented without such characteristics.

In addition, efficacy studies may include more contact time with subjects than is typically available in practice settings. For example, some empirically supported parent training programs have included as many as twenty 2-hour sessions with parents (e.g., Boggs et al., 2004). Some programs recommend home visits, frequent phone contact, or both. Yet many managed care insurance policies will not approve this amount of service. In addition, there is often insufficient time available in a practitioner's typical day to conduct follow-up phone calls with each client, let alone conduct home visits. This does not mean that there should not be more time allowed or that phone calls and home visits are not important, only that the day-to-day contingencies of actual practice may not support these types of services. Similarly, in a school setting, a practitioner may not have the time available to spend with individual families in a relatively intensive treatment protocol such as those described in the empirically supported parent training programs. Instead, the school psychologist may best be able to implement parent training in a group format that serves a larger number of parents and children in the same relative time frame as individual treatment. However, the only empirically supported parent training program that is group-based (The Incredible Years; Webster-Stratton, 1992; see also chap. 2, this volume) may be relatively expensive for many school districts.

Being aware of the differences and similarities of the practice setting relative to the setting in which research was conducted allows one to determine a level of confidence that a parent training program can be delivered with integrity. The extent to which the integrity of parent training is compromised by lack of time or resources means there will be less confidence that beneficial outcomes comparable to that found in the research will be attained. A poor match does not necessarily mean that parent training should not be implemented in a particular setting, but it does mean the practitioner will need to be cognizant of the variables that will affect the procedure's integrity and effectiveness. Subsequently there may be an increased need to monitor child and parent outcomes more closely to ensure that there is benefit for the child and family.

Client Characteristics

One particular challenge of evidence-based practice is adapting research to match the unique needs of the child and family. Practitioners must typically work with whoever presents to them and with the problems presented, assuming these are within the practitioner's scope of practice. In research, however, children and families are carefully screened to match the criteria for that parent training program. The result is a restricted problem sample and a restricted population sample. Translating research into practice requires consideration of the types of problems and populations served in the research protocol compared with those commonly seen in practice, in which identifying the unique needs of a child and family requires evaluation. Once obtained, information about the child and family can be compared with information about the participants included in research studies to determine the degree to which they match. This leads directly to the level of confidence the practitioner can have in attaining outcomes similar to those found in the research.

Restricted Problem Sample

When conducting efficacy research, it is common to restrict the sample of problems that are being addressed. The empirically supported parent training programs have the bulk of their research addressing oppositional behavior, noncompliance, and other forms of antisocial behavior, particularly in young children. Children with other problems are typically screened out of research protocols. Therefore, those who may have developmental delays or mental retardation, specific learning disabilities, autism spectrum disorder, anxiety, depression, obsessive–compulsive disorder, chronic illness, or other types of psychological, medical, or genetic problems may not be included in outcome studies evaluating the efficacy of parent training.

In actual practice, however, it is common for children to present with more than one type of problem. A child presenting with oppositional behavior may also have developmental delays, learning disabilities, an anxiety disorder, or medical adherence concerns. These comorbid problems must also be attended to when conducting parent training in practice but are rarely considered in research. For example, a child with autism who is also noncompliant may not find social attention to be reinforcing and may, in fact, find it aversive. As a result, the child may experience a timeout procedure as reinforcing because he or she escapes aversive social attention. In another example, consider a child who presents with both social anxiety and noncompliance. The parent may be more concerned about the social anxiety, but noncompliance may interfere with treatment adherence. Likewise, perhaps the social anxiety is contributing to the child's noncompliance. The practitioner would need to work with the parent to decide collaboratively where to start with treatment of each problem. Future research on the effectiveness of parent training to address comorbid child problems is needed. In the meantime, practitioners need to use their clinical expertise to implement empirically supported and evidence-based interventions to address multiple child problems (Chorpita, 2003; Kazdin, 2004).

Restricted Population Sample

In addition to a restricted problem sample, much of the research in parent training, as well as other psychological and medical research, is based on a restricted population sample and thus may not be representative of the children and families that practitioners in a school or community agency or clinic serve. Many research samples are overrepresentative of Caucasian, middle-income mothers (Tiano & McNeil, 2006). However, many of the families most in need of services are minority and low socioeconomic status; often they are from single-parent or other nontraditional situations, such as foster care or cases in which extended family members are the primary caregivers. The characteristics of the population served will affect how practitioners deliver services and require that practitioners carefully consider how parent training may best be used to meet the needs of the population with whom they are working. Further discussion of adapting parent training to meet child and family characteristics and cultural issues is provided in chapters 5 and 6 of this volume.

RESEARCH INTO PRACTICE IN EVIDENCE-BASED PARENT TRAINING

Translating research into practice is an integral aspect of evidence-based practice in parent training. Integrating research with clinical expertise in practice requires conscious planning and actions on the part of the practitioner. One aspect of integrating research with practice involves determining the scientific merit of the research, as described in chapters 2 and 3. Another aspect, presented in chapter 7, involves translating research into an organizing framework for parent training. A third consideration, described earlier in this chapter, is examining the match between research and practice.

In the remainder of this chapter, we integrate these steps for translating research into practice in evidence-based parent training with other steps inherent in a problem-solving approach to psychological service delivery. This comprehensive series of steps to evidence-based parent training is consistent with other models of behavioral consultation service delivery

(Bergan & Kratochwill, 1990; Shriver, 1998) and applied behavior analysis (Watson & Gresham, 1998) that place emphasis on integrating research with clinical expertise. These steps also align closely with the general procedures of the empirically supported parent training programs for child noncompliance. In short, these service delivery steps have been used successfully in parent training as well as other models to translate research into practice.

The steps are presented in Exhibit 8.1. We describe them generally first and then offer case examples to illustrate how they were used to deliver services in three problem areas. Note that the steps are meant to be implemented sequentially, but practitioners should be prepared to return to earlier steps in the sequence as dictated by the course of events when working with individual clients.

Step 1: Conduct a Comprehensive Assessment

Conducting a comprehensive assessment is considered an essential aspect of best practice in psychology (e.g., Sattler, 2002; Shapiro & Kratochwill,

---

EXHIBIT 8.1
Steps in Evidence-Based Practice in Parent Training

I. Conduct a comprehensive assessment of the problem including the following:
  A. parent interview,
  B. observation of parent–child interaction in the clinic or home,
  C. child interview,
  D. behavior rating forms,
  E. review of relevant records, and
  F. use of cultural sensitivity from first contact with parent and child (see chap. 6).
II. In collaboration with the parent, operationally define the target behavior and a goal behavior for treatment for the child and for the parent.
III. Teach parents to monitor target behavior.
  A. Use behavioral skills teaching strategies (see chap. 5).
  B. Have parents collect baseline data on target behavior and goal behavior.
IV. Identify and develop the intervention using the organizing framework for parent training (see chap. 7).
V. Train parents.
  A. Use behavioral skills training including instruction, modeling, rehearsal, and feedback (see chap. 5).
  B. Barriers to intervention implementation may be overcome by using clinical skills (see chap. 5) such as providing rationale, choosing language carefully, predicting outcomes, using reminders, recognizing the competition, developing rapport, using tangible incentives, using technology, using resources, and being flexible.
VI. Monitor treatment adherence and progress.
VII. Apply data-based decision making.
  A. Make changes in the intervention (i.e., what parent is being taught) as needed.
  B. Make changes in parent training (i.e., how parent is being taught) as needed.
  C. Fade intervention or incorporate strategies as part of the family's natural routine.

2000). A comprehensive evaluation before initiating treatment services provides practitioners with information about how a given child and family matches with those in the research literature. The empirically supported parent training programs for noncompliance each describe a comprehensive evaluation of the child and family, and the manuals for these programs may provide practitioners with specific guidance for the types of assessment procedures to conduct. Common components of an assessment in the empirically supported parent training programs include an extensive parent interview, completion of behavior rating forms, and parent and child observations.

It is suggested that, at a minimum, practitioners conduct an interview with the parent and observe parent–child interaction. A parent interview assists with gathering important information about the family and child and with defining problem behaviors and goals for service delivery. In addition, the parent interview serves as the first opportunity for the practitioner to begin to establish rapport with the parent and child. The interview thus provides an opening early on to overcome potential barriers to parent training, treatment implementation, and treatment effectiveness (see chap. 5). Likewise, from the first contact with the parent and child and throughout the parent training process, it is important that practitioners be culturally sensitive and consider how culture may influence parent and child behavior and adherence to treatment recommendations (see chap. 6). Assessment of parents' respective identification with particular cultural groups may assist in tailoring parent training to improve treatment integrity and effectiveness. Data from the interview help practitioners match characteristics of the child and family with those of children and families reported in research.

Observations of the parent and child are important to gather initial or baseline data regarding child behaviors of concern, as well as parent behaviors that may need to be changed. Observations may take place in the clinic (i.e., analogue settings and conditions), in the home, or both. Observations of parent–child interaction may include coding of predefined child and parent behaviors as described in two of the evidence-based parent training programs (Hembree-Kigin & McNeil, 1995; McMahon & Forehand, 2003). Home observations are often difficult to conduct because of logistical and reimbursement problems, but observations of parent–child interaction can be conducted in analogue settings and provide useful information (Peed, Roberts, & Forehand, 1977). Observations of parent–child interaction provide data to help practitioners match baseline levels of parent and child behaviors observed in their practice with that from observations in research. This comparison may provide practitioners information regarding the severity of the behaviors observed. Likewise, observation may reveal that parents are negatively reinforcing child behavior, consistent with a coercive interaction described in the empirically supported parent training programs.

Behavior rating forms, such as the Eyberg Child Problem Inventory (Eyberg & Pincus, 1999) or the Child Behavior Checklist (Achenbach, 1991) may assist with determining the severity of problems relative to a normative group. Child interviews can be of assistance in determining motivational variables. Children themselves can be important sources of information regarding what parents may want to use as potential rewards. In addition, they may provide additional information and perspective regarding problem situations (McConaughy, 2000). For example, parents may report that they ignore child misbehavior such as temper tantrums, but the child may report that the parents frequently yell at him or her in these situations. This discrepancy does not mean that the parent or child report is necessarily inaccurate. For example, the parents may perceive that they usually ignore tantrums, whereas the child perceives that they usually yell. The practitioner will want to gather additional information, perhaps through observation, to gain a more objective assessment. Finally, reviewing records respective to a child's medical and educational history can assist in obtaining information that may validate or expand on information gathered from the parent interview. For example, if a parent reports that a child has poor grades, a review of the child's records may indicate excessive absences from school. This information can be followed up with the parent to determine the cause of the absences, and perhaps parent training could include an intervention to improve the child's attendance.

On the basis of data from the evaluation, the practitioner makes decisions regarding the appropriateness of implementing parent training and whether to attend to other issues that may affect parenting (e.g., maternal depression, parental drug use) or to child problems such as school behavior problems. Attending to these other types of problems may not directly involve delivering treatment through parent training but providing services to parents or providing services in the classroom. An evaluation of the child and family assists in determining their current functioning, their need for services, and their similarity to other children and families with whom parent training has been conducted as demonstrated in published research.

Step 2: Operationally Define Target Problem Behavior and Goal

The empirically based parent training programs have explicit operational definitions for targeted child behaviors and parenting skills or behaviors. Likewise, in research the target dependent variable is usually well defined so that it can be readily measured or observed. In practice as well, it is important to define clearly the target child behaviors of concern and the goals for treatment so that the practitioner and parents are in agreement about the need for intervention and about whether parent training and intervention were effective in achieving identified goals. Operationally defining target behaviors and goals assists with matching problems presenting in practice with those addressed in the literature. Identifying problems and goals collaboratively with the parent also assists in reducing barriers to treatment implementation and effectiveness (see chap. 5).

Identification and definition of the primary child problem of concern is determined on the basis of the information gathered in the initial comprehensive evaluation. An operational definition requires that the behavior be observable and measurable in such a way that both the practitioner and the parent would agree upon observation that the child behavior occurred. Defining the behavior typically requires talking with the parent about what a particular behavior looks like and when it is most likely to occur. Even something as seemingly simple as child noncompliance can be a difficult behavior on which to come to agreement (e.g., Shriver & Allen, 1997). For example, it can be important to clarify whether a child is considered to be noncompliant 20, 10, or 5 seconds after a command has been given, or to agree about how long a child should be given to complete a task before he or she is considered not to have complied. The practitioner and parent must decide whether it is noncompliance if a child says "no" but does the task anyway, dawdles for half a minute before starting the requested task, or starts the task but becomes distracted and does not complete it. Similar considerations arise when discussing and defining child behaviors such as temper tantrums, stealing, lying, bedtime problems, and so forth. Guidance for making decisions regarding the definition of noncompliance can be found in the empirically supported parent training programs and in research. Likewise, guidance for defining other child behaviors may be found in the literature as well. However, many defining issues regarding child behaviors are not addressed by research. Practitioners need to rely on their expertise and on parents' expectations regarding behavior to develop definitions.

It is also important to identify parent behaviors that may be contributing or maintaining a child's problem behaviors. For example, perhaps during the initial assessment, a parent is found to be skilled at using differential attention but poor at implementing a time-out procedure. Observations may indicate that the parent appears to be providing an adequate level of differential reinforcement for compliance but is not effectively providing punishing consequences for noncompliance. In this case, it may be that the practitioner would not spend much, if any, time on teaching differential attention skills (e.g., those taught in child-directed interactions [Parent–Child Interaction Therapy; Eyberg & Robinson, 1982; see also chap. 2, this volume] or Child's Game [Helping the Noncompliant Child program; McMahon & Forehand, 2003; see also chap. 2, this volume]) but would focus instead on training parents to implement a more effective time-out procedure. In short, on the basis of data from the comprehensive assessment, decisions are made regarding the skills parents exhibit in interaction with their children and the skills they will need to learn.

Finally, practitioners also need to collaborate with parents in determining and then operationally defining treatment goals. Parents often have different ideas than practitioners about what is reasonable to expect from treatment. Defining goals for treatment up-front helps break down possible barriers to implementing treatment in parent training (see chaps. 5 and 6, this volume, for more information). The practitioner should operationally define with the parent what the child's behavior will look like if treatment is successful. Likewise, the practitioner may want to define operationally with the parent what the parent's behavior would look like after successful treatment. Knowledge of research findings regarding parenting skills and child behavior helps guide the practitioner–parent collaboration. For example, the criteria for parent skills training in Parent–Child Interaction Therapy (Hembree-Kigin & McNeil, 1995) and in the manual *Helping the Noncompliant Child* (McMahon & Forehand, 2003) are particularly helpful in this regard when working with parents to address child noncompliance. The degree to which these criteria or expectations for parent behavior may need to change to address parental expectations and cultural issues determines the degree to which the research matches practice.

Step 3: Monitor Target Behavior

After the target child behavior and goal for treatment have been identified, the parent is trained to monitor child behavior and collect data on problem or goal behavior (or both). It is at this point that the behavioral skills training strategies described in chapter 5 become more prominent. Training parents to monitor child behavior involves instruction, modeling, rehearsal, and feedback on the monitoring procedures. Training parents to monitor child behavior serves three important purposes in parent training: (a) It teaches the parent an important skill for achieving positive child outcomes, (b) it may provide the practitioner with information regarding a parent's ability to follow through with treatment recommendations with integrity, and (c) it assists with collecting important data to determine the child's baseline functioning and to monitor treatment effectiveness and progress toward goals.

Parental monitoring of child behavior is emerging as an important variable in research on positive child outcomes (Crouter & Head, 2002; Patterson, Reid, & Dishion, 1992). Parents need to be able to monitor child behavior accurately and consistently to respond differentially to it; if they are not able to do so, it will be difficult for them to make their responses contingent on the child's behavior. In such cases, a parent would be unable to implement effectively any of the recommended reinforcing or punishing consequences that may be taught.

Because monitoring children's behavior is the first skill taught to parents, it provides an initial assessment of the success of behavioral skills training. Parents' ability to learn and demonstrate the skill during sessions and collect data throughout the week provides information about whether they can monitor child behavior. Conversely, the parent's ability to learn and demonstrate the skill during the session is also directly reflective of the practitioner's ability to train the parent effectively. The practitioner acquires information about the amount of practice or repetition needed during sessions, the role of the child during practice, and the type of support needed, such as written protocols (data sheets) or phone calls throughout the week to the parent to assist with completing the homework assignment.

Finally, parental monitoring and the collection of data on the child's behavior, and perhaps the parent's behavior as well, provide the practitioner with baseline information which can be used later to judge the success of treatment. On the basis of these data, the practitioner can collaborate with the parent to develop realistic goals for short-term as well as longer term treatment success. The initial goals developed in Step 2 (described earlier) may well be revised here to better reflect realistic goals based on current baseline parent and child functioning. In addition, child and parent outcomes typically achieved in research may be used as initial benchmarks with which to develop initial intervention goals as well. Practitioners can compare the baseline data achieved with their respective clients relative to the baseline data of sample participants in research. The degree to which the child and family, their problems, and their baseline data match existing research provides practitioners a level of confidence regarding how the research outcomes achieved might be attainable for a given family.

Step 4: Identify and Develop Intervention and Plan for Parent Training

Data and information from the comprehensive evaluation, operationally defined child and parent behaviors, and baseline data collection guide the practitioner's search for empirically supported or evidence-based interventions that match the presenting child and family's needs and characteristics. If there is an empirically supported intervention with an accompanying manual, the practitioner will most likely be successful in choosing it to implement parent training. If there is not a clearly identified empirically supported parent training program, the practitioner needs to search the literature to identify and develop a parent training intervention. Practitioners' skills and expertise in reading and critically evaluating research are important here. When evidence-based interventions for child problems that can be implemented in parent training are identified, the organizing framework for parent training presented in chapter 7 will be useful to plan what to teach, as well as how to teach specific strategies.

Step 5: Train Parents

Parents are trained to deliver interventions for children that have the best available research support. Parent training requires clinical expertise in behavioral skills training and in addressing barriers to parent implementation of intervention. For each aspect of what to teach parents and why, the practitioner can use the organizing framework to identify how parents will be trained in each of the necessary components of the intervention. In chapters 5 and 6 we discussed specific issues related to culture and addressing barriers to treatment that are important to training parents effectively. Practitioners need to consider developing skills in providing rationales for intervention, choosing language carefully, predicting outcomes, using reminders, developing rapport, using tangible incentives, using technology to reduce effort, identifying resources, and being flexible. These skills will facilitate parents' adherence to implementing the intervention.

Step 6: Monitor Treatment Adherence and Progress

Collecting data on child and parent behavior is an integral aspect of the empirically supported parent training programs and of research examining the effects of interventions in parent training. Data that practitioners collect about child and parent functioning and progress during treatment are important to clinical decision making and to meeting the unique needs of children and families (Edwards, Dattilio, & Bromley, 2004; Hawkins & Hursh, 1992); such data also provide information about the effectiveness of practice. Two other types of data collection are important for any treatment addressing child problems. The first is data collection on the integrity with which the parent is implementing treatment recommendations, known as treatment adherence; the second is data collection on child outcomes or progress toward the identified goal.

Treatment Adherence

Practitioners need to collect data on whether parents are actually implementing the intervention as they were trained to do. If a parent is not implementing an intervention as recommended, positive changes in child behavior are unlikely to occur. Identifying and addressing problems with implementation as soon as each skill is taught is critical. With this information, practitioners can make decisions regarding the changes needed in training the parent to perform the intervention.

Data on treatment adherence can be obtained through homework assignments and data collection that parents are asked to undertake between sessions. Treatment adherence and integrity data are not commonly collected or reported in research (Gresham, 2005; Gresham, Gansle, & Noell, 1993); however, the empirically supported parent training programs can provide some guidance for practitioners on collecting treatment adherence data. For example, data on parent behavior may be collected through observations of parent–child interaction and comparisons with explicit criteria for parenting skills made before the practitioner decides to move to the next step in the parent training process (e.g., Hembree-Kigin & McNeil, 1995; McMahon & Forehand, 2003). Phone calls to parents are frequently used in parent training programs and may occur weekly, if not more often, to monitor parent implementation and child behavior (e.g., Patterson, Reid, Jones, & Conger, 1975; Webster-Stratton & Hancock, 1998). Given the time constraints many practitioners face, phone calls may be most efficiently used for those cases in which treatment adherence is a particular concern. Parents' completion of data sheets on their own behavior (i.e., self-monitoring) and on the child's behavior, or other means of tracking child behavior, such as wrist counters, can also provide some evidence regarding treatment adherence.

Progress Monitoring and Outcome Data

Data on child outcomes can be obtained through various methods but typically rely on observations in the clinic or parent training setting and on home observations, parent report, or other parental assessment of child behavior in the home. Not only are child outcome data important in practice, they are also one of the criteria described in chapter 3 regarding evaluation of the scientific merit of parent training programs. Similarly, research describing direct measurement of child and parent outcomes may also guide practice in collecting outcomes data. Typically, child and parent outcome data are obtained through the same homework assignments and data collection procedures used to monitor treatment adherence. Many methods and measures can be used to collect data (Hawkins, Mathews, & Hamdan, 1999). If children are not making progress toward defined goals, clinical decisions regarding changes in treatment strategies need to be made (Cone, 2001).

Step 7: Apply Data-Based Decision Making

As part of evidence-based practice in parent training, data are used to make decisions regarding changes in intervention and parent training strategies. If the data collected during parent training suggest that parents are not implementing intervention components with integrity, the practitioner needs to consider either how the intervention may be changed to facilitate ease of implementation or how the parent may be trained differently (e.g., provide daily phone reminders, rehearse more in session) to facilitate treatment integrity.

As the data begin to indicate that the child's behavior is progressing closer to the defined goal or achieves the defined goal, then the practitioner works with the parent either to fade the intervention or to incorporate it into the family's natural routine. The empirically supported parent training programs and research may provide some guidance on how to fade interventions, but for individual children and families, these decisions are largely based on clinical expertise informed by data collected during parent training. Evidence-based practice in parent training starts with data—the best available research evidence—and ends with data—parent and child outcomes.

CASE EXAMPLES

Three case examples are now provided that follow the evidence-based practice in parent training described in Exhibit 8.1.[1] The first case is that of a 6-year-old boy with problems of poor attention span, demonstrated by short duration of independent play, who presented to an outpatient clinic. The second case is that of an 8-year-old girl brought to a school psychologist by her parents for concerns about stealing. The third case is that of a 9-year-old girl with developmental disabilities who was brought to a primary care office to address toileting concerns.

CASE 1

A single mother brought her 6-year-old son, David, to a clinical psychologist in an outpatient psychology clinic. The mother and child were African American. David was described as very active and as constantly seeking her attention.

Comprehensive Assessment

On the basis of parent interview and review of records during the first meeting, the practitioner learned that David had a previous diagnosis of attention-deficit/hyperactivity disorder (ADHD). David's mother reported that he rarely played with toys available in his house and frequently interrupted her at home. He attended a full-day kindergarten and was in a before- and after-school day-care program while his mother worked a full-time job. She had no other children. Although she expressed no other concerns regarding his compliance, school behavior, socialization, or medical and developmental issues, the mother did note that he was very active and had a short attention span. Observations in the clinic supported that he rarely played with toys available and frequently interrupted his mother, but he was generally compliant with her redirection or commands. Behavior rating

---

[1]The cases presented in this chapter are provided for illustrative purposes only and do not represent a single actual case. Rather, they represent composites of actual cases presenting to our clinic.

forms were not administered in this particular case because there was previous documentation of behavior outside normative range given the diagnosis of ADHD. Discussion with his mother indicated that she was comfortable with learning skills that involved using reinforcement to teach David to play independently.

Operationally Define Target Problem Behavior and Goal

During the parent interview, the practitioner and David's mother decided that the problem behavior was the short duration of his independent play. The defined goal for intervention was to increase this duration. The goal for David's mother was to learn how to attend differentially to David to increase his duration of independent play.

Monitor Target Behavior

Following the initial intake of information, David's mother recorded data throughout the next week on the duration of time he would play independently when asked. Parent training occurred in the clinic regarding the data collection procedures and monitoring of David's independent play. The data collected from home indicated that he engaged in independent play in a range of 2 to 15 minutes, approximately 10 minutes on average.

Identify and Develop Intervention and Plan for Parent Training

A review of research regarding interventions to improve child attention or independent play behavior revealed no peer-reviewed studies. However, small N studies have used reinforcement to increase children's on-task or in-seat behavior and attending in classroom situations (Basile & Hintze, 1998; Rathvon, 1999). This research was adapted for use in developing an intervention for increasing independent play and in a plan to train David's mother to implement the intervention. The organizing framework for research and parent training was used for this purpose and is presented in Table 8.1. The match between research and practice in this case was poor regarding setting and child characteristics, but the practitioner had previous experience using differential reinforcement strategies to shape child behavior. The practitioner decided to adapt these strategies and basic science principles to a different setting for purposes of addressing the parent and child concerns in this case.

A reinforcement program was developed using David's mother's differential attention as the primary source of reinforcement. Initially, when told to play on his own, a timer was set for 10 minutes. During independent play, David frequently (i.e., every 2 minutes) received brief exposure

TABLE 8.1
Parent Training to Improve Independent Play

What to teach	Why to teach	How to teach: parent training
Teach parent to identify and monitor independent play behavior. Teach parent to provide social attention contingent on independent play during the child's play and reward following his attainment of criteria for duration of independent play.	Reinforcement: Social attention increases duration of independent play.	Instruction: Describe and provide rationale for positive social attention and reward for the child's independent play. Modeling: Demonstrate with the child or parent how to provide praise, positive touch, descriptions, and reflections during the child's play. Rehearsal: Have the parent practice providing social attention with the child as he plays independently in clinic. Feedback: Provide positive and corrective feedback during rehearsal to shape the parent's effective use of social attention during and after play.
Teach the parent to ignore minor misbehavior during play or when the child interrupts his mother.	Extinction: Removal of social attention contingent on non-compliance or interruption that reduces the probability of the behavior recurring. Note the possibility of an extinction burst.	Instruction: Describe and provide rationale for ignoring minor misbehavior as well as reducing social attention for interruptions. Predict the possibility of extinction burst. Modeling: Demonstrate the use of ignoring with the child. Rehearsal: Have the parent practice ignoring with the child during session. Feedback: Shape effective ignoring skills.
Teach parent to provide toys or activities with which the child typically prefers to play. Teach parent how to provide direct, one-step, developmentally appropriate commands and redirection that states the expectation of his independent play.	Stimulus control: The presence of preferred toys increases the likelihood of independent play. An effective parent command signals the availability of reinforcement for compliance—in this case, independent play.	Instruction: Describe and provide rationale for setting up the home environment to encourage independent play and for giving effective commands and redirection that specifies the expectation of independent play.

TABLE 8.1
Parent Training to Improve Independent Play

What to teach	Why to teach	How to teach: parent training
		Modeling: Demonstrate with the parent or child how to set up an independent play situation and provide a command or an expectation.
		Rehearsal: Have the parent practice how to give an effective command and redirection for independent play with the practitioner or child. Set up a practice session to include preferred toys and activities.
		Feedback: Shape the parent's use of effective commands.
The child loses access to a reward contingent on interrupting.	Punishment: Loss of reward decreases the probability of interruptions during independent play.	Instruction: Describe and provide rationale for loss of reward and using time-out.
Time-out may be used for noncompliant behavior, interruptions, or misbehavior that the parent cannot ignore.	Time-out decreases the probability of non-compliance and interruptions recurring.	Modeling: Model with the child how to implement time-out.
		Rehearsal: Have the parent practice time-out with the child in the clinic.
		Feedback: Shape the parent's use of time-out.

(less than 5 seconds) to positive labeled praise and touch from his mother during independent play. If he played 10 minutes without seeking her attention, he was provided 5 minutes of game time with his mother. One to two opportunities to practice independent play were planned each day at home.

Train Parents

The practitioner presented these procedures to David's mother with a rationale for why they were important to achieving the defined treatment goal. The intervention procedures were modeled directly with David in the clinic. David's mother had opportunities to practice the procedure in the clinic with immediate feedback.

Monitor Treatment Adherence and Progress

David's mother received a data sheet to monitor progress at home. She reviewed these with the practitioner at subsequent sessions, and together they solved problems with implementation. The practitioner conducted observations of David and his mother weekly to provide feedback on treatment implementation.

Apply Data-Based Decision Making

The intervention resulted in an immediate increase in the duration of David's independent play. He was consistently exceeding the initial expectation of 10 minutes of independent play and earned time with his mother. From these data, the criteria for earning time with his mother were slowly increased. Eventually, the time with his mother was faded, and differential attention during independent play was enough for David to sustain longer periods of play.

CASE 2

Kathleen was an 8-year-old Caucasian girl who was referred to the school psychologist at her school by her teacher and biological parents because of several incidents of stealing in the classroom and from friends' homes.

Comprehensive Assessment

The school psychologist interviewed both parents, conducted a brief parent–child observation, and interviewed Kathleen. In addition, the school psychologist also interviewed the teacher and conducted a classroom observation. An interview with Kathleen's parents indicated that Kathleen had stolen on at least four occasions over the past 2 months. Three of the occasions were from other students in her classroom, and one was from a friend's house. The items stolen were small toy items. Kathleen's parents had reprimanded her, made her return the toys, and removed privileges such as television consequent to each known episode but were concerned that stealing continued. Her parents were initially interested in individual counseling for Kathleen, but in conversation with the school psychologist, they agreed that they would also benefit from learning strategies to prevent stealing and provide more effective punishment when stealing occurred. The school psychologist conducted observations of parent–child interaction during the meeting. Observations suggested that Kathleen was generally compliant with parent commands. Individual interview with Kathleen indicated that she took the items because she liked them and did not readily consider the effect of her actions on her friends or peers at school. Also, she did not recall what consequences her parents had implemented for stealing. Behavior rating forms completed by her parents did not indicate any other clinically significant or elevated behavioral difficulties. An interview with Kathleen's teacher and classroom observation also indicated that there were no other difficulties in the classroom, and peer relations appeared generally positive.

Operationally Define Target Problem Behavior and Goal

The school psychologist decided in collaboration with Kathleen's parents that the primary problem behavior currently was stealing items. This was defined as possessing an item that was not originally Kathleen's without permission of the owner. The goal for parent training was for parents to implement strategies to reduce the frequency of Kathleen's stealing and eventually prevent stealing from occurring completely.

Monitor Target Behavior

Kathleen's parents received training in how to monitor Kathleen's stealing behavior. This basically required daily sweeps of her room and backpack to look for items that were not hers. The daily sweeps allowed Kathleen's parents to record whether stealing occurred on a daily basis.

Identify and Develop Intervention and Plan for Parent Training

Patterson and colleagues provided information for parent training to address stealing in their previous manual for clinicians, as well as in their books for parents (Patterson, 1975, 1976; Patterson et al., 1975). At that time, there was little research that specifically addressed stealing, and Patterson and colleagues appear to have relied on their clinical expertise and knowledge about scientific principles and parent training procedures to implement intervention for stealing. Since that time, there has been little research conducted that demonstrates the efficacy of interventions for stealing in school-age children (Venning, Blampied, & France, 2003). Review articles about stealing for teachers and parents suggest that contingency management may be an effective approach to reduce stealing (G. E. Miller & Klugness, 1986; Tremblay & Drabman, 1997; Williams, 1985). Based on Patterson's early work and considerations of conceptual principles outlined in subsequent review articles, the organizing framework for research and parent training presented in chapter 7 of this volume was used to help develop the intervention and parent training process to apply in this case (see Table 8.2). The school psychologist reviewed

TABLE 8.2
Parent Training to Address Stealing

What to teach	Why to teach	How to teach: parent training
Teach parents to define, identify, and monitor stealing behavior. Develop list of rewards (i.e., tangibles and privileges) that the child may earn. Develop a point system for earning rewards and criteria for reward exchange. Develop criteria for earning points contingent on not stealing. Teach parents to provide positive social attention contingent on earning points and rewards for not stealing.	Reinforcement: Social attention, points, and rewards increase the probability of non-stealing behavior recurring.	Instruction: Describe and provide rationale for using points and rewards for not stealing. Modeling: Demonstrate with the child or parent how to provide points and rewards. Rehearsal: Have parents practice providing points and rewards with the child through role-play. Feedback: Provide positive and corrective feedback during rehearsal to shape parents' effective use of reward and social attention.
Teach parents to ignore minor argumentative or other misbehavior that may occur in response to loss of points or punishment. Eliminate verbal reprimands and lectures.	Extinction: Removal of social attention for argumentative or other misbehavior reduces possible reinforcement of that behavior.	Instruction: Describe and provide rationale for ignoring minor misbehavior and eliminating reprimands and lecture. Modeling: Demonstrate the use of ignoring in role-play with the child or parents. Rehearsal: Have parents practice ignoring in role-play with the practitioner or child. Feedback: Shape effective ignoring skills.
Teach parents to develop and write a contract or point system with the child and post it in visible location at home. Teach parents to provide clear expectation for earning and losing points, earning rewards, and earning punishment/returning the item.	Stimulus control: Posting a plan and points earned signals availability of reinforcement.	Instruction: Describe and provide rationale for point, reward, and punishment intervention. Provide protocol or other example that shows parents how the point system or behavior contract may look. Modeling: Work with the parents to start a reward list and demon-
Teach parents to restrict access to rewards unless they are earned by the child.	Reduced access to preferred or reinforcing activities used for rewards increases the value of that reward (i.e., establishing operation).	strate how to provide points, rewards, and punishment.

TABLE 8.2
Parent Training to Address Stealing

What to teach	Why to teach	How to teach: parent training
		Rehearsal: Have parents practice how to provide points, rewards, and punishment and record data on point sheet or contract with practitioner or child.
		Feedback: Shape effective contract development and implementation.
Teach parents to take away points contingent on stealing (i.e., response cost).	Punishment: Removal of points reduces stealing.	Instruction: Describe and provide rationale for using response cost and time-out.
Teach parents how to apply punishment in the form of time-out or house chores contingent on loss of points and stealing.	House chores are applied contingent on stealing or point loss. The child is briefly removed from access to reinforcement through time-out contingent on stealing or point loss.	Modeling: Model or role-play with the parents and child how to implement the punishment. Rehearsal: Have parents role-play punishment in the clinic with the child. Feedback: Shape parental implementation of response cost and time-out.
Have the child return the stolen item to its owner.	Returning the item may function as loss of reinforcement, reducing likelihood of stealing recurring. Public notice of stealing may also be punishing.	

the intervention components and decided that she had the skills to train the parents to implement these procedures.

Kathleen's parents were provided instruction for setting up a behavior contract with her that incorporated losing points for stealing and earning points for the desired behavior—namely, not stealing. The points could be exchanged for rewards of interest to Kathleen. Her parents were taught to minimize social attention when stealing occurred. This meant that verbal reprimands and lecture were eliminated. The school psychologist provided several options for punishment to Kathleen's parents. For example, Kathleen could be grounded for 1 day or expected to provide 1 hour of useful work as a consequence for stealing items of small value. She could be grounded for 2 days or expected to provide 2 hours of work for stealing items of greater value. Other examples of punishment included completing chores or receiving a time-out contingent on stealing. Kathleen's parents decided to use time-out and loss of points as punishment. Kathleen was also expected to return the item she had stolen.

Train Parents

Kathleen's parents were provided with instruction, rationale, modeling, and opportunities for practice with feedback for all aspects of the intervention. Kathleen was included in this training, and completion of the point sheet and provision of rewards and time-out were practiced. In addition, her parents expressed concern regarding maintaining calm behavior and minimizing lecture and reprimand should stealing occur so that these parenting skills were emphasized in training through role-play with the school psychologist and practice with Kathleen.

Monitor Treatment Adherence and Progress

Data were gathered by Kathleen's parents over the next 2 weeks. Kathleen had one incident of stealing. She was placed in time-out and lost points. Her parents maintained a calm response and minimized their lecture and reprimand. She earned points on each of the other days, which she used to exchange for access to rewards, in particular, extra time playing video and computer games.

Apply Data-Based Decision Making

Kathleen's parents collected data for 1 month with the program implemented as initially planned. There were no more instances of stealing that month. With consultation from the school psychologist, the parents faded the program over the following month. They found the point system useful and decided to use it to address another problem that had begun to occur with more frequency with Kathleen. The school psychologist helped the parents change the program to address a new target behavior of talking respectfully to others in the family (no talking back, no name calling, no whining).

CASE 3

Jerry was a 6-year-old boy brought by his mother and father to a licensed mental health practitioner consulting in a primary care clinic. The family was of Latino heritage. Jerry's parents had seen his pediatrician regarding concerns with toileting, and the pediatrician had referred the family to the mental health practitioner.

Comprehensive Assessment

An interview with Jerry's parents revealed that he had never learned to use the toilet to urinate or for bowel movements. He was wearing pull-ups. He had a previous diagnosis of mild mental retardation and cerebral palsy, resulting in partial left hemiplegia. Medical evaluation indicated no other physical concerns that would impede toilet training. He was receiving special education services at school. Interview with the parents and observations in the clinic of parent–child interaction indicated that Jerry was frequently noncompliant with parental commands and often exhibited temper tantrums when told to do something he did not want to do. Discussion with Jerry's parents indicated they were comfortable with parent training and with the possible intervention components they might be taught to facilitate Jerry's toilet training.

Operationally Define Target Problem Behavior and Goal: Part I—Compliance

On the basis of the information gathered during the initial evaluation, discussion with Jerry's parents focused on the need first to improve Jerry's compliance before initiating toilet training. They were accepting of this recommendation. Because of Jerry's age and developmental delays, the practitioner decided to train the parents using the Helping the Noncompliant Child behavioral parent training program (McMahon & Forehand, 2003). This program has been used with children who have developmental disabilities. The practitioner was experienced with it, and the primary care office had resources and space available to conduct parent training to treat noncompliance (e.g., room to conduct parent–child observations and demonstrate time-out with toys available). Compliance and noncompliance were defined with Jerry's parents. He was observed to be compliant with less than 40% of parent commands. Tantrums occurred three to five times daily. A goal was established to improve compliance to greater than 70% and decrease tantrums to once daily. Jerry and his parents were seen in the clinic weekly. The practitioner and parents followed the program with close integrity. More time and practice were needed for Jerry to make progress with compliance relative to "typical" children. In approximately 3 months, Jerry's compliance had substantially increased, and temper tantrums were less frequent and more manageable. He was still wearing pull-ups, however, and not using the toilet for elimination.

Operationally Define Target Problem Behavior and Goal: Part II—Elimination

Following parent training for compliance, the practitioner and parents decided that the defined problem behavior at this time was elimination (i.e., urinary and bowel movements) in pull-ups. The defined goal for intervention was to have 90% or more eliminations in the toilet. Although both urinary continence and bowel movements were targets for improvement and intervention, urinary continence was chosen as the priority because it occurs more frequently and may be trained within a shorter time period.

Monitor Target Behavior

Jerry's parents were trained to collect data throughout the day on dry versus wet or soiled pants. These data provided information on the times of day that Jerry was most likely to void.

Identify and Develop Intervention and Plan for Parent Training

Toilet training for children with disabilities has tended to rely on techniques first described by Azrin and Foxx (1974). This is an intensive toilet training intervention that is conducted over the course of a short time period (e.g., a day, several days). Parents and teachers have been trained to teach children with disabilities to use the toilet for elimination (LeBlanc, Carr, & Crossett, 2005; Post & Kirkpatrick, 2004; Tarbox, Williams, & Friman, 2004), and reviews describe toilet training for parents and for professionals in primary care settings (Christophersen & Mortweet, 2003; Polaha, Warzak, & Dittmer-McMahon, 2002). The interventions rely on reinforcement to teach toileting skills (e.g., Cicero & Pfadt, 2002). Much of the research is small N studies. The subjects in the studies range in age from preschool through adolescence and adulthood. Children with mental retardation and autism have been studied as well. There appeared to be scientific merit of a reinforcement-based approach founded on Azrin and Foxx's procedure, and there was a match with child characteristics and setting characteristics. The practitioner also had previous experience teaching parents interventions for toilet training. A plan for parent training was developed on the basis of a review of the research and is presented in Table 8.3.

Train Parents

The practitioner described both the procedures and the rationale for them. Steps were clearly delineated for increasing fluids, scheduled toilet sits, checking pants, responding to accidents, and reinforcing compliance with toileting routine. The practitioner walked through the steps in role-play with Jerry and his parents to ensure that they accurately understood each component of the intervention. The parents implemented the procedure over a planned weekend with phone contact initiated by the practitioner to monitor treatment integrity and progress.

TABLE 8.3
Parent Training for Toilet Training

What to teach	Why to teach	How to teach: parent training
Teach parents to monitor and collect data on wet or soiled versus dry pants. Teach parents to develop a list of rewards (i.e., tangibles and privileges). Teach parents to provide positive social attention contingent on dry pants. Teach parents to provide positive social attention and rewards contingent on compliance with toileting routine, such as indicating need, sitting on the toilet, elimination, cleanup, and dressing.	Reinforcement: Social attention and reward increases targeted toileting behaviors.	Instruction: Describe and provide rationale for using positive social attention and a reward system for toileting. Modeling: Role-play with the parents or child how to provide positive social attention and reward. Rehearsal: Have parents role-play with the child how to provide social attention and reward. Feedback: Provide positive and corrective feedback to parents during rehearsal to shape effective monitoring and reinforcement.
Teach parents to reduce reprimand and lecture contingent on toileting accidents and noncompliance with toileting routine.	Extinction: Removal of social attention contingent on noncompliance or other defined misbehavior that reduces the probability of the behavior recurring.	Instruction: Describe and provide rationale for reducing verbal interaction contingent on accidents and noncompliance with routine. Modeling: Role-play with parent or child how to respond to accidents and noncompliance. Rehearsal: Have parents role-play with child during the Child's Game activity. Feedback: Shape parental ignoring skills.
Teach parents how to provide direct, one-step, developmentally appropriate commands. Have parents increase child's fluid intake. Teach parents to have the child sit on toilet at times the data indicate he is most likely to eliminate, such as after meals or after awakening in the morning.	Stimulus control: Clear commands signal availability of reinforcement. Increasing fluids increases the need to eliminate (i.e., establishing operation). Schedule sits on the toilet for times the child is most likely to eliminate.	Instruction: Describe and provide rationale for giving effective commands, increasing fluid intake, and scheduling toilet sits. Modeling: Demonstrate with parents or the child how to give effective commands. Rehearsal: Have parents practice with practitioner or child how to give effective commands. Feedback: Shape parental use of commands.

(continues)

TABLE 8.3
Parent Training for Toilet Training *(Continued)*

What to teach	Why to teach	How to teach: parent training
Have parents stop having the child wear pull-ups or diapers and begin wearing underwear.	Punishment: Underwear increases discomfort of accidental elimination.	Instruction: Describe and provide rationale for using time-out and wearing underwear.
Teach parents how to apply time-out contingent on noncompliance or other target misbehavior.	Time-out decreases the probability of non-compliance recurring.	Modeling: Model with parent and/or child how to implement time-out.
		Rehearsal: Have the parent practice time-out in the clinic with the child.
		Feedback: Shape parental time-out skills.

Monitor Treatment Adherence and Progress

Jerry's parents continued to collect data on wet or soiled versus dry pants. During the intensive training weekend, Jerry had several initial incidents of urinary accidents. He was successfully using the toilet and maintaining dry pants by the end of the day Saturday and throughout Sunday. He had bowel movements in his pants during the weekend but was having them in the toilet on Monday and everyday thereafter.

Apply Data-Based Decision Making

Jerry's parents continued to keep data on pants checks and toileting for 2 weeks and implemented reinforcement for that time. Occasional accidents occurred when the family was on an outing or if Jerry was busy with an activity such as video games, but these incidences decreased over time in frequency. The parents faded reinforcement and other procedural steps (e.g., scheduled sits) over the next 2 months with guidance from the parent trainer.

SUMMARY

Integrating research with clinical expertise requires translating research into practice. This translation involves examining the scientific merit of research support and the match between research and practice conditions. Much of the best available research evidence in parent training is based on efficacy research that may not translate readily into practice situations in which there are often unique practitioner, setting, and client variables affecting treatment integrity and outcomes. However, effectiveness studies and increased attention to issues inherent in translating research into practice can begin to address some of these variables. Practitioners are required to be cognizant of the differing types or levels of research support and need to take the initiative to stay abreast of current research. With this knowledge, they are in position to follow the steps in evidence-based parent training service delivery to improve outcomes for children. In the next chapter, we present issues for consideration in future research about parent training.

9

PARENT TRAINING: PREVENTION AND FUTURE RESEARCH

The parent training programs discussed throughout this book have focused on intervention for child problems. However, many practitioners are also interested in how such problems can be prevented. In fact, prevention was an impetus in the establishment of child guidance clinics across the country in the early 20th century (Horn, 1989). As noted in chapter 2 of this volume, research demonstrates that positive parent and child outcomes can be maintained over time following implementation of parent training. To a large degree, prevention has been and is an important goal of parent training. In this chapter, we look at some promising prevention programs that incorporate parent training as a core component. First it is important to understand some general differences between parent training for intervention and parent training for prevention.

Perhaps the most obvious difference between intervention and prevention is the time frame that is examined for measuring desired outcomes. Parent training conducted for intervention is largely focused on producing immediate changes in child and parent behavior. Attempts may be made to measure parent and child changes long term (DeGarmo, Patterson, & Forgatch, 2004), but the interest in these cases has generally been in measuring whether demonstrated intervention outcomes are maintained over time. However, researchers and practitioners conducting parent training for prevention are usually focused on child outcomes years in the future. Immediate changes are measured in both prevention and intervention, but long-term changes in parental behavior are the explicit goal in prevention strategies. Parents are taught skills to improve their current parenting behaviors and improve the parent–child relationship, but successful prevention is determined by positive outcomes for the child in the future. In short, the difference between intervention and prevention is dependent on the emphasis placed on short-term outcomes relative to long-term outcomes, respectively.

A second major difference between parent training for intervention and parent training for prevention is the target population. Intervention focuses on children who are already exhibiting problems; prevention focuses on children who are not exhibiting problems and who may or who may not be considered at risk for developing problems in the future. There are three levels of prevention that are largely defined by the population of children or families targeted. *Universal prevention strategies* target a general population of children or families who have not been identified on the basis of any assumed risk for a disorder or disability. *Selected prevention strategies* focus on individuals or groups of children or families who are assumed or identified to be at risk for developing a disorder on the basis of biological, psychological, or social risk factors associated with it. *Indicated prevention programs* target individuals or groups who are identified to be at high risk for developing a disorder (Weissberg, Kumpfer, & Seligman, 2003). Children targeted by indicated prevention programs may have subthreshold characteristics of a particular diagnosis or multiple risk factors for a particular disorder. There is clearly overlap between the target populations for indicated preventions and interventions; the latter may be provided to both indicated populations and children with diagnosed problems. However, there is less overlap in target populations between intervention and universal or selected prevention strategies because intervention is not typically delivered universally or even selectively.

OVERVIEW OF SELECTED PARENT TRAINING PREVENTION PROGRAMS

In the sections that follow, we describe three prevention programs that include parent training and summarize current research regarding the efficacy of each program (see chaps. 2 and 3, this volume, on criteria for scientific merit). Each of these prevention programs has a parent training component with ties to the empirically supported parent training programs described in chapter 2 of this volume. The prevention programs reviewed include FAST Track (Conduct Problems Prevention Research Group, 1992, 2000, 2004), Linking the Interests of Families and Teachers (LIFT; Eddy, Reid, & Fetrow, 2000;

J. B. Reid & Eddy, 2002), and the Adolescent Transitions Program (ATP; Dishion & Kavanagh, 2003). The practical implications of most of this research are still unknown, but we review these programs in some depth to illustrate the current state of the science in this area for practitioners interested in parent training for prevention purposes.

FAST Track

Overview of the Program

The FAST Track program is a multisite prevention program initiated in the early 1990s (Conduct Problems Prevention Research Group, 1992, 1999, 2000, 2004; McMahon & Forehand, 2003). The goal of the FAST Track program is to prevent the development of serious conduct problems in at-risk school-age children. The program includes parent training, home visits, social skills training, academic tutoring, and a classroom intervention delivered by teachers and designed to increase social and emotional competencies in the classroom. The program begins in first grade and continues through tenth grade. Two periods of child development and school transition are emphasized for intervention: school entry in first and second grades and transition to middle school in fifth and sixth grades. Initially the interventions target six domains: (a) disruptive behaviors in the home, (b) disruptive and off-task behaviors in the school, (c) social–cognitive skills related to emotional regulation and problem solving, (d) peer relations, (e) academic skills, and (f) family–school relations (McMahon & Forehand, 2003). As the children mature and transition to middle school, the target behaviors for intervention include parent or adult monitoring and positive involvement, peer affiliation and peer influence, social cognition and identity development, and academic achievement and orientation to school.

The classroom intervention is based on the PATHS (Promoting Alternative Thinking Strategies) curriculum (Kusche & Greenberg, 1994). The PATHS curriculum teaches self-control, emotional awareness, and problem-solving skills to children in elementary school. As part of the FAST Track program, the PATHS curriculum is taught approximately three times weekly. In addition, teachers are taught specific strategies for effective classroom management and for reducing disruptive behavior in the classroom. In Grades 1 and 2, children also participate in reading tutoring sessions individually with a tutor three times a week. A reading session with the parent is also included in the parent meeting described later in this section.

Review of the Parent Training Component

The FAST Track program has three family components: (a) a parenting skills group, (b) a parent–child relationship enhancement group, and (c) a home visiting program. The family-based interventions are delivered during the elementary school years of the children and families' participation in the program. Parent training is provided in a group format by family coordinators (FC). An FC typically has previous training in social work or another psychological discipline and extensive experience working with families. There are 22 weekly sessions throughout the first-grade year and 14 biweekly sessions throughout the second-grade year (McMahon, Slough, & the Conduct Problems Prevention Research Group, 1996). There are nine monthly meetings in Grades 3 through 5 with several meetings during the end of the fifth-grade year to prepare for the transition to middle school. The parent training component is modified to address developmental issues as children mature and to build on previous skills learned as children continue through second grade and beyond.

The parent training sessions are 1 hour each and address topics such as establishing positive family–school relationships, supporting children's anger control and problem-solving skills learned in the classroom social skills curriculum, using anger control and problem-solving skills to increase parental self-control, and effective parenting skills. The curriculum on effective parenting skills is adapted primarily from the program by Forehand and McMahon (1981). Select videotaped vignettes from the Parents and Children Series program by Webster-Stratton (1987) are used with the parent groups. Although this is a group-based program, the leader places an emphasis on demonstration and modeling, behavioral rehearsal of skills by the parent, and guided practice with the children. Child care is provided while the parents are in the group during the first hour. It is during this time that children participate in a social skills friendship group. Child care is also provided for siblings.

Following the parent group, there is a half hour of parent and child activity time in which opportunities for practicing skills learned in the parent group are provided. The focus of this activity time is to foster positive parent–child interactions. For children in first grade, there is also a half hour of parent–child reading time with a reading tutor to foster parent involvement in academic skill acquisition.

In studies of the program, the parent groups were offered weekly on Saturdays, and refreshments were provided. Transportation was provided for families if needed. Parents were paid $15 per session for their attendance. The FCs made biweekly home visits or phone contacts to monitor and practice implementation of parenting skills. In addition, the FCs worked with the parents to improve problem-solving competence related to life management issues, improve feelings of competence and confidence, and facilitate providing a safe and supportive environment for children.

Empirical Support

FAST Track is largely a selected prevention program in that it targets children at risk for conduct problems. It includes a universal prevention component in the school-based, teacher-implemented, classwide social–emotional skills curriculum. The program is currently under evaluation at four sites in the United States. A total of 891 children identified as high risk by their teachers or parents on the basis of displays of high levels of conduct problems in kindergarten are participating. At each site, children and families were matched by demographics into two sets. Sets were then randomly assigned to the intervention or control condition at the start of the program study. The four program sites are located in different geographic regions of the United States. The children represent urban, semiurban, and rural communities and also include representation of girls (31%) and African Americans (51%). There are no or negligible numbers of Latino or Hispanic child and family participants. Reports have been published on outcomes following the 1st year of implementation after Grade 1 (Conduct Problems Prevention Research Group, 1999), after 3 years of implementation after Grade 3 (Conduct Problems Prevention Research Group, 2002), and after Grade 5 or the end of elementary school (Conduct Problems Prevention Research Group, 2004). Attrition has been low, at approximately 10%, by the end of Grade 5.

At the end of Grade 3, significant differences were noted between groups in both teacher and parent ratings of child behavior change, and differences were noted between groups in parents' daily report of child behavior (Conduct Problems Prevention Research Group, 2002). Children in the intervention group were significantly less likely to be found eligible for special education services. However, it is unclear whether the special education labels were for learning disability, emotional and behavior disorders, or other diagnoses because these were not documented. Parents in the intervention group also rated themselves as less likely to use physical punishment. Parents described perceived improvement in their parenting skills over the previous year. The effect sizes for the differences noted between groups were low to moderate. There were no significant differences in children's social cognition; academic progress in reading, math, or language arts; or peer ratings of social preference. There were no differences noted in parent ratings of their competence or in teacher ratings of parent involvement in school (Conduct Problems Prevention Research Group, 2002).

At the end of Grade 5, measures were examined within four areas of functioning: (a) social cognition and social competence problems, (b) peer deviance, (c) home and community problems, and (d) school context academic and behavior problems (Conduct Problems Prevention Research Group, 2004). Children in the intervention group scored higher on a measure of social problem solving and were rated higher by teachers on a measure of social competence compared with the control group. The children in the intervention group were less likely to report having friends who engaged in deviant or antisocial behaviors. The children in the intervention group rated their own behavior as less deviant, and their parents rated fewer behavior problems, both at home and in the community. There were no statistically significant differences noted between the intervention and control groups on measures of classroom aggressive behavior and academic risk (Conduct Problems Prevention Research Group, 2004).

In summary, the FAST Track program appears to be having a modest positive effect on some aspects of children's behavior and on parenting skills. Most positive changes are based on teacher or parent report rather than direct observation of child functioning. The program is intensive and involves implementation of interventions across home and classroom settings. Continued evaluation over the next several years will provide important information about the effects of this project.

Linking the Interests of Families and Teachers

Overview of the Program

Linking the Interests of Families and Teachers (LIFT) is a universal prevention program delivered to elementary school children and their parents. Specifically, children in first and fifth grades are targeted in this program. Similar to the FAST Track program rationale, these grades are perceived as important transition times for children and families as they enter the schooling process and as they progress into middle school and adolescence.

The LIFT program is based on the model of coercive adult–child interaction developed by the clinicians and researchers at the Oregon Social Learning Center (OSLC). It is "hypothesized that the driving force in a child's conduct problems are the reinforcement processes that occur in his or her day-to-day relationships" (J. B. Reid & Eddy, 2002, p. 222). Therefore, Eddy et al. (2000) noted that

> the LIFT targets for change those child and parent behaviors thought to be most relevant to the development of adolescent delinquent and violent behaviors, namely opposition, defiance, and social ineptitude on the part of the child and disciplining and monitoring on the part of the parent (see Stoff et al., 1997).

The program is delivered in three contexts in the LIFT program: in the classroom, on the playground, and with the family or parents. The classroom program is delivered by the teacher or other classroom instructor and consists of teaching prosocial behaviors with peers. Two 30-minute sessions are held weekly for 10 weeks. Skills targeted include problem-solving skills, listening, emotional recognition and management, and group cooperation. In addition, fifth-grade students are taught study skills important for middle school success. Instruction includes lecture, discussion, and skill practices in small and large groups.

Following each classroom session, children participated in free play on the playground. Children were divided into small groups at the beginning of the program, and a modification of the Good Behavior Game was implemented (Barrish, Saunders, & Wolfe, 1969; Dolan et al., 1993). A LIFT instructor and playground monitors provided armbands and verbal praise for demonstrating positive social behaviors and docked points for negative behaviors. At the end of recess, armbands were collected and counted, and points were counted as well. The small groups as well as the class accessed rewards daily according to the number of armbands and points. The playground component allowed for practice and reinforcement of the skills learned during the classroom intervention.

Other aspects of the LIFT program include dissemination of a weekly newsletter to families, development of frequent parent–teacher communication through installation of a phone line and answering machine in each classroom, and weekly phone calls by the parent trainers to each family in their respective parent group.

Review of the Parent Training Component

Parent training was conducted in groups of 10 to 15 families. Sessions of 1.5 hours each were held weekly for 6 weeks. The group training process included lecture, discussion, role-play, videotaped vignettes, assignment of home practices, and review of home practice results. Child care was provided during these meetings. Parents could attend sessions during weekday evenings or on a weekday afternoon. If parents could not attend a session, a home visit was scheduled for the same week. If a home visit was not possible, written materials were delivered to the parents for review about that week's session content. Parent group leaders also called each parent weekly to monitor home practices and answer any questions the parent might have.

The content of the sessions for Grades 1 and 5 similar but emphasized developmentally appropriate topics such as positive play interactions for first-grade students and negotiation skills for fifth-grade students. The content of the parent training groups was also linked to the social skills taught in the classroom intervention. The parent groups and classroom and playground interventions were all conducted during the same period of time within the academic year. Specific topics covered during training are similar to what Patterson and colleagues developed in their evidence-based parent training program more than 30 years ago (Patterson, Reid, Jones, & Conger, 1975). These topics include disengagement; paying attention sooner; appearing calm; using small positive and negative consequences; listening and tracking; making effective requests; controlling negative emotions; giving encouragement; defining cooperation; developing behavior contracts; using time-out, work chores, and response cost (i.e., privilege removal); working with teachers; and problem solving.

Empirical Support

Twelve schools from high juvenile crime areas in the Eugene–Springfield, Oregon, area were randomly chosen to participate in the study. The program was implemented over 3 years from 1991 through 1994. Within the schools, first- and fifth-grade classrooms were randomly chosen to participate. There were 382 children in the intervention group and 289 children in the control group. Attrition over the 3 years was low, only 3%. Participants were mostly Caucasian and lower to middle income, which was generally representative of the geographic catchment area (Eddy et al., 2000). Immediate improvements were noted in observations of playground behavior, mother–child interactions, and teacher behavior ratings in the classroom. Significantly fewer aggressive incidents were observed for the children in the program than for control children on the playground.

Mothers in the treatment condition were observed to demonstrate greater reductions of aversive behaviors compared with mothers in the control condition. Teachers rated fewer behavior problems for children in the program compared with children in the control condition. These findings were consistent across the first- and fifth-grade samples. The effect sizes ranged from low to large and were greatest for children and mothers with the highest levels of negative behaviors during pretest evaluation. Longer term effects several years later indicate that children who participated in the program in first grade were less likely than the control group to evidence symptoms of attention-deficit disorder, according to teacher reports. Children who participated in the program in fifth grade were less likely to be arrested in the 30 months following completion of the program compared with children in the control group. Fifth-grade students in the LIFT program were also less likely to report patterned alcohol use, and teachers reported they were less likely to affiliate with defiant peer groups (J. B. Reid & Eddy, 2002).

In summary, the LIFT program appears to have immediate positive effects on child behavior with observed changes in parent and child outcomes, in addition to ratings by parents and teachers. Long-term effects in child functioning were also noted. Replication of this program in other settings and with other samples of children and families, as well as teachers and clinicians, would be helpful to determine how well it may be implemented in practice.

Adolescent Transitions Program

Overview of the Program

ATP is a multilevel prevention and intervention strategy that is targeted to preadolescents and adolescents in middle schools. A book for clinicians on development and implementation of ATP (Dishion & Kavanagh, 2003) describes its logistical aspects, as well as the clinical skills necessary for interviewing children and families, intervening directly with adolescents, and training parents individually or in groups. It also provides a summary of empirical research on the program.

ATP focuses on providing services to parents and families within a school context. There are three levels, or "tiers," in the program. Tier 1 is described as a universal prevention strategy and involves development of a family resource center (FRC) within a middle school or high school. The FRC is staffed by a full-time professional with expertise in parent training and classroom consultation. The FRC provides a parent orientation meeting at the beginning of the school year and has media on effective parenting and normative information available for parents. The FRC staff members work in classrooms to provide instruction and exercises for adolescents to improve parent–child interaction and promote family management practices. The FRC staff facilitates communication with parents regarding adolescents' behavior, school attendance, academic work completion, and academic performance. If necessary, parents and adolescents may be referred to a higher level of intervention.

Tier 2 is described as a selected prevention strategy and is the initial stage of direct intervention work with a family. Parents and their adolescents may be referred for this level of intervention by school personnel through contact with the FRC staff or by self-referral. Referrals typically occur because of concerns regarding the adolescent's adjustment or behavior at home or at school. The primary strategy of intervention at this level consists of a "family check-up" (FCU). The FCU is a three-session intervention that consists of an initial interview with the adolescent and participating family members (parents), a comprehensive assessment of individual and family functioning, and a feedback session to review assessment results and encourage maintenance of positive behaviors and systematic changes in negative or problematic behaviors.

Tier 3 is an indicated prevention or intervention strategy that provides direct intervention services to parents and adolescents to remediate problems that cannot be addressed during Tier 2, or that were addressed unsuccessfully. The intervention strategies in this tier are dependent on assessment information gathered during the FCU. The book by Dishion and Kavanagh (2003) provides a menu of intervention strategies. Examples of interventions at this tier include participation in a family management group, a home–school note program, one to two sessions focused on a particular topic, monthly monitoring, individual family management therapy, or referral to more intensive services in the community.

Review of the Parent Training Component

Whereas the FAST Track and LINK programs include multiple components within multiple settings, ATP is largely focused on improving parenting skills as the prevention strategy. There are no systematic intervention components targeting behavior and academic problems in the classroom or targeting peer relations. Parent training in the ATP largely occurs in Tier 3 and is derived from the Family Management Curriculum (FMC; Dishion et al., 2003). The FMC is a 12-session parent training program. It is designed for groups of 8 to 16 parents. It is focused primarily on parents of children in middle school with mild to moderate behavior problems. Weekly phone calls are conducted to monitor parent progress with homework. Home visits are also encouraged as necessary to encourage or further train parent skills.

There are three broad content areas within the curriculum: (a) the use of incentives for behavior change, (b) limit setting and monitoring, and (c) relationship skills. The curriculum includes an active skills teaching approach with didactic presentation, group discussion, modeling, videotapes, role-play and practice, and homework for parents; it is based on the theoretical and empirical research developed at the OSLC by Patterson and colleagues (1975). There appears to be overlap with the two-part manual titled *Parents and Adolescents: Living Together* (Forgatch & Patterson, 1987, 2005; Patterson & Forgatch, 1987, 2005; see also chap. 2, this volume).

Empirical Support

Research to date is supportive of the FMC for reducing child problem behaviors and improving parenting skills (Dishion & Andrews, 1995; Irvine, Biglan, Smolkowski, Metzler, & Ary, 1999). As a prevention program, ATP has been evaluated for its effects on adolescent substance use. Data indicate that youth who had contact with the ATP were less likely to report substance use such as tobacco, alcohol, marijuana, and other illicit drugs over the previous month. This was true whether the youth were categorized as at risk or typically developing. Because the typically developing youth were not as likely to have had Tier 3 services or even Tier 2 service, this finding provides some indirect support for the FRC services as a universal prevention (Dishion, Kavanagh, Schneiger, Nelson, & Kaufman, 2002).

At this time, the data appear promising for ATP as a prevention and intervention strategy. Additional research using stronger experimental designs is needed, as is research targeting more direct measures of youth functioning. Replication in other settings and additional research on immediate and long-term effects of this prevention approach are needed. Of particular question may be the differential effect of the various levels of parent education and parent training in this program on parent and child outcomes.

Summary of Prevention Strategies

The descriptions of these prevention programs reveal that parent training is but one component of these comprehensive prevention programs. In addition, the programs rely on multiple staff members and practitioners. There is extensive attention paid to intervening in multiple contexts in which children and parents function, such as the school, playground, and community, so that changes in child and parent behavior may be better maintained over time. Much more research regarding the effects of these programs for the prevention of child and adolescent problems needs to be conducted before conclusions can be drawn regarding efficacy. However, parenting skills are clearly a key variable in these prevention efforts (Forgatch & Knutson, 2002; Kumpfer & Alvarado, 2003). If these programs are demonstrated to be efficacious, future research replicating them in other settings and with other populations will be needed. In addition, future research examining the differential effects of the individual components of these programs will be necessary. Effectiveness research will also be needed before implementing these programs in practice. Prevention research is costly in terms of time, money, and other resources, and as noted by Biglan, Mrazek, Carnine, and Flay (2003, p. 433), the pace and success of prevention programs will be dependent on the "actions that scientific and funding organizations take to facilitate the process." Although much work remains, the promise of preventing later child, adolescent, and adult problems seems worth the price for continued research at this time.

FUTURE RESEARCH WITH IMPLICATIONS FOR PRACTICE

Prevention is but one area of research in parent training that may have important implications for practitioners in the future. Although many excellent resources provide up-to-date reviews of research in parenting and parent training (e.g., Bornstein, 2002; Hoghughi & Long, 2004; J. B. Reid, Patterson, & Snyder, 2002), it can be difficult for practitioners to keep abreast of research with practical implications for parent training. It might be said that all research has some potential value to affect practice positively, but it is clear that some research has more direct implications than other research. In the sections that follow, we present some research areas and questions with particular practical relevance for the day-to-day practice of parent training that may be addressed in future research.

The topics and questions presented here are largely derived from the parent training research and practice guidelines presented in previous chapters. We seek to highlight for practitioners and researchers some of the topics and questions that still need to be addressed relevant to the day-to-day practice of parent training. Topics and questions are organized under specific areas of research, including ongoing research regarding (a) empirically supported parent training programs, (b) parent training for the treatment of other child problems, (c) how to train parents, (d) models of child development and parenting, and (e) examination of disseminating research for practice. Ongoing and preliminary research is occurring in each of these areas, and we attempt to note some of the relevant and recent research in addition to proposing questions that remain to be addressed. Areas, topics, and some questions for future research in parent training are summarized in Table 9.1.

Research on the Empirically Supported Parent Training Programs

Although the empirically supported parent training programs are considered to be well supported or even exemplary, many topics and questions still need to be addressed (Forehand & Kotchick, 2002). Three topics of particular importance to practitioners stand out: (a) examination of the efficacy and effectiveness of these programs with different populations or in different settings, (b) analysis of components of the programs to improve the efficacy and effectiveness of the programs, and (c) comparison of the programs with each other and as a standard for other parent training programs addressing child noncompliance.

Other Populations and Settings

Many practitioners work in clinical, school, and other community agency settings and with a diverse population of children and families, but the empirically supported parent training programs were developed and tested largely in university-affiliated clinics with middle-class Caucasian families. Continued research on the application of these programs to address child noncompliance in other settings and with other populations of children and families is needed.

The Incredible Years and the Helping the Noncompliant Child (HNC) and Parent–Child Interaction Therapy (PCIT) parent training programs have some initial research support for their efficacy with other populations and in other settings. The Incredible Years has been evaluated for its efficacy when applied in a Head Start setting and with other ethnic groups (M. J. Reid, Webster-Stratton, & Beauchaine, 2001; Webster-Stratton, 1998; Webster-Stratton, Reid, & Hammond, 2001) and in clinical practice settings (Scott, 2005). As described in chapter 7 of this volume, the HNC program has been applied in the treatment of noncompliance for other populations, such as children with developmental disabilities and attention-deficit/hyperactivity disorder and children who have been abused and neglected (Wells, 2003). In addition, the program has been used in inpatient settings and adopted for use in prevention programs in school settings (Conduct Problems Prevention Research Group, 2004; Wells, 2003). The PCIT program has been implemented with other populations of parents, such as fathers (Bagner & Eyberg, 2003) and parents who have abused or neglected their children (Timmer, Urquiza, & Zebell, 2005). The PCIT program has initial research support for use with

TABLE 9.1
Research Directions in Parent Training Important for Practice

Area	Topics	Examples of research questions
Empirically supported parent training programs	Efficacy Effectiveness Extending populations and settings Component analyses Program comparisons	Is the program efficacious for other child or parent populations? Is the program efficacious in settings other than the clinic, such as schools or community agencies? What adaptations are needed for the program to be effective with other populations or in other settings? What components of commands are most important to increase the probability of child compliance? Which time-out procedures are most effective to reduce child noncompliance? What are the additive effects of commands relative to reinforcement and punishment? Does the order of presentation of components affect child or parent outcomes? Which assessment procedures and data contribute best to treatment decisions in parent training? Is one program more efficacious or effective (or both) relative to another program? Are more recent programs as efficacious or effective as the empirically supported parent training programs?
Extensions to other child problems	Efficacy and effectiveness of the empirically supported parent training programs in treating other child problems Efficacy and effectiveness of training parents to implement evidence-based interventions for other child problems	Is the program efficacious in treating other child problems, such as depression, bedtime problems, academic problems, stealing, etc.? Can parents be trained to deliver evidence-based interventions to address child depression, bedtime problems, stealing, etc., and is this training efficacious or effective in treating the child problems?
How to train parents	Defining adherence Identifying strategies to improve adherence	How much adherence to treatment recommendations is necessary or sufficient to obtain beneficial child outcomes? What level or type of practitioner support is needed for parents to meet necessary or sufficient levels of parental adherence? Is videotaped modeling as effective as live modeling for changing parent behavior? Is group-based parent training as efficacious as individualized training? Is clinic- or school-based parent training as efficacious as home-based parent training?

foster parents (Fricker-Elhai, Ruggiero, & Smith, 2005; Timmer, Sedlar, & Urquiza, 2004) and in Head Start workshops for African American parents (Lipson, Eisenstadt, & Hembree-Kigin, 1993).

Each of the studies described represents good initial efforts to address the efficacy of the programs in other settings and with other populations of children and families. However, continued research, including replications, is needed. One study demonstrating efficacy with a particular sample of parents and children or in a particular setting is helpful, but two studies demonstrating efficacy, particularly if conducted by other researchers, leads to more confidence that the programs are beneficial across settings and populations.

In addition to studies of efficacy, examination of issues related to the effectiveness of the parent training programs with other populations and in other settings is also important. Whereas efficacy research may examine whether a particular program works with an identified population or setting, effectiveness research may examine particular adaptations in the program that are made for the program to work in particular settings or with particular populations of families and children. It may be expected that implementation of the empirically supported programs in other settings or with other populations of children and families may require some changes or adaptations (see chaps. 5 and 6).

The Living With Children parent training program (Patterson, 1976) may be particularly suited for modification to match setting and client characteristics. The Living With Children program emphasizes the identification and teaching of behavioral principles for parents to use in solving behavior problems. This emphasis has resulted in a parent training program that has gradually evolved since its inception in the 1970s. Recent research from the OSLC is extending parent training to other populations, including foster parents, divorced parents, and stepparents (Chamberlain, Fisher, & Moore, 2002; Forgatch & DeGarmo, 2002; Forgatch, DeGarmo, & Beldavs, 2005). In addition, parent training has been used to address problems presented by other populations (e.g., Latino; Martinez & Eddy, 2005) and to adolescents (Dishion & Kavanagh, 2003). Practitioner manuals have been developed for some of these populations (e.g., Forgatch, 1994).

A recent meta-analysis suggests that low family income and maternal mental health may be important predictors of whether there are beneficial outcomes of parent training (Reyno & McGrath, 2006). Parents of lower family income and poor maternal mental health appear less likely to benefit from parent training. It also appears that parent training can lead to lower reported maternal depression (Bunting, 2004; DeGarmo et al., 2004). Further research examining how maternal depression may affect child outcomes in parent training, and how training may affect maternal depression, is needed. Specific to practice, researchers may address how best to involve mothers with depression in training. For example, mothers who are depressed may be less likely to initiate attending to and praise with their children contingent on compliant behavior. Explicit prompting procedures, such as timers and predetermined time intervals to deliver differential attention, may be examined for their effectiveness in improving parental adherence and child outcomes. Researchers may also examine whether adjunct therapy for maternal depression improves parent training outcomes. This is consistent with recent extensions of parent training as part of behavioral family intervention (Sanders, 1996). The role of fathers in parent training with mothers with depression has not been examined (Ramchandani & McConachie, 2005). Researchers might address whether greater father involvement in parent training sessions may facilitate child outcomes relative to mother involvement only, particularly for mothers with depression.

Parents of low-income status typically have fewer resources, and this may impede effective implementation of certain procedures in parent training. For example, parents in low-income housing are more likely to have limited space in their home or apartment or have neighbors nearby that make it difficult to allow a child to scream and throw a tantrum during time-out or as part of an extinction burst because the child's screaming disrupts others in the family or neighborhood. Researchers may examine other forms of punishment such as response cost relative to time-out in parent training or implementation of reinforcement programs for children to comply quietly with time-out procedures as part of parent training. In addition, researchers might examine whether parent training that is provided in community agencies in low-income areas relative to other clinical settings outside these communities improves attendance, adherence, and outcomes (e.g., Webster-Stratton, 1997). The practitioner in an agency within the low-income community may be more aware of local problems (e.g., inaccessibility of resources) or barriers (e.g., cultural) that may impede adherence to parent training. In addition, services provided locally or in the neighborhood reduce problems with transportation and encourage consistent attendance. Other variables related to implementation of parent training for low-income families may include provision of transportation and child care or helping parents access other social service agencies, such as employment or social security, that may provide support for making the behavioral changes expected during parent training.

Because most children attend school, school settings may provide more of a community-centered approach for low-income families because they may be more comfortable with their local school, relative to a clinic setting, and the school may be more likely to be in their neighborhood. A few researchers have examined the efficacy and effectiveness of parent training in school settings (Cunningham et al., 2000; Marchant, Young, & West, 2004; Markey, Markey, Quant, Santelli, & Turnbull, 2002), but there has been a paucity of peer-reviewed research evaluating evidence-based parent training programs in school settings (Valdez, Carlson, & Zanger, 2005). Because many practitioners in schools have a large number of children for whom they are responsible, it seems probable that parent training by practitioners in schools can be accomplished most effectively in a group-training format. The Incredible Years is the only group-based parent training program with empirical support. However, the HNC and PCIT programs have been adapted for use in group formats (McMahon & Forehand, 2003; Niec, Hemme, Yopp, & Brestan, 2005). Researchers may compare outcomes of the HNC or PCIT group-based parent training programs delivered in a school setting with a parent education (no behavioral skills training) group delivered in the same school setting. Researchers might also address whether the group parent training format of The Incredible Years is comparable in outcomes to the group parent training format of the HNC or PCIT program in a school setting.

In clinical settings, time is often constrained by managed care policies. All of the empirically supported parent training programs require numerous sessions and extensive time with individual parents. In addition, the HNC and PCIT program have established criteria that parents are expected to meet before moving on to the next phase of treatment. The number of sessions and the criteria may influence the effectiveness of the programs in clinical practice by increasing the parent dropout rate (e.g., Boggs et al., 2004). Researchers may address the effect of implementing abbreviated versions of the empirically supported programs in terms of duration of sessions or frequency of sessions. For example, one study found that an abbreviated version of PCIT may have outcomes comparable to the standard PCIT program (Nixon, Sweeney, Erickson, & Touyz, 2003). Replication of this study is needed, and further investigations of abbreviated programs for each of the empirically supported parent training programs are needed. Researchers may address which minimal criteria lead to most beneficial outcomes for children. Lower criteria for mastery would assist parents' completion of the program within a shorter period of time, perhaps reducing dropout rates.

Component Analyses

Practitioners often have constraints that impede implementation of time- and resource-intensive interventions. For this reason, it is important that the empirically supported parent training programs continue to be examined to determine the components that are most important to positive parent and child outcomes. The authors of the HNC parent training program have devoted much effort to researching the various aspects of parent training and child intervention to reduce noncompliance. For example, these researchers and others have examined the effectiveness of attending and rewards (Kotler & McMahon, 2004), effective instructions (Roberts, 1982, 1988; Roberts, McMahon, Forehand, & Humphreys, 1978) and timeout (Bean & Roberts, 1981; Hobbs, Forehand, & Murray, 1978). It is important not only to demonstrate the differential effect of each program component but also to determine how they should be implemented in relation to each other. For example, previous research on the PCIT program suggests that the order in which child-directed and parent-directed interaction are presented does not differentially affect child outcomes in terms of improving compliance (Eisenstadt, Eyberg, McNeil, Newcomb, & Funderburk, 1993).

Although this previous research serves an important role in demonstrating the efficacy of individual components of the parent training programs, replication is needed. Many of the previous studies were conducted in clinical settings with a small number of referred or recruited children and their mothers. Replication would advance confidence regarding use of these component procedures in other clinics and settings and with different populations of children and parents. For example, there are still important questions regarding the most effective procedures for providing commands. Parents often do not naturally provide effective commands and must be taught how to do so. Researchers have noted that the proximity of the parent to the child is important when giving commands to increase child compliance (Hudson & Blane, 1985). Likewise, eye contact before a command may increase compliance (Hamlet, Axelrod, & Kuerschner, 1984). The rate and type of commands may also influence compliance (Houlihan, Vincent, & Ellison, 1994). Researchers may examine the differential or additive effects of these variables on child compliance as part of training parents to provide effective commands. Practitioners would benefit from further research demonstrating the most effective components of good commands to improve child compliance.

In addition, each of the empirically supported parent training programs uses different procedures for time-out and for enforcing the procedure with children who are resistant to it. Researchers may continue to explore the effectiveness of various time-out procedures and, particularly, to address the identification of effective techniques enforcing time-out.

Researchers may also examine the additive effects of specific components on treatment outcomes. For example, the additive effect of teaching parents effective commands relative to reinforcement and punishment procedures is still unknown. Specific differential and additive effects of parental skills such as reflections or imitation in PCIT may also be examined. If these are skills that do not contribute to positive child outcomes, then it is questionable whether practitioners should spend time and effort training parents in them. A difficulty with examining the additive effects of components is determining how much a particular component should add to the outcomes to be considered worthwhile. Researchers and practitioners need to examine the additive effects from a cost–benefit perspective. For example, teaching parents effective commands may not provide substantially improved child outcomes, but it may be a relatively simple task that is determined to be worth the time and effort for the benefit gained.

The treatment validity of the evaluation procedures administered before initiation of parent training programs has not yet been evaluated. *Treatment validity* refers to whether an assessment measure or procedure provides data that contributes to the development of effective treatments (Hayes, Nelson, & Jarrett, 1987). The manuals for the empirically supported parent training programs provide descriptions of evaluation procedures that include interviews, observations, and rating forms, but it is not known how or whether data from these measures contribute to decision making in the programs. For example, it is unclear which information from parents is most useful in determining how to proceed in parent training or which behavior rating forms are most useful to determining which interventions to teach and how to teach them or which child behaviors to target. Knowing which assessment methods are most informative or useful for decision making regarding treatment could help reduce practitioners' time and costs in assessment. For example, if behavior rating forms do not provide useful information regarding treatment, it is not worth the practitioner's time and cost to have parents complete behavior rating forms. There are specific research designs that can be used to examine the differential effect of assessment measures on treatment decisions (Hayes et al., 1987).

Observations of parent–child interaction are recommended in all of the programs, but the procedures for observation vary. Research identifying the most efficient procedures for observation leading to effective treatment decisions would be helpful to practitioners. This type of research may involve comparing the treatment utility of data obtained from the various observational procedures, as well as the relative costs in time and resources for each observation procedure. There is also minimal research directly comparing data from clinical observations and home observations of parent–child interaction. It is still unclear to what degree data from clinical observations agree or accurately represent data from home observations. Additional studies on the validity of analogue or clinical observations are needed (Gardner, 2000; Haynes, 1991).

Research demonstrates the utility of functional behavior assessment for identifying and developing effective treatment components (Watson & Steege, 2003). A functional behavior assessment is conducted to identify relations or contingencies (e.g., positive or negative reinforcement) that maintain behavior. However, little research is specific to the empirically supported parent training programs regarding the role that functional behavior assessment may play in parent training. Although coercion theory assumes escape is the primary function of noncompliance, the empirically supported parent training programs have procedures in place to address both attention and escape as possible functions for child noncompliance. The programs are not universally effective for all children who are noncompliant, however. For children who are "treatment resistors," functional behavior assessment may provide data that lead to more effective outcomes. Of course, this would seemingly require changes in the parent training program, and future research should examine what changes based on functional behavior assessment data would lead to better child outcomes.

Comparisons Between Programs

The empirically supported parent training programs have derived some of their research support by showing beneficial outcomes relative to control or wait-list parent groups or other types of child treatment. These programs have not yet been compared with each other to determine whether one may provide better child and parent outcomes relative to another. This is important, because the programs include different procedures and may involve different costs in terms of time and resources. For example, Living With Children uses a point system and tangible rewards, whereas PCIT and HNC rely more on social attention for reinforcement. Each of the programs also has different procedures for punishment, whether it be time-out or a response cost system. In addition, the skill level expected of practitioners may differ between programs. Direct comparisons would examine the duration of time and amount of resources needed to implement the programs relative to the benefits accrued. This information would be helpful for practitioners to determine which program may best suit their needs and the needs of the children and families they serve. Researchers may also examine the resources and time required to bring practitioners to the point that they can implement each program with integrity. This would allow practitioners to judge which programs may best fit with their current skill level and training needs.

Several promising parent training programs address child problems of noncompliance and oppositional behaviors; these include Triple P (Sanders, 1999), Parent Management Training (Kazdin, 2005), Barkley's Defiant Child (Barkley, 1997), and Common Sense (Burke, Herron, & Schuchmann, 2004). Triple P and Common Sense are reviewed in chapter 3 of this volume; the other two programs are not reviewed. Each of these newer parent training programs has good initial research support. Questions arise, however, regarding why practitioners might choose one of these programs over one of the empirically supported parent training programs. It may be that these newer parent training programs produce better child and parent outcomes or that they are more time-, resource-, or cost-efficient. Perhaps they are more effective with particular parent or child populations or particular types of child problems. Certainly, comparison of these programs with control or other types of child treatment groups provides information about the efficacy of the program and is the first step for research. In addition, research comparing these parent training programs with the empirically supported parent training programs is needed to determine whether these up-and-coming programs may be more efficacious and effective.

Research on Parent Training for the Treatment of Other Child Problems

Practitioners typically work with children who present with a wide variety of problems beyond noncompliance. Although PCIT, Living With Children, and The Incredible Years all make claims regarding the efficacy of the programs in the treatment of other problems, there is minimal research in these areas. The reliance of each of the programs on behavioral principles and a behavioral skills training model suggests that they may be useful for solving other problems. A pilot study has been conducted examining the use of PCIT to address separation anxiety (Choate, Pincus, & Eyberg, 2005). Certainly, additional research should be conducted to examine whether and how the empirically supported parent training programs for noncompliance may be used to address the other types of child problems that program developers claim are appropriate targets for their programs.

Rather than taking a parent training program for noncompliance and adapting it to address other child problems, it may be best to take effective interventions for other child problems and adapt them to a parent training model. This second approach is largely the focus of chapter 7. Numerous studies have demonstrated effective interventions for other child problems, but a need to demonstrate effective application of these interventions in parent training remains. Development and empirical testing of manuals or protocols for parent training to address child problems of sleep, toileting, eating, and other child concerns is needed. Along this line, replication of studies supporting interventions to address other child problems should be conducted with particular emphasis placed on procedural aspects of how parents were trained to implement the procedures. For example, research may support interventions for picky eating that intersperse preferred with less preferred foods, but additional research that demonstrates exactly how parents should be trained to deliver this intervention effectively is lacking. Specific procedures for parent training to address picky eating need to be developed, empirically examined, and disseminated, and these efforts need to be replicated to develop parent training for other child problems.

Research on How to Train Parents

Behavioral skills training including instruction, modeling, rehearsal, and feedback has empirical support as an effective teaching strategy (Miltenberger, 2001) and is an integral part of empirically supported parent training programs. However, this does not necessarily mean that there is clear consensus about the most effective methods to use to instruct parents or model skills, how much rehearsal to include, or even how to provide feedback most effectively. There are excellent books on how to collaborate with parents and engage parents in parent training (Webster-Stratton & Herbert, 1994). There are also some journal articles describing examples of how to teach intervention procedures such as time-out, job card grounding (e.g., assigning chores as discipline), or behavior contracts (e.g., Eaves, Sheperis, & Blanchard, 2005). However, little solid empirical information exists about how best to collaborate with parents to engage them in the behavioral skills training.

Delineating variables regarding how we teach is important because the teaching strategies used in parent training can affect parents' adherence to treatment recommendations. Some researchers have examined variables that may increase adherence and completion of parent training, such as using audio cueing to increase parents' rate of attending behaviors (Hupp & Allen, 2005) or examining practitioners' verbal behavior at the beginning of treatment (M. D. Harwood & Eyberg, 2004). However, there is a paucity of empirical research on how to train parents to ensure adequate adherence to treatment recommendations so that parent training and child interventions will be effective.

Two topics for future research related to how we teach parents have particular implications for practitioners. The first relates to defining and determining what adherence means and to what degree parents need to adhere to treatment recommendations for beneficial treatment outcomes. The second topic is identifying effective strategies for teaching parents that increase adherence and outcomes.

Defining Adherence

Treatment adherence, fidelity, and *integrity* are terms that refer to whether interventions are implemented as intended (Allen & Warzak, 2000; Detrich, 1999; Gresham, 2005). On the one hand, *treatment integrity* and *fidelity* generally refer to whether the practitioner implemented an intervention as intended. In parent training, this would mean that the practitioner closely followed the procedures outlined in the empirically supported parent training programs or other manualized treatments. Treatment integrity is a particularly important subject for research because it is necessary to describe procedures clearly and in sufficient detail so that others can replicate them. In practice, however, variation or adaptation of treatment protocols on the basis of clinical expertise is common.

On the other hand, *treatment adherence* generally refers to whether the parent implements the intervention as recommended or taught by the practitioner. Parental adherence is a particularly difficult subject because it is unclear what parents should be expected to do in terms of adherence. It is not reasonable to expect parents to adhere to 100% of treatment recommendations with 100% integrity for 100% of the time (e.g., Detrich, 1999).

Researchers need to address what level of adherence is necessary or sufficient for beneficial child outcomes in parent training. In addition, the level of support needed for parental adherence to treatment recommendations appears relatively high in many research-based protocols and in the empirically supported parent training programs for noncompliance. Researchers may examine the least level of support a practitioner can provide to a parent that will still result in adequate parental adherence and positive child outcomes. Researchers may examine differences in child outcomes between groups of parents trained to different levels of or provided different levels of support for adherence. Measuring adherence is difficult because it is necessary to measure parent and child behavior in the home setting. Video cameras, live observations, parent self-reports, spouse reports, and child reports of parent behavior are possible methods for measuring adherence.

Teaching Strategies

Many questions remain in parent training regarding how practitioners can most effectively provide instructions, model skills, rehearse, and provide feedback to parents to increase parental adherence with intervention recommendations. For example, researchers may address whether parents benefit from reading instructional materials or written protocols in implementing treatments and what type of materials or protocol formats lead to greater treatment adherence (e.g., Danforth, 1999). Previous research reviews suggest that videotape modeling of skills in groups may be just as effective as modeling in individual-based parent training (Behan & Carr, 2000). Research replicating these findings would assist practitioners in making decisions regarding the purchase of videos and decisions for how to use them in practice. It would seem that videotaped modeling could be a more cost-efficient method and involve less response effort on the part of the practitioner relative to live modeling, possibly improving practitioners' treatment integrity.

Some parent training programs use dolls in role-play with parents, and researchers might address whether this results in comparable parental adherence to intervention relative to role-play with their child. It may be expected that, for some parents, their child would come to function as a discriminative stimulus from rehearsal in the clinic, and this could facilitate generalization of parent skills to the home setting. In addition, researchers may examine how often parents should practice skills at home to achieve performance standards necessary for attaining treatment goals. Researchers may also examine whether spouses or parent partners can provide feedback to one another during practice at home to improve adherence.

Other research that may be conducted includes examining whether group parent training produces greater adherence to recommendations relative to individualized parent training. Perhaps parents in group situations will be more likely to adhere to practitioner recommendations to avoid corrective feedback in front of other parents, or perhaps parents in individualized parent training may have more opportunities for rehearsal of skills and feedback from the practitioner that increases adherence relative to parents in groups.

The setting in which training takes place may well affect treatment adherence and generalization of skills. Researchers may examine whether parents trained in a clinic setting adhere to recommendations as well as parents trained in a home setting. On the basis of what we know about stimulus control and generalization (see chap. 4), the expectation would be that parents trained at home should adhere better to recommended treatment relative to parents trained in the clinic, but this has not been systematically investigated. This information may be important for practitioners in school or clinical settings who are not having success with a family and who might make referrals to community agencies that provide home-based treatment services.

Research on how to teach seems to have immediate practical implications for practitioners, and many questions need to be addressed. An area of research with less immediate implications for practitioners but still highly important is that on causal models of child development and parenting.

Research on Models of Child Development and Parenting

It is possible to develop and implement intervention techniques and teaching strategies without reference to basic science principles and empirical models and theories. However, it has been our premise throughout this book, and it is an implicit premise of a scientist–practitioner model and evidence-based practice, that knowledge of the science underlying practice will improve practice. Some previous research suggests that training parents in basic learning principles as part of a parent training program results in better parent and child outcomes relative to parents who are not trained in these principles (McMahon, Forehand, & Griest, 1981). Additional research, particularly related to what content knowledge is needed by parents to achieve the best child outcomes and how best this content may be taught, is necessary. On a related note, little attention has been paid to what practitioners need to know about the empirical models and conceptual underpinnings of child development and parent training. Researchers may address whether practitioners' knowledge of the conceptual foundations of parent training leads to better parent and child outcomes. Along this line, they may address what conceptual principles practitioners should know to improve parent training practice.

For the past several decades, Patterson and colleagues at the OSLC have been at the forefront in developing models based on empirical research to explain child behavior, particularly antisocial behavior and parent influences on child development and antisocial behavior (J. B. Reid, Patterson, & Snyder, 2002). In particular, coercion theory has informed the development of the empirically supported parent training programs. Models of behavior provide description of variables that correlate with each other and demonstrate some level of predictability. Such models can often appear complex and esoteric with little immediate implication for practice. However, coercion theory has helped inform development of parent training programs, and there may be other practical implications derived from current models of parent–child interaction. Two examples of how an empirical model of child development and parent–child interaction may inform research and practice include time-out implementation and teaching parental monitoring.

Consider that the use of time-out appears conceptually inconsistent with a coercion theory account of disruptive behavior. Coercion theory suggests that escalating child behavior is negatively reinforced by the removal (i.e., escape) of a demand, yet time-out, which is implemented contingent on undesired child behavior, often results in escape from some demand. One might hypothesize that time-out could actually increase problem behavior through negative reinforcement. How, then, is time-out found to be an effective component of the empirically supported treatments? It may be the addition of an escape–extinction procedure in which the child is expected to comply or otherwise engage in desired behavior shortly following the implementation of time-out, which results in immediate reinforcement of compliance. Thus, although the time-out component affords brief escape from a demand, the requirement to comply after the time-out, followed by praise for compliance, adds escape extinction and differential reinforcement components. Researchers may consider comparing time-out procedures with and without expectations for compliance following the time-out. They might also address the type of expectation following time-out that may lead to better compliance. For example, researchers have not established whether the task following time-out needs to be the same task expected of the child before going to time-out or whether any task may be directed to the child and reinforced.

It may be that time-out is effective because the loss of access to reinforcement while sitting in time-out is more punishing relative to any reinforcement related to the removal of the demand when a child is sent to time-out. This possibility would require that the child have access to a relatively rich reinforcement environment. Research on relative rates of reinforcement provides some support for this contention (Snyder & Patterson, 1995), suggesting that child behavior is affected by the reinforcement obtained contingent on that behavior relative to reinforcement obtained for other behavior the child exhibits. This means that a child's negative behavior will be exhibited proportional to the reinforcement obtained for that behavior relative to the reinforcement obtained for other behavior the child may exhibit (see chap. 4, this volume, on choice). Continued research on the rates of reinforcement available for compliance and noncompliance and the role that time-out plays in affecting the relative rates of reinforcement may provide additional information about why time-out works and how to make the procedure more effective.

A second issue of potential importance to the practice of parent training that is derived from empirical models of parent–child interaction is the issue of parental monitoring (Dishion & McMahon, 1998; Patterson, Reid, &

Dishion, 1992). Parental monitoring has yet to be defined in a manner acceptable for general professional consensus (Crouter & Head, 2002), but parental monitoring can be viewed as "a broad construct comprising a set of more specific, but highly correlated parenting behaviors" (Dishion & McMahon, 1998, p. 66). These behaviors include "both structuring the child's home, school, and community environment and tracking the child's behavior in those environments" (Dishion & McMahon, 1998, p. 66). As a parental behavior, monitoring would appear to be a necessary skill for differentially reinforcing appropriate child behaviors and responding with punishment to negative child behaviors. Researchers may examine whether parents who are trained to monitor specific child behaviors implement interventions based on differential attention better than parents who have not been taught this skill. Researchers might also examine how practitioners can teach parents to increase parental monitoring behavior (Dishion & McMahon, 1998). Increasing reinforcement for this skill may be one solution, and researchers may examine effective techniques to increase monitoring that can be readily implemented in practice.

Disseminating Research for Practice

Much of the research of interest to practitioners that remains to be conducted falls within the purview of what has previously been termed *effectiveness studies* and *translating research into practice* (see chap. 8, this volume). In addition to conducting effectiveness research, there is a need to disseminate research findings effectively so that practitioners can integrate it with their clinical expertise to address unique child and family problems. Although researchers may publish their work, it is up to practitioners to take the initiative to search for, adapt, and apply research findings in their own practice. Research that is not effectively disseminated so that practitioners can read and apply it in practice is not useful to them. Publications in journals intended to report findings to scholars may not be helpful to practitioners who have more practical needs (Schoenwald & Hoagwood, 2001). Some ideas for better dissemination of research to practice have included putting empirically supported interventions on Web pages (e.g., the What Works Clearinghouse: http://www.strengtheningfamilies.org); publishing research-to-practice journals (Shriver & Watson, 2005); and providing support (i.e., time and money) for practitioners to attend workshops, conventions, and in-services (Riley-Tillman, Chafouleas, Eckert, & Kelleher, 2005). Unfortunately, current contingencies do not seem to support researchers publishing in outlets other than scholarly journals or employers providing increased opportunities, resources, or benefits to practitioners to access research. Further exploration of the barriers and possible solutions to address the research-to-practice gap is needed.

The empirically supported parent training programs are relatively accessible to practitioners, with the exception of the Living With Children program. There has been less emphasis over the years for the OSLC to research and update the original parent training program from 1975 (Patterson et al., 1975). For practitioners, it remains unclear what effect, if any, the prodigious ongoing research at OSLC may have had on the core content of this parent training program for child noncompliance. Given OSLC's continuing leadership in the field of parent training, practitioners may benefit from a revision of the 1975 clinician's manual for parent training, one that takes into account the research and clinical expertise that has accumulated in the interim. This would not only benefit practitioners, it would also allow other researchers to conduct studies using the Living With Children program. Currently, it is difficult for other researchers studying Living With Children to examine issues related to replication, analysis of components, and extensions to other populations or settings because there is little detail available regarding what exactly the Living With Children parent training program currently entails.

SUMMARY

A substantial amount of research has taken place since the mid-1960s on the topics of parenting and parent training. This research has led to the development of empirically supported parent training programs to treat noncompliance and social aggression. In addition, there is research support for the use of parent training to address other child problems. Nevertheless, important questions remain. Perhaps most important are those regarding how best to translate parent training from a controlled research environment into the relatively uncontrolled environment of the everyday practitioner. Indeed, the life of a practitioner presents significant challenges that are not easily overcome and are, in some ways, exacerbated by programs with standardized procedures not easily replicated or even appropriate for a diverse population of children and parents. At the same time, researchers striving to conduct effectiveness studies and translate research-to-practice find many challenges in disseminating their findings to those most interested.

Despite these challenges, parent training represents one of the most well-established approaches to dealing with the common child behavior problems seen in daily practice. Practitioners can have considerable confidence in knowing what basic skills to teach parents and how to go about teaching them. This confidence is enhanced by understanding that these practices are built on a common conceptual foundation with its own considerable empirical support. For these reasons, parent training is currently and should continue to be an essential part of an evidence-based practice.

REFERENCES

Aanstoos, C. M., Serlin, I., & Greening, T. (2000). A history of Division 32 (Humanistic Psychology) of the American Psychological Association. In D. A. Dewsbury (Ed.), *Unification through division: Histories of the divisions of the American Psychological Association* (Vol. V, pp. 85–112). Washington, DC: American Psychological Association.

Achenbach, T. M. (1991). *Manual for the Child Behavior Checklist and 1991 profile*. Burlington: Department of Psychiatry, University of Vermont.

Administration for Children and Families. (2002, October). Outcomes being documented for Parent–Child Interaction Therapy. *Children's Bureau Express, 3*(8). Retrieved December 12, 2007, from http://cbexpress.acf.hhs.gov

Ainsworth, M. D. S., & Bowlby, J. (1991). An ethological approach to personality development. *American Psychologist, 46,* 333–341.

Alexander, J. F., & Parsons, B. V. (1973). Short-term behavioral intervention with delinquent families: Impact of family process and recidivism. *Journal of Abnormal Psychology, 81,* 219–225.

Allen, K. D., & Warzak, W. J. (2000). The problem of parental nonadherence in clinical behavior analysis: Effective treatment is not enough. *Journal of Applied Behavior Analysis, 33,* 373–391.

Althen, G., Doran, A. R., & Szmania, S. J. (2002). *American ways: A guide for foreigners in the United States.* Yarmouth, ME: Intercultural Press.

American Psychological Association. (2002). Ethical principles of psychologists and code of conduct. *American Psychologist, 57,* 1060–1073.

American Psychological Association. (2003). Guidelines on multicultural education, training, research, practice, and organizational change for psychologists. *American Psychologist, 58,* 377–402.

American Psychological Association. (2005). *Policy statement on evidence-based practice in psychology.* Retrieved December 12, 2007, from http://www2.apaorg/practice/ebpstatement.pdf

Armenta, F. (1993). Latinos and group parent training: A research study with implications for increasing parental participation in group parent training. *Dissertation Abstracts International, 54* (1-B), 482.

Arndorfer, R. E., Allen, K. D., & Aljazireh, L. (1999). Behavioral health needs in pediatric medicine and the acceptability of behavioral solutions: Implications for behavioral psychologists. *Behavior Therapy, 30,* 137–148.

Azrin, N. H., & Foxx, R. M. (1974). *Toilet training in less than a day.* New York: Simon and Schuster.

Azrin, N. H., Sneed, T. J., & Foxx, R. M. (1974). Dry-bed training: Rapid elimination of childhood enuresis. *Behaviour Research and Therapy, 12,* 147–156.

Baer, D. M., Wolf, M. M., & Risley, T. R. (1968). Some current dimensions of applied behavior analysis. *Journal of Applied Behavior Analysis, 1,* 91–97.

Baer, D. M., Wolf, M. M., & Risley, T. R. (1987). Some still-current dimensions of applied behavior analysis. *Journal of Applied Behavior Analysis, 20,* 313–327.

Bagner, D. M., & Eyberg, S. M. (2003). Father involvement in parent training: When does it matter? *Journal of Clinical Child and Adolescent Psychology, 32,* 599–605.

Bailey, J. S. (1991). Marketing behavior analysis requires different talk. *Journal of Applied Behavior Analysis, 24,* 445–448.

Bakken, J., Miltenberger, R. G., & Schauss, S. (1993). Teaching parents with mental retardation: Knowledge versus skills. *American Journal on Mental Retardation, 97,* 405–417.

Bakken, J., Miltenberger, R. G., & Schauss, S. (2002). Teaching parents with mental retardation: Knowledge versus skills. In J. Blacher & B. L. Baker (Eds.), *Best of AAMR: Families and mental retardation: A collection of notable AAMR journal articles across the 20th century* (pp. 247–257). Washington, DC: American Association on Mental Retardation.

Balsam, P. D., & Bondy, A. S. (1983). The negative side effects of reward. *Journal of Applied Behavior Analysis, 16,* 283–296.

Barkley, R. A. (1997). *Defiant children: A clinician's manual for assessment and parent training* (2nd ed.). New York: Guilford Press.

Barlow, D. H., & Hersen, M. (1984). Single case experimental designs: Strategies for studying behavior change (2nd ed.). Elmsford, NY: Pergamon Press.

Barrish, H. H., Saunders, M., & Wolfe, M. D. (1969). Good behavior game. Effects of individual contingencies for group consequences and disruptive behavior in the classroom. *Journal of Applied Behavior Analysis, 2*, 119–124.

Bartz, K. W., & Levine, E. S. (1978). Childrearing by Black parents: A description and comparison to Anglo and Chicano parents. *Journal of Marriage and the Family, 40*, 709–720.

Basile, I. M., & Hintze, J. M. (1998). Combined effects of differential reinforcement of low rate (DRL) and alternative (DRA) schedules on out-of-seat behavior. *Proven Practice: Prevention and Remediation Solutions for Schools, 1*, 22–27.

Baumrind, D. (1971). Current patterns of parental authority. *Developmental Psychology Monographs, 4*(1, Pt. 2).

Bean, A. W., & Roberts, M. W. (1981). The effect of time-out release contingencies on changes in child noncompliance. *Journal of Abnormal Child Psychology, 9*, 95–105.

Bear, G. G. (1998). School discipline in the United States: Prevention, correction and long term social development. *Educational and Child Psychology, 15*, 15–39.

Begin, G. (1978). Sex makes a difference: Evidence from a modeling study conducted in a natural setting. *Psychological Reports, 43*, 103–109.

Behan, J., & Carr, A. (2000). Oppositional defiant disorder. In A. Carr (Ed.), *What works with children and adolescents? A critical review of psychological interventions with children, adolescents and their families* (pp. 102–130). Florence, KY: Taylor & Francis/Routledge.

Behavior Analyst Certification Board. (2004). *Behavior analyst certification board guidelines for responsible conduct for behavior analysts*. Retrieved December 12, 2007, from http://www.bacb.com/consum_frame.html

Benjet, C., & Kazdin, A. E. (2003). Spanking children: The controversies, findings, and new directions. *Clinical Psychology Review, 23*, 197–224.

Bergan, J. R., & Kratochwill, T. R. (1990). *Behavioral consultation and therapy*. New York: Plenum Press.

Bernal, M. E. (1984). Consumer issues in parent training. In R. F. Dangel & R. A. Polster (Eds.), *Parent training: Foundations of research and practice* (pp. 477–503). New York: Guilford Press.

Bernal, M. E., Klinnert, M. D., & Schultz, L. A. (1980). Outcome evaluation of behavioral parent training and client-centered parent counseling for children with conduct problems. *Journal of Applied Behavior Analysis, 13*, 677–691.

Bernhardt, A. J., & Forehand, R. L. (1975). The effects of labeled and unlabeled praise upon lower and middle class children. *Journal of Experimental Child Psychology, 19*, 536–543.

Berrett, R. D. (1975). Adlerian mother study groups: An evaluation. *Journal of Individual Psychology, 31*, 179–182.

Biglan, A., Mrazek, P. J., Carnine, D., & Flay, B. R. (2003). The integration of research and practice in the prevention of youth problem behaviors. *American Psychologist, 58*, 433–440.

Blum, I. H., & Koskinen, P. S. (1991). Repeated reading: A strategy for enhancing fluency and fostering experience. *Theory into Practice, 30,* 195–200.

Boggs, S. R., Eyberg, S., Edwards, D., Rayfield, A., Jabos, J., Bagner, D., & Hood, K. (2004). Outcomes of Parent–Child Interaction Therapy: A comparison of treatment completers and study dropouts one to three years later. *Child & Family Behavior Therapy, 26,* 1–22.

Bor, W., Sanders, M. R., & Markie-Dadds, C. (2002). The effects of the Triple P-Positive Parenting Program on preschool children with co-occurring disruptive behavior and attentional/hyperactive difficulties. *Journal of Abnormal Child Psychology, 30,* 571–587.

Borkowski, J. G., Landesman Ramey, S., & Bristol-Power, M. (2002). *Parenting and the child's world: Influences on academic, intellectual, and social-emotional development.* Mahwah, NJ: Erlbaum.

Bornstein, M. H. (Ed.). (2002). *Handbook of parenting* (2nd ed.; Vols. 1–5. Mahwah, NJ: Erlbaum.

Bradley, R. H. (2002). Environment and parenting. In M. H. Bornstein (Ed.), *Handbook of parenting: Vol. 2. Biology and ecology of parenting* (2nd ed., pp. 281–314). Mahwah, NJ: Erlbaum.

Brady, J. V. (1978). Foreword. In W. W. Henton & I. H. Iversen (Eds.), *Classical conditioning and operant conditioning* (pp. v–vii). New York: Springer-Verlag.

Brestan, E. V., & Eyberg, S. M. (1998). Effective psychosocial treatments of conduct disordered children and adolescents: 29 years, 82 studies, and 5272 kids. *Journal of Clinical Child Psychology, 27,* 180–189.

Briesmeister, J. M., & Schaefer, C. E. (Eds.). (1998). *Handbook of parenting training: Parents as co-therapists for children's behavior problems* (2nd ed.). New York: Wiley.

Brink, P. J. (1982). An anthropological perspective on parenting. In J. Horowitz, C. Hughes, & B. Perdue (Eds.), *Parenting reassessed: A nurse perspective* (pp. 66–84). Englewood Cliffs, NJ: Prentice-Hall.

Bromberg, D. S., & Johnson, B. T. (1997). Behavioral versus traditional approaches to prevention of child abduction. *School Psychology Review, 26,* 622–633.

Bronfenbrenner, U. (1986). Ecology of the family as a context for human development: Research perspectives. *Developmental Psychology, 22,* 723–742.

Bruch, M. A. (1978). Type of cognitive modeling, imitation of modeled tactics, and modification of test anxiety. *Cognitive Therapy and Research, 2,* 147–164.

Budd, K. S., Chugh, C. S., & Berry, S. L. (1998). Parents as therapists for children's food refusal problems. In J. M. Briesmeister & C. E. Schaefer (Eds.), *Handbook of parent training: Parents as co-therapists for children's behavior problems* (2nd ed., pp. 418–444). New York: Wiley.

Budzynski, T. H., & Stoyva, J. M. (1969). An instrument for producing deep muscle relaxation by means of analog information feedback. *Journal of Applied Behavior Analysis, 2,* 231–237.

Bugental, J. (1964). The third force in psychology. *Journal of Humanistic Psychology, 4,* 19–25.

Bunting, L. (2004). Parenting programmes: The best available evidence. *Child Care in Practice, 10*, 327–343.

Burke, R., Herron, R., & Schuchmann, L. F. (2004). *Common Sense Parenting: Learn at home workbook and DVD*. Boys Town, NE: Boys Town Press.

Caldwell, J. C. (1996). The demographic implications of West African family systems. *Journal of Comparative Family Studies, 27*, 331–352.

Cameron, J., & Pierce, W. D. (2002). *Rewards and intrinsic motivation: Resolving the controversy*. Westport, CT: Bergin & Garvey.

Canales, G. (2000). Gender as subculture: The first division of multicultural diversity. In I. Cuellar & F. A. Paniagua (Eds.), *Handbook of multicultural mental health: Assessment and treatment of diverse populations* (pp. 63–77). New York: Academic Press.

Capage, L. C., Bennett, G. M., & McNeil, C. B (2001). A comparison between African American and Caucasian children referred for treatment of disruptive behavior disorders. *Child & Family Behavior Therapy, 23*, 1–14.

Carter, J. H. (2002). Religion/spirituality in African-American culture: An essential aspect of psychiatric care. *Journal of the National Medical Association, 94*, 371–375.

Cauce, A. M., & Domenech-Rodriguez, M. (2002). Latino families: Myth and realities. In J. M. Contreras, K. A. Kerns, & A. M. Neal-Barnett (Eds.), *Latino children and families in the United States: Current research and future directions* (pp. 3–25). Westport, CT: Greenwood Press.

Cedar, B., & Levant, R. F. (1990). A meta-analysis of Parent Effectiveness Training. *American Journal of Family Therapy, 18*, 373–384.

Chamberlain, P., & Baldwin, D. V. (1988). Client resistance to parent training: Its therapeutic management. In T. R. Kratochwill (Ed.), *Advances in school psychology* (Vol. VI, pp. 131–171). Hillsdale, NJ: Erlbaum.

Chamberlain, P., Fisher, P. A., & Moore, K. J. (2002). Multidimensional treatment foster care: Applications of the OSLC intervention model to high-risk youth and their families. In J. B. Reid, G. R. Patterson, & J. J. Snyder (Eds.), *Antisocial behavior in children and adolescents: A developmental analysis and model for intervention* (pp. 203–218). Washington, DC: American Psychological Association.

Chambless, D. L., & Hollon, S. D. (1998). Defining empirically supported therapies. *Journal of Consulting and Clinical Psychology, 66*, 7–18.

Chao, R., & Tseng, V. (2002). Parenting of Asians. In M. H. Bornstein (Ed.), *Handbook of parenting: Vol. 4. Social conditions and applied parenting* (2nd ed., pp. 59–93). Mahwah, NJ: Erlbaum.

Chin, T., & Phillips, M. (2004). Social reproduction and child-rearing practices: Social class, children's agency, and the summer activity gap. *Sociology of Education, 77*, 185–210.

Choate, M. L., Pincus, D. B., & Eyberg, S. M. (2005). Parent–child interaction therapy for treatment of separation anxiety disorder in young children: A pilot study. *Cognitive and Behavioral Practice, 12*, 126–135.

Chorpita, B. F. (2003). The frontier of evidence-based practice. In A. E. Kazdin & J. R. Weisz (Eds.), *Evidence-based psychotherapies for children and adolescents* (pp. 42–59). New York: Guilford Press.

Christenson, S. L., & Sheridan, S. M. (2001). *Schools and families: Creating essential connections for learning*. New York: Guilford Press.

Christophersen, E. R., & Mortweet, S. L. (2001). *Treatments that work with children: Empirically supported strategies for managing childhood problems*. Washington, DC: American Psychological Association.

Christophersen, E. R., & Mortweet, S. L. (2003). Facilitating toilet training. In E. R. Christopherson & S. L. Mortweet (Eds.), *Parenting that works: Building skills that last a lifetime* (pp. 229–265). Washington, DC: American Psychological Association.

Cicero, F. R., & Pfadt, A. (2002). Investigation of a reinforcement-based toilet training procedure for children with autism. *Research in Developmental Disabilities, 23*, 319–331.

Clancy, P. M. (1986). The acquisition of communicative style in Japanese. In B. B. Schieffelin and E. Ochs (Eds.), *Language socialization across cultures* (pp. 213–250). New York: Cambridge University Press.

Cleary, A., & Packham, D. (1968). A touch-detecting teaching machine with auditory reinforcement. *Journal of Applied Behavior Analysis, 1*, 341–345.

Condry, J. (1977). Enemies of exploration: Self-initiated versus other-initiated learning. *Journal of Personality and Social Psychology, 35*, 459–477.

Conduct Problems Prevention Research Group. (1992). A developmental and clinical model for the prevention of conduct disorder: The FAST Track Program. *Development and Psychopathology, 4*, 509–527.

Conduct Problems Prevention Research Group. (1999). Initial impact of the FAST Track prevention trial for conduct problems: I. The high-risk sample. *Journal of Consulting and Clinical Psychology, 67*, 631–647.

Conduct Problems Prevention Research Group. (2000). Merging universal and indicated prevention programs: The FAST Track model. *Addictive Behaviors, 25*, 913–927.

Conduct Problems Prevention Research Group. (2002). Evaluation of the first three years of the FAST Track prevention trial with children at high risk for adolescent conduct problems. *Journal of Abnormal Child Psychology, 30*, 19–35.

Conduct Problems Prevention Research Group. (2004). The effects of the FAST Track program on serious problem outcomes at the end of elementary school. *Journal of Clinical Child and Adolescent Psychology, 33*, 650–661.

Cone, J. D. (2001). *Evaluating outcomes: Empirical tools for effective practice*. Washington, DC: American Psychological Association.

Conley, C. S., Caldwell, M. S., Flynn, M., Dupre, A. J., & Rudolph, K. D. (2004). Parenting and mental health. In M. Hoghughi & N. Long (Eds.), *Handbook of parenting: Theory and research for practice* (pp. 276–295). London: Sage.

Cortes, D. E. (1995). Variations in familism in two generations of Puerto Ricans. *Hispanic Journal of Behavioral Sciences, 17*, 249–255.

Costa, I. G. D., Rapoff, M. A., Lemanek, K., & Goldstein, G. L. (1997). Improving adherence to medication regimens for children with asthma and its effect on clinical outcome. *Journal of Applied Behavior Analysis, 30*, 687–691.

Cox, D. J., Tisdelle, D. A., & Culbert, J. P. (1988). Increasing adherence to behavioral homework assignments. *Journal of Behavioral Medicine, 11*, 519–522.

Crane, D. R. (1995). Introduction to behavioural family therapy for families with young children. *Journal of Family Therapy, 17*, 229–242.

Croake, J. W. (1983). Adlerian parent education. *The Counseling Psychologist, 11*, 65–71.

Crouter, A. C., & Head, M. R. (2002). Parental monitoring and knowledge of children. In M. H. Bornstein (Ed.), *Handbook of parenting: Vol. 3. Being and becoming a parent* (2nd ed., pp. 461–483). Mahwah, NJ: Erlbaum.

Cunningham, C., Davis, J., Bremner, R., Dunn, K., & Rzasa, T. (1993). Coping modeling problem solving versus mastery modeling: Effects on adherence, in-session process, and skill acquisition in a residential parent-training program. *Journal of Consulting and Clinical Psychology, 61*, 871–877.

Cunningham, C. E., Boyle, M., Offord, D., Racine, Y., Hundert, J., Secord, M., & McDonald, J. (2000). Tri-ministry study: Correlates of school-based parenting course utilization. *Journal of Clinical and Consulting Psychology, 68*, 928–933.

Danforth, J. S. (1998). The outcome of parent training using the behavior management flow chart with mothers and their children with oppositional defiant disorder and attention-deficit hyperactivity disorder. *Behavior Modification, 22*, 443–473.

Danforth, J. S. (1999). The outcome of parent training using the Behavior Management Flow Chart with a mother and her twin boys with oppositional defiant disorder and attention-deficit hyperactivity disorder. *Child & Family Behavior Therapy, 21*, 59–80.

Dangel, R. F., & Polster, R. A. (Eds.). (1984). *Parent training: Foundations of research and practice*. New York: Guilford Press.

Davies, P. T., McMahon, R. J., Flessati, E., & Tiedemann, G. L. (1984). Verbal rationales and modeling as adjuncts to a parenting technique for child compliance. *Child Development, 55*, 1290–1298.

DeGarmo, D. S., Patterson, G. R., & Forgatch, M. S. (2004). How do outcomes in a specified parent training intervention maintain or wane over time? *Prevention Science, 5*, 73–89.

Dembo, M. H., Sweitzer, M., & Lauritzen, P. (1985). An evaluation of group parent education: Behavioral, PET, and Adlerian programs. *Review of Educational Research, 55*, 155–200.

Detrich, R. (1999). Increasing treatment fidelity by matching interventions to contextual variables within the educational setting. *School Psychology Review, 28*, 608–620.

Dickinson, A. M. (1989). The detrimental effects of extrinsic reinforcement in "intrinsic motivation." *Behavior Analyst, 12*, 1–15.

Dillard, D., & Manson, S. (2000). Native American and Alaskans: Assessment and treatment. In I. Cuellar & F. A. Paniagua (Eds.), *Handbook of multicultural mental health: Assessment and treatment of diverse populations* (pp. 225–248). New York: Academic Press.

Dinkmeyer, D., & McKay, G. D. (1977). *Systematic Training for Effective Parenting.* Circle Pines, MN: American Guidance Service.

Dinkmeyer, D., & McKay, G. D. (1983). *The parent's guide: STEP—Systematic Training for Effective Parenting.* Circle Pines, MN: American Guidance Service.

Dinkmeyer, D., & McKay, G. D. (1997). *Systematic Training for Effective Parenting: Leader's resource guide.* Shoreview, MN: AGS Publishing.

Dishion, T. J., & Andrews, D. W. (1995). Preventing escalation in problem behaviors with high-risk young adolescents: Immediate and 1-year outcomes. *Journal of Consulting and Clinical Psychology, 63,* 538–548.

Dishion, T. J., & Kavanagh, K. (2003). *Intervening in adolescent problem behavior: A family-centered approach.* New York: Guilford Press.

Dishion, T. J., Kavanagh, K., Schneiger, A., Nelson, S., & Kaufman, N. (2002). Preventing early adolescent substance use: A family-centered strategy for the public middle school ecology. *Prevention Science, 3,* 191–201.

Dishion, T. J., Kavanagh, K., Veltman, M., McCartney, T., Soberman, L., & Stormshak, E. A. (2003). *Family management curriculum: Vol. 20. Leader's guide.* Eugene, OR: Child and Family Center.

Dishion, T. J., & McMahon, R. J. (1998). Parental monitoring and the prevention of child and adolescent problem behavior: A conceptual and empirical formulation. *Clinical Child and Family Psychology Review, 1,* 61–75.

Dolan, L. J., Kellam, S. G., Brown, C. H., Werthamer-Larsson, L., Rebok, G. W., Mayer, L. S., et al. (1993). The short-term impact of two classroom-based preventive interventions on aggressive and shy behaviors and poor achievement. *Journal of Applied Developmental Psychology, 14,* 317–345.

Doleys, D. M., Ciminero, A. R., Tollison, J. W., Williams, D. L., & Wells, K. C. (1977). Dry-bed training and retention control training: A comparison. *Behavior Therapy, 8,* 541–548.

Donohue, B., Hersen, M., & Ammerman, R. T. (2000). Historical overview. In M. Hersen & R. T. Ammerman (Eds.), *Advanced abnormal child psychology* (2nd ed., pp. 3–14). Mahwah, NJ: Erlbaum.

Dunst, C. J., Lee, H. E., & Trivette, C. M. (1988). Family resources, personal well-being, and early intervention. *Journal of Special Education, 22,* 108–116.

Eaves, S. H., Sheperis, C. J., & Blanchard, T. (2005). Teaching time-out and job card grounding procedures to parents: A primer for family counselors. *Family Journal: Counseling and Therapy for Couples and Families, 13,* 252–258.

Eddy, J. M., & Chamberlain, P. (2000). Family management and deviant peer association as mediators of the impact of treatment condition on youth antisocial behavior. *Journal of Consulting and Clinical Psychology, 5,* 857–863.

Eddy, J. M., Reid, J. B., & Fetrow, R. A. (2000). An elementary school-based prevention program targeting modifiable antecedents of youth delinquency and violence: Linking the Interests of Families and Teachers (LIFT). *Journal of Emotional and Behavioral Disorders, 8,* 165–176. Retrieved May 6, 2004, from http://www.ebscohost.com/titleLists/pb-journals.htm

Edwards, D. J. A., Dattilio, F. M., & Bromley, D. B. (2004). Developing evidence-based practice: The role of case-based research. *Professional Psychology: Research and Practice, 35,* 589–597.

Eisenstadt, T., Eyberg, S., McNeil, C., Newcomb, K., & Funderburk, B. (1993). Parent–child interaction therapy with behavior problem children: Relative effectiveness of two stages and overall treatment outcome. *Journal of Clinical Child Psychology, 22,* 42–51.

Erion, J. (2006). Parent tutoring: A meta-analysis. *Education and Treatment of Children, 29,* 79–106.

Eyberg, S. M., & Boggs, S. R. (1998). Parent–Child Interaction Therapy: A psychosocial intervention for the treatment of young conduct-disordered children. In J. M. Briesmeister & C. E. Schaefer (Eds.), *Handbook of Parent training: Parents as co-therapists for children's behavior problems* (2nd ed., pp. 61–97). New York: Wiley.

Eyberg, S. M., Funderburk, B., Hembree-Kigin, T., McNeil, C., Querido, J., & Hood, K. (2001). Parent–child interaction therapy with behavior problem children: One and two year maintenance of treatment effects in the family. *Child & Family Behavior Therapy, 23(4),* 1–20.

Eyberg, S. M., & Johnson, S. M. (1974). Multiple assessment of behavior modification with families. *Journal of Consulting and Clinical Psychology, 42,* 594–606.

Eyberg, S. M., & Matarazzo, R. G. (1980). Training parents as therapists: A comparison between individual parent–child interaction training and parent group didactic training. *Journal of Clinical Psychology, 36,* 492–499.

Eyberg, S. M., & Pincus, D. B. (1999). *Professional manual for the Eyberg Child Behavior Inventory and Sutter–Eyberg Student Behavior Inventory—Revised.* Odessa, FL: Psychological Assessment Resources.

Eyberg, S. M., & Robinson, E. A. (1982). Parent–child interaction training: Effects on family functioning. *Journal of Clinical Child Psychology, 11,* 130–137.

Fallone, G., Owens, J. A., & Deane, J. (2002). Sleepiness in children and adolescents: Clinical implications. *Sleep Medicine Reviews, 6,* 287–306.

Ferster, C. B., & Skinner, B. F. (1957). *Schedules of reinforcement.* New York: Appleton-Century-Crofts.

Firestone, P., Kelly, M. J., & Fike, S. (1980). Are fathers necessary in parent training groups? *Journal of Clinical Child Psychology, 9,* 44–47.

Fisher, P. A., Gunnar, M. R., Chamberlain, P., & Reid, J. B. (2000). Preventive intervention for maltreated preschoolers: Impact of children's behavior, neuroendocrine activity, and foster parent functioning. *Journal of the American Academy of Child and Adolescent Psychiatry, 39,* 1356–1364.

Fiske, S. T. (1998). Stereotyping, prejudice, and discrimination. In D. T. Gilbert & S. T. Fiske (Eds.), *Handbook of social psychology* (4th ed., Vol. 2, pp. 357–411). New York: McGraw-Hill.

Flannagan, D. (1996). Mothers' and kindergartners' talk about interpersonal relationships. *Merrill-Palmer Quarterly, 42,* 519–536.

Fleischman, M. J. (1979). Using parenting salaries to control attrition and cooperation in therapy. *Behavior Therapy, 10,* 94–102.

Follette, W. C. (1995). Correcting methodological weaknesses in the knowledge base used to derive practice standards. In S. C. Hayes, V. M. Follette, R. M. Dawes, & K. E. Grady (Eds.), *Scientific standards of psychological practice: Issues and recommendations* (pp. 229–247). Reno, NV: Context Press.

Forehand, R. L., Armistead, L., Neighbors, B., & Klein, K. (1994). *Parent training for the noncompliant child: A guide for training therapists* [Motion picture]. South Burlington, VT: Child Focus.

Forehand, R. L., & Atkeson, B. M. (1977). Generality of treatment effects with parents as therapists: A review of assessment and implementation procedures. *Behavior Therapy, 8,* 575–593.

Forehand, R. L., Griest, D. L., & Wells, K. C. (1979). Parent behavioral training: An analysis of the relationship among multiple outcome measures. *Journal of Abnormal Child Psychology, 7,* 229–242.

Forehand, R. L., & King, H. E. (1974). Pre-school children's non-compliance: Effects of short-term behavior therapy. *Journal of Community Psychology, 2,* 42–44.

Forehand, R. L., & King, H. E. (1977). Noncompliant children: Effects of parent training on behavior and attitude change. *Behavior Modification, 1,* 93–108.

Forehand, R. L., & Kotchick, B. A. (1996). Cultural diversity: A wake-up call for parent training. *Behavior Therapy, 27,* 187–206.

Forehand, R. L., & Kotchick, B. A. (2002). Behavioral parent training: Current challenges and potential solutions. *Journal of Child and Family Studies, 11,* 377–384.

Forehand, R. L., & Long, N. (2002). *Parenting the strong-willed child: The clinically proven five week program for parents of two to six year olds.* Chicago: Contemporary Books.

Forehand, R. L., & McMahon, R. J. (1981). *Helping the Noncompliant Child: A clinician's guide to parent training.* New York: Guilford Press.

Forgatch, M. S. (1994). *Parenting through change: A training manual.* Eugene: Oregon Social Learning Center.

Forgatch, M. S., & DeGarmo, D. S. (2002). Extending and testing the social interaction learning model with divorce samples. In J. B. Reid, G. R. Patterson, & J. J. Snyder (Eds.), *Antisocial behavior in children and adolescents: A developmental analysis and model for intervention* (pp. 235–256). Washington, DC: American Psychological Association.

Forgatch, M. S., DeGarmo, D. S., & Beldavs, Z. G. (2005). An efficacious theory-based intervention for stepfamilies. *Behavior Therapy, 36,* 357–365.

Forgatch, M. S., & Knutson, N. M. (2002). Linking basic and applied research in a prevention science process. In H. A. Liddle, D. A. Santisteban, R. F. Levant, & J. H. Bray (Eds.), *Family psychology: Science-based interventions* (pp. 239–258). Washington, DC: American Psychological Association.

Forgatch, M. S., & Martinez, C. R. (1999). Parent management training: A program linking basic research and practical application. *Journal of the Norwegian Psychological Association, 36,* 923–937.

Forgatch, M. S., & Patterson, G. R. (1987). *Parents and adolescents: Living together: Part 2. Family problem solving.* Eugene, OR: Castalia.

Forgatch, M. S., & Patterson, G. R. (2005). *Parents and adolescents: Living together: Part 2. Family problem solving* (2nd ed.). Champaign, IL: Research Press.

Freeman, C. W. (1975). Adlerian mother study groups: Effects on attitudes and behavior. *Journal of Individual Psychology, 31,* 37–50.

French, V. (2002). History of parenting: The ancient Mediterranean world. In M. H. Bornstein (Ed.), *Handbook of parenting, Vol. 2: Biology and ecology of parenting* (2nd ed., pp. 345–376). Mahwah, NJ: Erlbaum.

Freud, S. (1955). The analysis of a phobia in a 5-year-old boy. In J. Strachey (Ed. & Trans.), *The standard edition of the complete psychological works of Sigmund Freud* (Vol. 10, pp. 149–289). London: Hogarth Press. (Original work published 1909)

Fricker-Elhai, A. E., Ruggiero, K. J., & Smith, D. W. (2005). Parent–child interaction therapy with two maltreated siblings in foster care. *Clinical Case Studies, 4,* 13–39.

Friman, P. C., Allen, K. D., Kerwin, M. L. E., & Larzelere, R. (1993). Changes in modern psychology: A citation analysis of the Kuhnian displacement thesis. *American Psychologist, 48,* 658–664.

Friman, P. C., & Jones, K. M. (1998). Elimination disorders in children. In T. S. Watson & F. Gresham (Eds.), *Handbook of child behavior therapy* (pp. 239–260). New York: Plenum Press.

Friman, P. C., & Poling, A. (1995). Making life easier with effort: Basic findings and applied research on response effort. *Journal of Applied Behavior Analysis, 28,* 583–590.

Frosh, S. (2004). Religious influences on parenting. In M. Hoghughi & N. Long (Eds.), *Handbook of parenting: Theory and research for practice* (pp. 98–109). London: Sage.

Fuligni, A. J. (1998). Authority, autonomy, and parent-adolescent conflict and cohesion: A study of adolescents from Mexican, Chinese, Filipino, and European family backgrounds. *Developmental Psychology, 34,* 782–792.

Fuligni, A. J., Tseng, V., & Lam M. (1999). Attitudes toward family obligations among American adolescents with Asian, Latin American, and European family backgrounds. *Child Development, 70,* 1030–1044.

Funderburk, B., Eyberg, S. M., Newcomb, K., McNeil, C., Hembree-Kigin, T., & Capage, L. (1998). Parent–child interaction therapy with behavior problem children: Maintenance of treatment effects in the school setting. *Child & Family Behavior Therapy, 20,* 17–38.

Gallagher, N. (2003). Effects of parent–child interaction therapy on young children with disruptive behavior disorders. *Bridges: Practice-Based Research Syntheses, 1,* 1–17.

Garcia, J. L. A. (1992). African American perspectives, cultural relativism, and normative issues: Some conceptual questions. In H. Flack & E. Pelligrino (Eds.), *African American perspectives on biomedical ethics* (pp. 11–73). Washington, DC: Georgetown University Press.

Garcia-Coll, C., & Pachter, L. M. (2002). Ethnic and minority parenting. In M. H. Bornstein (Ed.), *Handbook of parenting: Vol. 4. Social conditions and applied parenting* (2nd ed., pp. 1–20). Mahwah, NJ: Erlbaum.

Gardner, F. (2000). Methodological issues and the direct observation of parent–child interactions: Do observational findings reflect the natural behavior of participants? *Clinical Child and Family Psychology Review, 3,* 185–198.

Glogower, F., & Sloop, E. W. (1976). Two strategies of group training of parents as effective behavior modifiers. *Behavior Therapy, 7,* 177–184.

Gone, J. P. (2004). Mental health services for Native Americans in the 21st century United States. *Professional Psychology, 35,* 10–18.

Gordon, T. (1970). *Parent Effectiveness Training.* New York: Peter Wyden.

Gordon, T. (1975). *P. E. T.: Parent Effectiveness Training.* New York: New American Library.

Gordon, T. (1997). *Family effectiveness training* [Video]. Solana Beach, CA: Gordon Training International.

Gottman, J. M., Coan, J., & Carrere, S. (1998). Predicting marital happiness and stability from newlywed interactions. *Journal of Marriage & the Family, 60,* 5–22.

Gresham, F. M. (2005). Treatment integrity and therapeutic change: A commentary on Perepletchikova and Kazdin. *Clinical Psychology: Science and Practice, 12,* 391–394.

Gresham, F. M., Gansle, K. A., & Noell, G. H. (1993). Treatment integrity in applied behavior analysis with children. *Journal of Applied Behavior Analysis, 26,* 257–263.

Gross, D., Fogg, L., Webster-Stratton, C., Garvey, C., Julion, W., & Grady, J. (2003). Parent training with families of toddlers in day care in low-income urban communities. *Journal of Consulting and Clinical Psychology, 71,* 261–278.

Hall, C. S. (1979). *A primer of Freudian psychology.* New York: New American Library.

Hall, E. T., & Hall, M. R. (1990). *Understanding cultural differences: Germans, French & Americans.* Yarmouth, ME: Intercultural Press.

Hamlet, C. C., Axelrod, S., & Kuerschner, S. (1984). Eye contact as an antecedent to compliant behavior. *Journal of Applied Behavior Analysis, 17,* 553–557.

Hanf, C. (1969). *A two-stage program for modifying maternal controlling during mother–child (M-C) interaction.* Paper presented at the meeting of the Western Psychological Association, Vancouver, British Columbia, Canada.

Hansen, D. J., & MacMillan, V. M. (1990). Behavioral assessment of child abusive and neglectful families: Recent developments and current issues. *Behavior Modification, 14,* 255–278.

Harkness, S., & Super, C. M. (2002). Culture and parenting. In M. H. Bornstein (Ed.), *Handbook of parenting: Vol. 2. Biology and ecology of parenting* (2nd ed., pp. 253–280). Mahwah, NJ: Erlbaum.

Hart, B., & Risley, T. R. (1995). *Meaningful differences in the everyday experience of young American children.* Baltimore: Brookes.

Harwood, M. D., & Eyberg, S. M. (2004). Therapist verbal behavior early in treatment: Relation to successful completion of Parent–Child Interaction Therapy. *Journal of Clinical Child and Adolescent Psychology, 33,* 601–612.

Harwood, R. L., Leyendecker, B., Carlson, V., Ascencio, M., & Miller, A. (2002). Parenting among Latino families in the U.S. In M. H. Bornstein (Ed.), *Handbook of parenting: Vol. 4. Social conditions and applied parenting* (2nd ed., pp. 21–46). Mahwah, NJ: Erlbaum.

Harwood, R. L., Scholmerich, A., Schulze, P. A., & Gonzalez, Z. (1999). Cultural differences in maternal beliefs and behaviors: A study of middle-class Anglo and Puerto Rican mother-infant pairs in four everyday situations. *Child Development, 70,* 1005–1016.

Haugaard, J., & Hazan, C. (2002). Foster parenting. In M. H. Bornstein (Ed.), *Handbook of parenting: Vol. 1. Children and parenting* (2nd ed., pp. 313–328). Mahwah, NJ: Erlbaum.

Hawkins, R. P., & Hursh, D. E. (1992). Levels of research for clinical practice: It isn't as hard as you think. *West Virginia Journal of Psychological Research and Practice, 1,* 61–71.

Hawkins, R. P., Mathews, J. R., & Hamdan, L. (1999). *Measuring behavioral health outcomes: A practical guide.* New York: Plenum Press.

Hayes, S. C., Nelson, R. O., & Jarrett, R. B. (1987). The treatment utility of assessment: A functional approach to evaluating assessment quality. *American Psychologist, 42,* 963–974.

Haynes, S. N. (1991). Behavioral assessment. In M. Hersen, A. E. Kazdin, & A. S. Bellack (Eds.), *The clinical psychology handbook* (pp. 430–464). New York: Pergamon Press.

Hembree-Kigin, T. L., & McNeil, C. B. (1995). *Parent–Child Interaction Therapy.* New York: Plenum Press.

Herrnstein, R. J. (1970). On the law of effect. *Journal of the Experimental Analysis of Behavior, 13,* 243–266.

Herschell, A. D., Calzada, E., Eyberg, S., & McNeil, C. (2002a). Clinical issues in parent–child interaction therapy. *Cognitive and Behavioral Practice, 9,* 16–27.

Herschell, A. D., Calzada, E., Eyberg, S., & McNeil, C. (2002b). Parent–child interaction therapy: New directions in research. *Cognitive and Behavioral Practice, 9,* 9–16.

Herwig, J. E., Wirtz, M., & Bengel, J. (2004). Depression, partnership, social support, and parenting: Interaction of maternal factors with behavioral problems of the child. *Journal of Affective Disorders, 80,* 199–208.

Hill, S. A. (1999). *African-American children: Socialization and development in families*. Thousand Oaks, CA: Corwin Press.

Ho, D. Y. F. (1996). Filial piety and its psychological consequences. In M. H. Bond (Ed.), *The handbook of Chinese psychology* (pp. 155–165). Hong Kong: Oxford University Press.

Ho, M. K. (1992). *Minority children and adolescents in therapy*. Newberry Park, CA: Sage.

Hobbs, S. A., & Forehand, R. L. (1975). Effects of differential release from time-out on children's deviant behavior. *Journal of Behavior Therapy and Experimental Psychiatry, 6*, 256–257.

Hobbs, S. A., Forehand, R. L., & Murray, R. G. (1978). Effects of various durations of time-out on the noncompliant behavior of children. *Behavior Therapy, 9*, 652–656.

Hobbs, S. A., Walle, D. L., & Hammersly, G. A. (1990). The relationship between child behavior and acceptability of contingency management procedures. *Child & Family Behavior Therapy, 12*, 95–102.

Hoff, E., Laursen, B., & Tardif, T. (2002). Socioeconomic status and parenting. In M. H. Bornstein (Ed.), *Handbook of parenting: Vol. 2. Biology and ecology of parenting* (2nd ed., pp. 231–252). Mahwah, NJ: Erlbaum.

Hoffman, E. (1994). *The drive for self: Alfred Adler and the founding of individual psychology*. Upper Saddle River, NJ: Addison-Wesley.

Hoghughi, M., & Long, N. (Eds.). (2004). *Handbook of parenting: Theory and research for practice*. London: Sage.

Hojat, M., Gonella, J., & Caelleigh, A. (2003). Impartial judgment by the "gatekeepers" of science: Fallibility and accountability in the peer review process. *Advances in Health Sciences Education, 8*, 75–96.

Holden, G. W. (1997). *Parents and the dynamics of child rearing*. Boulder, CO: Westview Press.

Honig W. K., & Staddon, J. E. R. (1977). *Handbook of operant behavior*. Englewood Cliffs, NJ: Prentice-Hall.

Hood, K. K., & Eyberg, S. M. (2003). Outcomes of parent–child interaction therapy: Mothers' reports of maintenance three to six years after treatment. *Journal of Clinical Child and Adolescent Psychology, 32*, 419–429.

Horn, M. (1989). *Before it's too late: The child guidance movement in the United States, 1922–1945*. Philadelphia: Temple University Press.

Houlihan, D., Vincent, J., & Ellison, P. J. (1994). Assessing childhood noncompliance: Subtle differences in one-step commands and their effects on response topography. *Journal of Applied Behavior Analysis, 16*, 9–20.

Houts, A. C., Liebert, R. M., & Padawer, W. (1983). A delivery system for the treatment of primary enuresis. *Journal of Abnormal Child Psychology, 11*, 513–519.

Hudson, A., & Blane, M. (1985). The importance of non verbal behavior in giving instructions to children. *Child & Family Behavior Therapy, 7*, 1–10.

Hughes, J. R., & Gottlieb, L. N. (2004). The effects of the Webster-Stratton parenting program on maltreating families: Fostering strengths. *Child Abuse & Neglect, 28*, 1081–1097.

Hupp, S. D. A., & Allen, K. D. (2005). Using an audio cueing procedure to increase rate of parental attention during parent training. *Child & Family Behavior Therapy, 27*, 43–49.

Innocenti, M. S., Huh, K., & Boyce, G. (1992). Families of children with disabilities: Normative data and other considerations on parenting stress. *Topics in Early Childhood Special Education, 12*, 403–427.

Irvine, A. B., Biglan, A., Smolkowski, K., Metzler, C. W., & Ary, D. V. (1999). The effectiveness of a parenting skills program for parents of middle school students in small communities. *Journal of Clinical and Consulting Psychology, 67*, 811–825.

Iwata, B. (1987). Negative reinforcement in applied behavior analysis: An emerging technology. *Journal of Applied Behavior Analysis, 20*, 361–378.

Jackson, M. D., & Brown, D. (1986). Use of Systematic Training for Effective Parenting (STEP) with elementary school parents. *School Counselor, 34*, 100–104.

Jankowiak, W. (1992). Father–child relations in urban China. In B. S. Hewlett (Ed.), *Father–child relations: Cultural and biosocial contexts* (pp. 345–363). New York: De Gruyter.

Jason, L. A. (1985). Using a token-actuated timer to reduce television viewing. *Journal of Applied Behavior Analysis, 18*, 269–272.

Jensen, W. R., Rhode, G., & Reavis, H. K. (1994). *The tough kid tool box.* Longmont, CO: Sopris West.

Johnson, S., & Brown, R. (1969). Producing behavior change in parents of disturbed children. *Journal of Child Psychology and Psychiatry, 10*, 107–121.

Johnston, J. M., & Pennypacker, H. S. (1993). *Strategies and tactics of behavioral research* (2nd ed.). Hillsdale, NJ: Erlbaum.

Jones, F. H., Fremouw, W., & Carples, S. (1977). Pyramid training of elementary school teachers to use a classroom management skill package. *Journal of Applied Behavior Analysis, 10*, 239–253.

Jones, M. L., Eyberg, S. M., & Adams, C. D. (1998). Treatment acceptability of behavioral interventions for children: An assessment by mothers of children with disruptive behavior disorders. *Child & Family Behavior Therapy, 20*, 15–26.

Jones, R. R., Reid, J. B., & Patterson, G. R. (1975). Naturalistic observation in clinical assessment. In P. McReynolds (Ed.), *Advances in psychological assessment* (Vol. 3, pp. 42–95). San Francisco: Jossey-Bass.

Kazdin, A. E. (2001). *Behavior modification in applied settings* (6th ed.). Belmont, CA: Wadsworth/Thompson Learning.

Kazdin, A. E. (2003). Publishing your research. In M. J. Prinstein & M. D. Patterson (Eds.), *Portable mentor: Expert guide to a successful career in psychology* (pp. 85–99). New York: Kluwer Academic/Plenum Press.

Kazdin, A. E. (2004). Evidence-based treatments: Challenges and priorities for practice and research. *Child and Adolescent Psychiatric Clinics of North America, 13,* 923–940.

Kazdin, A. E. (2005). *Parent management training: Treatment for oppositional, aggressive, and antisocial behavior in children and adolescents.* New York: Oxford University Press.

Kelley, M. L. (1990). *School–home notes: Promoting children's classroom success.* New York: Guilford Press.

Knight, G. P., Cota, M. K., & Bernal, M. E. (1993). The socialization of cooperative, competitive, and individualistic preferences among Mexican American children: The mediating role of ethnic identity. *Hispanic Journal of Behavioral Sciences, 15,* 291–309.

Kohn, A. (2001). Five reasons to stop saying, "good job!" *Young Children, 56,* 24–30.

Kohn, A. (2005). *Unconditional parenting: Moving from rewards and punishment to love and reason.* New York: Simon & Schuster.

Kotler, J. S., & McMahon, R. J. (2004). Compliance and noncompliance in anxious, aggressive, and socially competent children: The impact of the child's game on child and maternal behavior. *Behavior Therapy, 35,* 494–512.

Kratochwill, T. R., & Shernoff, E. S. (2004). Evidence-based practice: Promoting evidence-based interventions in school psychology. *School Psychology Review, 33,* 34–48.

Krebs, L. (1986). Current research on theoretically based parenting programs. *Individual Psychology: Journal of Adlerian Theory, Research, and Practice, 42,* 375–387.

Kubany, E. S., Richard, D. C., & Bauer, G. B. (1992). Impact of assertive and accusatory communication of distress and anger: A verbal component analysis. *Aggressive Behavior, 18,* 337–347.

Kuhn, B. R., & Elliott, A. J. (2003). Treatment efficacy in behavioral pediatric sleep medicine. *Journal of Psychosomatic Research, 54,* 587–597.

Kuhn, B. R., & Weidinger, D. (2000). Interventions for infant and toddler sleep disturbance: A review. *Child & Family Behavior Therapy, 22,* 33–50.

Kumpfer, K. L. (1999). *Strengthening America's families: Exemplary parenting and family strategies for delinquency prevention.* Retrieved December 12, 2007, from http://www.strengtheningfamilies.org

Kumpfer, K. L., & Alvarado, R. (2003). Family-strengthening approaches for the prevention of youth problem behaviors. *American Psychologist, 58,* 457–465.

Kusche, C., & Greenberg, M. T. (1994). *The PATHS curriculum.* Seattle, WA: Developmental Research and Programs.

Larzelere, R. E. (1999). [Review of the book *Parents and the dynamics of child rearing*]. *Family Relations, 48,* 339.

Lawson, A. B. (2001). *Statistical methods in spatial epidemiology.* Chichester, England: Wiley.

LeBlanc, L. A., Carr, J. E., & Crossett, S. E. (2005). Intensive outpatient behavioral treatment of primary urinary incontinence of children with autism. *Focus on Autism and Other Developmental Disabilities, 20,* 98–105.

Lepper, M. R., & Greene, D. (Eds.). (1978). *The hidden costs of reward: New perspectives on the psychology of human motivation.* Hillsdale, NJ: Erlbaum.

Lepper, M. R., & Henderlong, J. (2000). Turning "play" into "work" and "work" into "play": 25 years of research on intrinsic versus extrinsic motivation. In C. Sansone & J. Harackiewicz (Eds.), *Intrinsic and extrinsic motivation: The search for optimal motivation and performance* (pp. 257–307). San Diego, CA: Academic Press.

Lerman, D. C., & Vorndran, C. M. (2002). On the status of knowledge for using punishment: Implications for treating behavior disorders. *Journal of Applied Behavior Analysis, 35,* 431–464.

Lerner, R. M., Rothbaum, F., Boulos, S., & Castellino, D. R. (2002). Developmental systems perspective on parenting. In M. H. Bornstein (Ed.), *Handbook of parenting: Vol. 2. Biology and ecology of parenting* (2nd ed., pp. 315–344). Mahwah, NJ: Erlbaum.

Levine, M., & Levine, A. (1992). *Helping children: A social history.* New York: Oxford University Press.

Linscheid, T. R. (1998). Behavioral treatment of feeding disorders in children. In T. S. Watson & F. M. Gresham (Eds.), *Handbook of child behavior therapy* (pp. 357–368). New York: Plenum Press.

Lipson, K., Eisenstadt, T., & Hembree-Kigin, T. (1993). *Parent–child interaction therapy conducted in a Head Start workshop for at-risk African American preschoolers.* Paper presented at the National Head Start Conference, Washington, DC.

Long, P., Forehand, R. L., Wierson, M., & Morgan, A. (1994). Moving into adulthood: Does parent training with young noncompliant children have long term effects? *Behavior Research and Therapy, 32,* 101–107.

Lowry, M. A., & Whitman, T. L. (1989). Generalization of parenting skills: An early intervention program. *Child & Family Behavior Therapy, 11,* 45–65.

Luiselli, J. K., & Cameron, M. J. (Eds.). (1998). *Antecedent control: Innovative approaches to behavioral support.* Baltimore: Brookes.

Luiselli, J. K., & Pine, J. (1999). Social control of childhood stealing in a public school: A case study. *Journal of Behavior Therapy and Experimental Psychiatry, 30,* 231–239.

Lundquist, L. M., & Hansen, D. J. (1998). Enhancing treatment adherence, social validity, and generalization of parent-training interventions with physically abusive and neglectful families. In J. R. Lutzker (Ed.), *Handbook of child abuse research and treatment* (pp. 449–471). New York: Plenum Press.

Magen, R. H., & Rose, S. D. (1994). Parents in groups: Problem solving versus behavioral skills training. *Research on Social Work Practice, 4,* 172–191.

Mahoney, C. R., Taylor, H. A., Kanarek, R. B., & Samuel, P. (2005). Effect of breakfast composition on cognitive processes in elementary school children. *Physiology and Behavior, 85,* 635–645.

Marchant, M., Young, R. K., & West, R. P. (2004). The effects of parental teaching on compliance behavior of children. *Psychology in the Schools, 41,* 337–350.

Markey, U., Markey, D. J., Quant, B., Santelli, B., & Turnbull, A. (2002). Operation positive change: PBS in an urban context. *Journal of Positive Behavior Interventions, 4*, 218–230.

Markus, H. R., & Kitayama, S. (1991). Culture and the self: Implications for cognition, emotion, and motivation. *Psychological Review, 98*, 224–253.

Markus, H. R., & Kitayama, S. (2001). The cultural construction of self and emotion: Implications for social behavior. In W. G. Perrod (Ed.), *Emotions in social psychology: Essential reading* (pp. 119–137). Philadelphia: Brunner-Routledge.

Martinez, C. R., Jr., & Eddy, J. M. (2005). Effects of culturally adapted parent management training on Latino youth behavioral health outcomes. *Journal of Consulting and Clinical Psychology, 73*, 841–851.

Martinez, C. R., Jr., & Forgatch, M. S. (2001). Preventing problems with boys' noncompliance: Effects of a parent training intervention for divorcing mothers. *Journal of Consulting and Clinical Psychology, 69*, 416–428.

McAdoo, H. P. (2002). African American parenting. In M. H. Bornstein (Ed.), *Handbook of parenting: Vol. 4. Social conditions and applied parenting* (2nd ed., pp. 46–58). Mahwah, NJ: Erlbaum.

McCabe, O. L. (2004). Crossing the quality chasm in behavioral health care: The role of evidence-based practice. *Professional Psychology: Research and Practice, 35*, 571–579.

McCain, A. P., & Kelley, M. L. (1994). Improving classroom performance in underachieving preadolescents: The additive effects of response cost to a school–home note system. *Child & Family Behavior Therapy, 16*, 27–41.

McConaughy, S. H. (2000). Self-report: Child clinical interviews. In E. S. Shapiro & T. R. Kratochwill (Eds.), *Conducting school-based assessments of child and adolescent behavior* (pp. 170–202). New York: Guilford Press.

McIntire, R., & McIntire, C. (1991). *Teenagers and parents: Ten steps for a better relationship.* Amherst, MA: Human Resource Development Press.

McKendry, J. B., Stewart, D. A., Khanna, F., & Netley, C. (1975). Primary enuresis: Relative success of three methods of treatment. *Canadian Medical Association Journal, 113*, 953–955.

McMahon, R. J. (1999). Parent training. In S. W. Russ & T. H. Ollendick (Eds.), *Handbook of Psychotherapies with children and adolescents* (pp. 153–180). New York: Kluwer Academic/Plenum Press.

McMahon, R. J., & Forehand, R. L. (2003). *Helping the Noncompliant Child: Family-based treatment for oppositional behavior* (2nd ed.). New York: Guilford Press.

McMahon, R. J., Forehand, R. L., & Griest, D. L. (1981). Effects of knowledge of social learning principles on enhancing treatment outcome and generalization in a parent training program. *Journal of Consulting and Clinical Psychology, 49*, 526–532.

McMahon, R. J., Forehand, R., & Tiedemann, G. (1985, November). *Relative effectiveness of a parent training program with children of different ages.* Paper presented at the meeting of the Association for Advancement of Behavior Therapy, Houston, TX.

McMahon, R. J., Slough, N. M., & the Conduct Problems Prevention Research Group. (1996). Family-based intervention in the Fast Track program. In R. DeV. Peters & R. L. McMahon (Eds.), *Preventing childhood disorders, substance use, and delinquency* (pp. 90–110). Thousand Oaks, CA: Sage.

McNeil, C., Capage, L., Bahl, A., & Blanc, H. (1999). Importance of early intervention for disruptive behavior problems: Comparison of treatment and waitlist-control groups. *Early Education and Development, 10,* 445–454.

McNeil, C., Eyberg, S., Eisenstadt, T., Newcomb, K., & Funderburk, B. (1991). Parent–child interaction therapy with behavior problem children: Generalization of treatment effects to the school setting. *Journal of Clinical Child Psychology, 20,* 140–151.

Meichenbaum, D., & Turk, D. C. (1987). *Facilitating treatment adherence: A practitioner's guidebook.* New York: Plenum Press.

Mellon, M. W., & Houts, A. C. (1998). Home-based treatment for primary enuresis. In J. M. Briesmeister & C. E. Schaefer (Eds.), *Handbook of parent training: Parents as co-therapists for children's behavior problems* (2nd ed., pp. 384–417). New York: Wiley.

Messer, S. B. (2004). Evidence-based practice: Beyond empirically supported treatments. *Professional Psychology: Research and Practice, 35,* 580–588.

Miller, D. L., & Kelley, M. L. (1992). Treatment acceptability: The effects of parent gender, marital adjustment and children behavior. *Child & Family Behavior Therapy, 14,* 11–23.

Miller, G. E., & Klugness, L. (1986). Treatment of nonconfrontative stealing in school-age children. *School Psychology Review, 15,* 24–35.

Miltenberger, R. G. (2001). *Behavior modification: Principles and procedures* (2nd ed.). Belmont, CA: Wadsworth/Thomson Learning.

Mindell, J. A. (1999). Empirically supported treatments in pediatric psychology: Bedtime refusal and night awakenings in young children. *Journal of Pediatric Psychology, 24,* 465–481.

Moore, K. J., & Patterson, G. R. (2003). Parent training. In W. O'Donohue, J. E. Fisher, & S. Hayes (Eds.), *Cognitive behavior therapy: Applying empirically supported techniques in your practice* (pp. 280–287). Hoboken, NJ: Wiley.

Morelli, G. A., Rogoff, B., Oppenheim, D., & Goldsmith, D. (1992). Cultural variation in infants' sleeping arrangements: Questions of independence. *Developmental Psychology, 28,* 604–613.

Mrazek, P. J., & Haggerty, R. J. (1994). Illustrative preventive intervention research programs. In P. J. Mrazek & R. J. Haggerty (Eds.), *Reducing risks for mental disorders: Frontiers for preventive intervention research* (pp. 215–313). Washington, DC: National Academy Press.

Mueller, C. T., Hager, W., & Heise, E. (2001). On the effectiveness of Parent Effectiveness Training: A meta-evaluation. *Gruppendynamik, 32,* 339–364.

Mueller, M. M., Piazza, C. C., Moore, J. W., Kelley, M. E., Bethke, S. A., Pruett, A. E., et al. (2003). Training parents to implement pediatric feeding protocols. *Journal of Applied Behavior Analysis, 34,* 511–515.

Myers, L. B., & Midence, K. (Eds.). (1998). *Adherence to treatment in medical conditions*. Amsterdam: Harwood Academic.

Naylor, J. C., & Briggs, G. E. (1963). Effect of rehearsal of temporal and spatial aspects on the long-term retention of a procedural skill. *Journal of Applied Psychology, 47*, 120–126.

Neef, N. A. (1995). Pyramidal parent training by peers. *Journal of Applied Behavior Analysis, 28*, 333–337.

Nelson, R. O., & Hayes, S. C. (1986). *Conceptual foundations of behavioral assessment*. New York: Guilford Press.

Nezu, A. M., & Nezu, C. M. (2005). Comments on "Evidence-based behavioral medicine: What is it and how do we achieve it?": The interventionist does not always equal the intervention—The role of therapist competence. *Annals of Behavioral Medicine, 29*, 80.

Niec, L. N., Hemme, J. M., Yopp, J. M., & Brestan, E. V. (2005). Parent–Child Interaction Therapy: The rewards and challenges of a group format. *Cognitive and Behavioral Practice, 12*, 113–125.

Nixon, R. (2001). Changes in hyperactivity and temperament in behaviourally disturbed preschoolers after parent–child interaction therapy (PCIT). *Behavior Change, 18*, 168–176.

Nixon, R., Sweeney, L., Erickson, D., & Touyz, S. (2003). Parent–Child Interaction Therapy: A comparison of standard and abbreviated treatments for oppositional defiant preschoolers. *Journal of Consulting and Clinical Psychology, 71*, 251–260.

Nystul, M. S. (1982). The effects of systematic training for effective parenting on parental attitudes. *Journal of Psychology, 112*, 63–66.

Okazaki, S. (2000). Assessing and treating Asian Americans—Recent advances. In I. Cuellar & F. A. Paniagua (Eds.), *Handbook of multicultural mental health: Assessment and treatment of diverse populations* (pp. 171–193). New York: Academic Press.

Pachter, L. M., & Dumont-Mathieu, T. (2004). Parenting in culturally diverse settings. In M. Hoghughi & N. Long (Eds.), *Handbook of parenting: Theory and research for practice* (pp. 88–97). London: Sage.

Packard, T., Robinson, E. A., & Grove, D. (1983). The effect of training procedures on the maintenance of parental relationship building skills. *Journal of Clinical Child Psychology, 12*, 181–186.

Paniagua, F. A. (1994). *Assessing and treating culturally diverse clients: A practical guide*. Thousand Oaks, CA: Sage.

Parrish, J. M. (1986). Parent compliance with medical and behavioral recommendations. In N. Krasnegor, J. Arasteh, & M. Cataldo (Eds.), *Child health behavior: A behavioral pediatrics perspective* (pp. 453–501). New York: Wiley.

Patterson, G. R. (1975). *Families: Applications of social learning to family life* (Rev. ed.). Champaign, IL: Research Press.

Patterson, G. R. (1976). *Living With Children: New methods for parents and teachers* (Rev. ed.). Champaign, IL: Research Press.

Patterson, G. R. (1979). Treatment for children with conduct problems: A review of outcome studies. In S. Feshbach & A. Fraczek (Eds.), *Aggression and behavior change: Biological and social process* (pp. 83–132). New York: Praeger.

Patterson, G. R. (1980). Treatment for children with conduct problems: A review of outcome studies. In S. Feshback & A. Fraczek (Eds.), *Aggression and behavior change*. New York: Praeger.

Patterson, G. R. (1982). *A social learning approach: Vol. 3. Coercive family process*. Eugene, OR: Castalia.

Patterson, G. R. (2002). The early development of coercive family process. In J. B. Reid, G. R. Patterson, & J. Snyder (Eds.), *Antisocial behavior in children and adolescents: A developmental analysis and model for intervention* (pp. 25–44). Washington, DC: American Psychological Association.

Patterson, G. R., Chamberlain, P., & Reid, J. B. (1982). A comparative evaluation of a parent-training program. *Behavior Therapy, 13,* 638–650.

Patterson, G. R., & Fisher, P. A. (2002). Recent developments in our understanding of parenting: Bidirectional effects, causal models, and the search for parsimony. In M. H. Bornstein (Ed.), *Handbook of parenting, Vol. 5: Practical issues in parenting* (2nd ed., pp. 59–88). Mahwah, NJ: Erlbaum.

Patterson, G. R., & Forgatch, M. S. (1985). Therapist behavior as a determinant for client noncompliance: A paradox for the behavior modifier. *Journal of Consulting and Clinical Psychology, 53,* 846–851.

Patterson, G. R., & Forgatch, M. S. (1987). *Parents and adolescents: Living together: Part 1. The basics*. Eugene, OR: Castalia.

Patterson, G. R., & Forgatch, M. S. (2005). *Parents and adolescents: Living together: Part 1. The basics* (2nd ed.). Champaign, IL: Research Press.

Patterson, G. R., & Narrett, C. M. (1990). The development of a reliable and valid treatment program for aggressive young children. *International Journal of Mental Health, 19,* 19–26.

Patterson, G. R., Reid, J. B., & Dishion, T. J. (1992). *A social interactional approach: Vol. 4. Antisocial boys*. Eugene, OR: Castalia.

Patterson, G. R., Reid, J. B., Jones, R. R., & Conger, R. E. (1975). *A social learning approach to family intervention: Families with aggressive children* (Vol. 1). Eugene, OR: Castalia.

Pedersen, P. B. (1997). *Culture-centered counseling interventions: Striving for accuracy* (pp. 62–69). Thousand Oaks, CA: Sage.

Peed, S., Roberts, M., & Forehand, R. L. (1977). Evaluation of the effectiveness of a standardized parent training program in altering the interactions of mothers and their noncompliant children. *Behavior Modification, 1,* 323–350.

Peterson, R. F. (1979). The effects of teacher use of I-messages on student disruptive and study behavior. *Psychological Record, 29,* 187–199.

Piaget, J. (1976). *The child and reality: Problems of genetic psychology*. New York: Penguin.

Piazza, C. C., Patel, M. R., Santana, C. M., Goh, H. L., Delia, M. D., & Lancaster, B. M. (2002). An evaluation of simultaneous and sequential presentation of preferred and nonpreferred food to treat food selectivity. *Journal of Applied Behavior Analysis, 35,* 259–270.

Pierce, W. D., Cameron, J., Banko, K. M., & So, S. (2003). Positive effects of rewards and performance standards on intrinsic motivation. *Psychological Record, 53,* 561–578.

Polaha, J., Warzak, W., & Dittmer-McMahon, K. (2002). Toilet training in primary care: Current practice and recommendations from behavioral pediatrics. *Journal of Developmental and Behavioral Pediatrics, 23,* 424–429.

Popkin, M. H. (1983). *Active Parenting.* Marietta, GA: Active Parenting.

Popkin, M. H. (2002a). *Active Parenting now.* Kennesaw, GA: Active Parenting.

Popkin, M. H. (2002b). *Active Parenting now: Leader's guide.* Kennesaw, GA: Active Parenting.

Post, R. A., & Kirkpatrick, M. A. (2004). Toilet training for a young boy with pervasive developmental disorder. *Behavioral Interventions, 19,* 45–50.

Prince, K. (1997). Black family and Black liberation. *Psychological Discourse, 238,* 4–7.

Puckering, C. (2004). Parenting in social and economic adversity. In M. Hoghughi & N. Long (Eds.), *Handbook of parenting: Theory and research for practice* (pp. 38–54). London: Sage.

Raajpoot, U. A. (2000). Multicultural demographic developments: Current and future trends. In I. Cuellar & F. A. Paniagua (Eds.), *Handbook of multicultural mental health: Assessment and treatment of diverse populations* (pp. 79–94). New York: Academic Press.

Ramchandani, P., & McConachie, H. (2005). Mothers, fathers and their children's health. *Child: Care, Health and Development, 31,* 5–6.

Rapp, J. T., Miltenberger, R. G., & Long, E. S. (1998). Augmenting simplified habit reversal with an awareness enhancement device: Preliminary findings. *Journal of Applied Behavior Analysis, 31,* 665–668.

Rathvon, N. (1999). *Effective school interventions: Strategies for enhancing academic achievement and social competence.* New York: Guilford Press.

Reid, J. B., & Eddy, J. M. (2002). Preventive efforts during the elementary school years: The Linking the Interests of Families and Teachers project. In J. B. Reid, G. R. Patterson, & J. J. Snyder (Eds.), *Antisocial behavior in children and adolescents: A developmental analysis and model for intervention* (pp. 219–234). Washington, DC: American Psychological Association.

Reid, J. B., Patterson, G. R., & Snyder, J. J. (2002). *Antisocial behavior in children and adolescents: A developmental analysis and model for intervention.* Washington, DC: American Psychological Association.

Reid, M. J., Webster-Stratton, C., & Baydar, N. (2004). Halting the development of conduct problems in Head Start children: The effects of parent training. *Journal of Clinical Child and Adolescent Psychology, 33,* 279–291.

Reid, M. J., Webster-Stratton, C., & Beauchaine, T. (2001). Parent training in Head Start: A comparison of program response among African American, Asian American, Caucasian, and Hispanic mothers. *Prevention Science, 2,* 209–227.

Reid, M. J., Webster-Stratton, C., & Hammond, M. (2003). Follow-up of children who received The Incredible Years intervention for oppositional defiant disorder: Maintenance and prediction of 2-year outcome. *Behavior Therapy, 34,* 471–491.

Reiss, S. (2005). Extrinsic and intrinsic motivation at 30: Unresolved scientific issues. *Behavior Analyst, 28,* 1–14.

Resetar, J. L., Noell, G. H., & Pellegrin, A. L. (2006). Teaching parents to use research-supported systematic strategies to tutor their children in reading. *School Psychology Quarterly, 21,* 241–261.

Reyno, S. M., & McGrath, P. J. (2006). Predictors of parent training efficacy for child externalizing behavior problem—A meta-analytic review. *Journal of Child Psychology and Psychiatry, 47,* 99–11.

Riley-Tillman, T. C., Chafouleas, S. M., Eckert, T. L., & Kelleher, C. (2005). Bridging the gap between research and practice: A framework for building research agendas in school psychology. *Psychology in the Schools, 42,* 459–473.

Ringeisen, H., Henderson, K., & Hoagwood, K. (2003). Context matters: Schools and the "research to practice gap" in children's mental health. *School Psychology Review, 32,* 153–168.

Rinn, R. C., & Markle, A. (1977). Parent Effectiveness Training: A review. *Psychological Reports, 41,* 95–109.

Ritchie, M. H., & Partin, R. L. (1994). Parent education and consultation activities of school counselors. *School Counselor, 41,* 165–170.

Roberts, M. W. (1982). The effects of warned versus unwarned time-out procedures on child noncompliance. *Child & Family Behavior Therapy, 4,* 37–53.

Roberts, M. W. (1988). Enforcing chair timeouts with room timeouts. *Behavior Modification, 12,* 353–370.

Roberts, M. W., McMahon, R., Forehand, R. L., & Humphreys, L. (1978). The effects of parental instruction giving on child compliance. *Behavior Therapy, 9,* 793–798.

Roberts, M. W., & Powers, S. W. (1990). Adjusting chair timeout enforcement procedures for oppositional children. *Behavior Therapy, 21,* 257–271.

Robinson, P. W., Robinson, M. P., & Dunn, T. W. (2003). STEP parenting: A review of the research. *Canadian Journal of Counseling, 37,* 270–278.

Rogers, T. R., Forehand, R. L., Griest, D., Wells, K., & McMahon, R. (1981). Socioeconomic status: Effects on parent and child behaviors and treatment outcome of parent training. *Journal of Clinical Child Psychology, 10,* 98–101.

Rolider, A., Axelrod, S., & Van Houten, R. (1998). Don't speak behaviorism to me: How to clearly and effectively communicate behavioral interventions to the general public. *Child & Family Behavior Therapy, 20,* 39–56.

Rolison, M. R., & Scherman, A. (2002). Factors influencing adolescents' decisions to engage in risk-taking behavior. *Adolescence, 37,* 585–597.

Romero, A. J. (2000). Assessing and treating Latinos. In I. Cuellar & F. A. Paniagua (Eds.), *Handbook of multicultural mental health: Assessment and treatment of diverse populations* (pp. 209–223). New York: Academic Press.

Sanders, M. R. (1982). The generalization of parent responding to community settings: The effects of instructions, plus feedback, and self-management training. *Behavioural Psychotherapy, 10,* 273–287.

Sanders, M. R. (1996). New directions in behavioral family intervention with children. *Advances in Clinical Child Psychology, 18,* 283–330.

Sanders, M. R. (1999). Triple P—Positive Parenting Program: Toward an empirically validated multilevel parenting and family support strategy for the prevention of behavior and emotional problems in children. *Clinical Child and Family Psychology Review, 2,* 71–90.

Sanders, M. R., & Dadds, M. R. (1993). *Behavioral family intervention.* Needham Heights, MA: Allyn & Bacon.

Sanders, M. R., & Glynn, T. (1981). Training parents in behavioral self-management: An analysis of generalization and maintenance. *Journal of Applied Behavior Analysis, 14,* 223–237.

Sanders, M. R., Markie-Dadds, C., Tully, L., & Bor, W. (2000). The Triple P—Positive Parenting Program: A comparison of enhanced, standard, and self-directed behavioral family intervention for parents of children with early onset conduct problems. *Journal of Consulting and Clinical Psychology, 68,* 624–640.

Sanders, M. R., Markie-Dadds, C., & Turner, K. (2003). *Theoretical, scientific and clinical foundations of the Triple P—Positive Parenting Program: A population approach to the promotion of parenting competence* (Parenting Research and Practice Monograph No. 1). Brisbane, Australia: The Parenting and Family Support Centre, University of Queensland.

Sanders, M. R., Pidgeon, A., Gravestock, F., Connors, M. D., Brown, S., & Young, R. (2004). Does parental attribution retraining and anger management enhance the effects of the Triple P—Positive Parenting Program with parents at risk of child maltreatment? *Behavior Therapy, 35,* 513–535.

Sattler, J. M. (2002). *Assessment of children: Behavioral and clinical applications* (4th ed.). San Diego, CA: Jerome M. Sattler.

Schlinger, H. D. (1992). Theory in behavior analysis: An application to child development. *American Psychologist, 47,* 1396–1410.

Schoenwald, S. K., & Hoagwood, K. (2001). Effectiveness, transportability, and dissemination of interventions: What matters when? *Psychiatric Services, 52,* 1190–1197.

Schrepferman, L., & Snyder, J. J. (2002). Coercion: The link between treatment mechanisms in behavioral parent training and risk reduction in child antisocial behavior. *Behavior Therapy, 33,* 339–359.

Schroeder, C. S., Gordon, B. N., Kanoy, K., & Routh, D. K. (1983). Managing children's behavior problems in pediatric practice. *Advances in Developmental & Behavioral Pediatrics, 4,* 25–86.

Schuhmann, E., Foote, R., Eyberg, S., Boggs, S. R., & Algina, J. (1998). Efficacy of parent–child interaction-therapy: Interim report of a randomized trial with short-term maintenance. *Journal of Clinical Child Psychology, 27*, 34–45.

Schulman, J. L., Stevens, T. M., Suran, B. G., Kupst, M. J., & Naughton, M. J. (1978). Modification of activity level through biofeedback and operant conditioning. *Journal of Applied Behavior Analysis, 11*, 145–152.

Scott, S. (2005). Do parenting programmes for severe antisocial behaviour work over the longer term, and for whom? One year follow-up of a multi-centre controlled trial. *Behavioural and Cognitive Psychotherapy, 33*, 403–421.

Seideman, R. Y., Williams, R., & Burns, P. (1994). Culture sensitivity in assessing urban Native American parenting. *Public Health Nursing, 11*, 98–103.

Shapiro, E. S., & Kratochwill, T. R. (2000). *Behavioral assessment in schools: Theory, research, and clinical foundations* (2nd ed.). New York: Guilford Press.

Sheridan, S. M. (1997). Conceptual and empirical bases of conjoint behavioral consultation. *School Psychology Quarterly, 12*, 119–133.

Sheridan, S. M., Kratochwill, T. R., & Bergan, J. R. (1996). *Conjoint behavioral consultation: A procedural manual.* New York: Plenum Press.

Shriver, M. D. (1998). Teaching parenting skills. In T. S. Watson & F. Gresham (Eds.), *Handbook of child behavior therapy* (pp. 165–182). New York: Plenum Press.

Shriver, M. D., & Allen, K. D. (1996). The time-out grid: A guide to effective time-out implementation in the classroom. *School Psychology Quarterly, 11*, 67–75.

Shriver, M. D., & Allen, K. D. (1997). Defining child noncompliance: An examination of temporal parameters. *Journal of Applied Behavior Analysis, 30*, 173–176.

Shriver, M. D., & Watson, T. S. (2005). Bridging the great divide: Linking research to practice in scholarly publications. *Journal of Evidence-Based Practices for Schools, 6*, 5–18.

Sidman, M. (1989). *Coercion and its fallout.* Boston, MA: Authors Cooperative.

Sims, H., & Manz, C. (1982). Modeling influences on employee behavior. *Personnel Journal, 61*, 58–65.

Skinner, B. F. (1938). *The behavior of organisms: An experimental analysis.* New York: Appleton-Century.

Skinner, B. F. (1953). *Science and human behavior.* New York: Macmillan.

Skinner, B. F. (1957). *Verbal behavior.* Englewood Cliffs, NJ: Prentice-Hall.

Skinner, B. F. (1974). *About behaviorism.* New York: Random House.

Smith, P. K., & Drew, L. M. (2002). Grandparenthood. In M. H. Bornstein (Ed.), *Handbook of parenting: Vol. 3. Being and becoming a parent* (2nd ed., pp. 141–172). Mahwah, NJ: Erlbaum.

Snyder, J. J., & Patterson, G. R. (1995). Individual differences in social aggression: A test of a reinforcement model of socialization in the natural environment. *Behavior Therapy, 26*, 371–391.

Snyder, J. J., & Stoolmiller, M. (2002). Reinforcement and coercion mechanisms in the development of antisocial behavior: The family. In J. B. Reid, G. R. Patterson, & J. J. Snyder (Eds.), *Antisocial behavior in children and adolescents: A developmental analysis and model for intervention* (pp. 65–100). Washington, DC: American Psychological Association.

Spaccarelli, S., Cotler, S., & Penman, D. (1992). Problem-solving skills training as a supplement to behavioral parent training. *Cognitive Therapy and Research, 16*, 1–18.

Sprott, J. E. (1994). One person's "spoiling" in another's freedom to become: Overcoming ethnocentric views about parental control. *Social Science Medicine, 38*, 1111–1124.

Stein, H. T., & Edwards, M. E. (1998). Alfred Adler: Classical theory and practice. In P. Marcus and A. Rosenberg (Eds.), *Psychoanalytic versions of the human condition: Philosophies of life and their impact on practice* (pp. 64–93). New York: New York University Press.

Stewart-Brown, S., Patterson, J., Mockford, C., Barlow, J., Klimes, I., & Pyper, C. (2004). Impact of a general practice based group parenting programme: Quantitative and qualitative results from a controlled trial at 12 months. *Archives of Diseases for Children, 89*, 519–525.

Stoff, D. M., Breiling, J., & Masters, J. D. (1997). *The handbook of antisocial behavior*. New York: Wiley.

Stokes, T. F., & Osnes, P. G. (1989). An operant pursuit of generalization. *Behavior Therapy, 20*, 337–355.

Strain, P. S., & Joseph, G. E. (2004). A not so good job with "Good Job": A response to Kohn 2001. *Journal of Positive Behavior Interventions, 6*, 55–59.

Strauss, M. A. (1994). Should the use of corporal punishment by parents be considered child abuse? Yes. In M. A. Mason & E. Gambrill (Eds.), *Debating children's lives* (pp. 195–203, 219–222). Thousand Oaks, CA: Sage.

Streisand, R., Kazak, A. E., & Tercyak, K. P. (2003). Pediatric-specific parenting stress and family functioning in parents of children treated for cancer. *Children's Health Care, 32*, 245–256.

Stuart, R. B. (2004). Twelve practical suggestions for achieving multicultural competence. *Professional Psychology: Research and Practice, 35*, 3–9.

Sue, D. W. (2004). Whiteness and ethnocentric monoculturalism: Making the "invisible" visible. *American Psychologist, 59*, 761–769.

Sue, D. W., & Sue, D. (1990). *Counseling the culturally different: Theory and practice* (2nd ed.). New York: Wiley.

Tarbox, R. S. F., Williams, L. W., & Friman, P. C. (2004). Extended diaper wearing: Effects on continence in and out of the diaper. *Journal of Applied Behavior Analysis, 37*, 97–100.

Taylor, T. K., & Biglan, A. (1998). Behavioral family interventions for improving child-rearing: A review for clinician and policy makers. *Clinical Child and Family Psychology Review, 1*, 41–60.

Teti, D. M., & Candelaria, M. A. (2002). Parenting competence. In M. H. Bornstein (Ed.), *Handbook of parenting: Vol. 4. Social conditions and applied parenting* (2nd ed., pp. 149–180). Mahwah, NJ: Erlbaum.

Thompson, R. W., Ruma, P., Brewster, A., Besetsney, L., & Burke, R. (1997). Evaluation of an Air Force child physical abuse prevention project using the reliable change index. *Journal of Child and Family Studies, 6,* 421–434.

Thompson, R. W., Ruma, P. R., & Schuchmann, L. F. (1996). A cost-effectiveness evaluation of parent training. *Journal of Child and Family Studies, 5,* 415–429.

Thompson, V. L., Bazile, A., & Akbar, M. (2004). African Americans' perceptions of psychotherapy and psychotherapists. *Professional Psychology: Research and Practice, 35,* 19–26.

Tiano, J. D., & McNeil, C. B. (2006). The inclusion of fathers in behavioral parent training: A critical evaluation. *Child & Family Behavior Therapy, 27,* 1–28.

Timmer, S. G., Sedlar, G., & Urquiza, A. J. (2004). Challenging children in kin versus nonkin foster care: Perceived costs and benefits to caregivers. *Child Maltreatment: Journal of the American Professional Society on the Abuse of Children, 9,* 251–262.

Timmer, S. G., Urquiza, A. J., & Zebell, N. M. (2005). Parent–child interaction therapy: Application to maltreating parent–child dyads. *Child Abuse & Neglect, 29,* 825–842.

Tremblay, G. C., & Drabman, R. S. (1997). An intervention for childhood stealing. *Child & Family Behavior Therapy, 19,* 33–40.

Tseng, W. S. (2003). *Clinician's guide to cultural psychiatry.* New York: Academic Press.

Urdan, T. (2003). Intrinsic motivation, extrinsic rewards, and divergent views of reality. *Educational Psychology Review, 15,* 311–325.

Urquiza, A. J., & McNeil, C. B. (1996). Parent–Child Interaction Therapy: An intensive dyadic intervention for physically abusive families. *Child Maltreatment, 1,* 134–144.

Utting, D., & Pugh, G. (2004). The social context of parenting. In M. Hoghughi & N. Long (Eds.), *Handbook of parenting: Theory and research for practice* (pp. 19–37). London. Sage.

Valdez, C. R., Carlson, C., & Zanger, D. (2005). Evidence-based parent training and family interventions for school behavior change. *School Psychology Quarterly, 20,* 403–433.

Valleley, R. J., Begeney, J. C., & Shriver, M. D. (2005). Collaborating with parents to improve children's reading. *Journal of Evidence Based Practices for Schools, 6,* 19–41.

Valleley, R. J., Evans, J. H., & Allen, K. D. (2002). Parent implementation of an oral reading intervention. *Child & Family Behavior Therapy, 24,* 39–50.

Van Dijken, S., Van Der Veer, R., Van Ijzendoorn, M., & Kuipers, H. (1998). Bowlby before Bowlby: The sources of an intellectual departure in psychoanalysis and psychology. *Journal of the History of the Behavioral Sciences, 34,* 247–269.

van Londen, A., van Londen-Barentsen, M. W., van Son, M. J., & Mulder, G. A. (1993). Arousal training for children suffering from nocturnal enuresis: A 2½ year follow-up. *Behaviour Research and Therapy, 31,* 613–615.

VandenBos, G. R., Cummings, N. A., & DeLeon, P. H. (1992). A century of psychotherapy: Economic and environmental influences. In D. K. Freedheim (Ed.), *History of psychotherapy: A century of change* (pp. 65–102). Washington, DC: American Psychological Association.

Venning, H. B., Blampied, N. M., & France, K. G. (2003). Effectiveness of a standard parenting-skills program in reducing stealing and lying in two boys. *Child & Family Behavior Therapy, 25,* 31–44.

Vigilante, V. A., & Wahler, R. G. (2005). Covariations between mothers' responsiveness and their use of "do" and "don't" instructions: Implications for child behavior therapy. *Behavior Therapy, 36,* 207–212.

Volmink, J., Matchaba, P., & Garner, P. (2000). Directly observed therapy and treatment adherence. *Lancet, 355,* 1345–1350.

Wade, S. M. (2004). Parenting influences on intellectual development and educational achievement. In M. Hoghughi & N. Long (Eds.), *Handbook of parenting: Theory and research for practice* (pp. 198–212). London: Sage.

Wahler, R. G., & Hann, D. M. (1986). A behavioral systems perspective in childhood psychopathology: Expanding the three-term operant contingency. In N. Krasnegor, J. Anasteh, & M. Cataldo (Eds.), *Child Health Behavior: A behavioral pediatrics perspective* (pp. 146–167). New York: Wiley.

Wahler, R. G., Vigilante, V. A., & Strand, P. S. (2004). Generalization in a child's oppositional behavior across home and school settings. *Journal of Applied Behavior Analysis, 37,* 43–51.

Walter, H. I., & Gilmore, S. K. (1973). Placebo versus social learning effects in parent training procedures designed to alter the behaviors of aggressive boys. *Behavior Therapy, 4,* 361–377.

Wampold, B. E., & Bhati, K. S. (2004). Attending to the omissions: A historical examination of evidence-based practice movements. *Professional Psychology: Research and Practice, 35,* 563–570.

Watson, T. S., & Gresham, F. M. (Eds.). (1998). *Handbook of child behavior.* New York: Plenum Press.

Watson, T. S., & Steege, M. W. (2003). *Conducting school-based functional behavioral assessments: A practitioner's guide.* New York: Guilford Press.

Webster-Stratton, C. (1981). Videotaped modeling: A method of parent education. *Journal of Clinical Child Psychology, 10,* 93–98.

Webster-Stratton, C. (1984). A randomized trial of two parent training programs for families with conduct-disordered children. *Journal of Consulting and Clinical Psychology 52,* 666–678.

Webster-Stratton, C. (1987). *The parents and children series.* Eugene, OR: Castalia.

Webster-Stratton, C. (1990). Enhancing the effectiveness of self-administered videotape parent training for families with conduct problem children. *Journal of Abnormal Child Psychology, 18,* 479–492.

Webster-Stratton, C. (1992). *The Incredible Years: A trouble-shooting guide for parents of children aged 3–8.* Toronto, Ontario, Canada: Umbrella Press.

Webster-Stratton, C. (1994). Advancing videotape parent training: A comparison study. *Journal of Consulting and Clinical Psychology, 62,* 583–593.

Webster-Stratton, C. (1997). From parent training to community building. *Families in Society, 78,* 156–171.

Webster-Stratton, C. (1998). Preventing conduct problems in Head Start children: Strengthening parenting competencies. *Journal of Consulting and Clinical Psychology, 66,* 715–730.

Webster-Stratton, C., & Hancock, L. (1998). Training for parents of young children with conduct problems: Content, methods, and therapeutic processes. In J. M. Briesmeister & C. E. Schaefer (Eds.), *Handbook of parent training: Parents as co-therapists for children's behavior problems* (2nd ed., pp. 98–152). New York: Wiley.

Webster-Stratton, C., & Herbert, M. (1994). *Troubled families—problem children: Working with parents: A collaborative process.* New York: Wiley.

Webster-Stratton, C., Kolpacoff, M., & Hollingsworth, T. (1988). Self-administered videotape therapy for families with conduct problem children: Comparison with two cost-effective treatments and a control group. *Journal of Consulting and Clinical Psychology, 56,* 558–566.

Webster-Stratton, C., & Reid, M. J. (2003). The Incredible Years parents, teachers, and children training series: A multifaceted treatment approach for young children with conduct problems. In A. E. Kazdin & J. R. Weisz (Eds.), *Evidence-based psychotherapies for children and adolescents* (pp. 224–241). New York: Guilford Press.

Webster-Stratton, C., Reid, M. J., & Hammond, M. (2001). Preventing conduct problems, promoting social competence: A parent and teacher training partnership in Head Start. *Journal of Clinical Child Psychology, 30,* 283–302.

Webster-Stratton, C., & Taylor, E. T. (1998). Adopting and implementing empirically supported interventions: A recipe for success. In A. Buchanan (Ed.), *Parenting, schooling, and children's behavior* (pp. 127–160). Hampshire, England: Ashgate.

Weinraub, M., Horvath, D. L., & Gringlas, M. B. (2002). Single parenthood. In M. H. Bornstein (Ed.), *Handbook of parenting: Vol. 3. Being and becoming a parent* (2nd ed., pp. 109–140). Mahwah, NJ: Erlbaum.

Weiss, L., & Wolchik, S. (1998). New beginnings: An empirically-based intervention program for divorced mothers to help their children adjust to divorce. In J. M. Briesmeister & C. E. Schaefer (Eds.), *Handbook of parent training: Parents as co-therapists for children's behavior problems* (2nd ed., pp. 445–478). New York: Wiley.

Weissberg, R. P., Kumpfer, K. L., & Seligman, M. E. P. (2003). Prevention that works for children and youth. *American Psychologist, 58,* 425–432.

Weisz, J. R., Weiss, B., & Donenberg, G. R. (1992). The lab versus the clinic: Effects of child and adolescent psychotherapy. *American Psychologist, 47,* 1578–1585.

Wells, K. C. (2003). Adaptations for specific populations. In R. J. McMahon & R. L. Forehand, *Helping the Noncompliant Child: Family-based treatment for oppositional behavior* (2nd ed., pp. 182–200). New York: Guilford Press.

Wells, K. C., & Egan, J. (1988). Social learning and systems family therapy for childhood oppositional disorder: Comparative treatment outcome. *Comprehensive Psychiatry, 29,* 138–146.

Wells, K. C., Griest, D. L., & Forehand, R. L. (1980). The use of a self-control package to enhance temporal generality of a parent training program. *Behavior Research and Therapy, 18,* 347–353.

Wells, K. C., Pfiffner, L., Abramowitz, A., Abikoff, H., Courtney, M., Cousins, L., et al. (1996). *Parent training for attention-deficit/hyperactivity disorder: The MTA study.* Unpublished manual.

Wertsch, J. V. (1985). *Vygotsky and the social formation of mind.* Cambridge, MA: Harvard University Press.

Wesnes, K. A., Pincock, C., Richardson, D., Helm, G., & Hails, S. (2003). Breakfast reduces declines in attention and memory over the morning in school children. *Appetite, 41,* 329–331.

Whitcomb, M. E. (2005). Why we must teach evidence-based medicine. *Academic Medicine, 80,* 1–2.

Williams, R. M. (1985). Children's stealing: A review of theft-control procedures for parents and teachers. *RASE: Remedial and Special Education, 6,* 17–23.

Wiltz, N. A., & Patterson, G. R. (1974). An evaluation of parent training procedures designed to alter inappropriate aggressive behavior of boys. *Behavior Therapy, 5,* 215–221.

Witt, J. C., Moe, G., Gutkin, T. B., & Andrews, L. (1984). The effect of saying the same thing in different ways: The problem of language and jargon in school-based consultation. *Journal of School Psychology, 22,* 361–367.

Wolfson, A. R. (1998). Working with parents on developing efficacious sleep/wake habits for infants and young children. In J. M. Briesmeister & C. E. Schaefer (Eds.), *Handbook of parent training: Parents as co-therapists for children's behavior problems* (2nd ed., pp. 347–383). New York: Wiley.

Wolfson, A. R., & Carskadon, M. A. (2003). Understanding adolescents' sleep patterns and school performance: A critical appraisal. *Sleep Medicine Reviews, 7,* 491–506.

Woods, D. W., & Miltenberger, R. G. (Eds.). (2001). *Tic disorders, trichotillomania and other repetitive behavior disorders.* Boston: Kluwer.

Woolfolk, A. E., & Woolfolk, R. L. (1979). Modifying the effect of the behavior modification label. *Behavior Therapy, 10,* 575–578.

AUTHOR INDEX

Baumrind, D., 21
Baydar, N., 49
Bazile, A., 145
Bean, A. W., 234
Bear, G. G., 159
Beauchaine, T., 49, 230
Begeney, J. C., 180
Begin, G., 120
Behan, J., 240
Behavior Analyst Certification Board, 165
Bejet, C., 109
Beldavs, Z., 232
Bennett, G. M., 64
Bergan, J. R., 177, 195–196
Bernal, M. E., 39, 72, 132, 134, 147
Bernhardt, A. J., 56
Berrett, R. D., 81
Berry, S. L., 174
Besetsney, L., 86
Bhati, K. S., 190, 191
Biglan, A., 26, 30, 49, 82, 191, 228, 229
Blampied, N. M., 209
Blanc, H., 64
Blanchard, T., 239
Blane, M., 235
Blum, I. H., 182
Boggs, S. R., 18, 64, 65, 193, 234
Bondy, A. S., 130
Bor, W., 88
Borkowski, J. G., 3, 14
Bornstein, M. H., 4, 14, 229
Boulos, S., 17
Bowlby, J., 18
Boyce, G., 135
Bradley, R. H., 22
Brady, J. V., 94
Bremner, R., 120
Brestan, E. V., 26, 30, 31, 234
Brewster, A., 86
Briesmeister, J. M., 26, 160, 183
Briggs, G. E., 121
Brink, P. J., 150
Bristol-Power, M., 3, 14
Bromberg, D. S., 118
Bromley, D. B., 202
Bronfenbrenner, U., 22

Brown, D., 82
Brown, R., 120
Bruch, M. A., 120
Budd, K. S., 174
Budzynski, T. H., 134
Bugental, J., 17
Bunting, L., 232
Burke, P., 86
Burke, R., 86, 237
Burns, P., 151

Caelleigh, A., 70
Caldwell, J. C., 144
Caldwell, M. S., 21, 135
Calzada, E., 63, 65
Cameron, J., 108
Cameron, M. J., 94
Canales, G., 144
Candelaria, M. A., 18, 21
Capage, L., 64
Carlson, C., 233–234
Carlson, V., 146
Carnine, D., 26, 30, 229
Carr, A., 240
Carr, J. E., 214
Carrere, S., 77
Carskadon, M. A., 166
Carter, J. H., 145
Castellino, D. R., 17
Cauce, A. M., 145, 146
Cedar, B., 78
Chafouleas, S. M., 243
Chamberlain, P., 26, 39, 40, 99, 99–100, 232
Chambless, D. L., 29, 30, 160
Chao, R., 148, 149
Chin, T., 135
Choate, M. L., 238
Chorpita, B. F., 195
Christensen, S. L., 177
Christophersen, E. R., 170, 214
Chugh, C. S., 174
Cicero, F. R., 214
Ciminero, A. R., 170
Clancy, P. M., 148
Cleary, A., 134
Coan, J., 77

Freeman, C. W., 81
Fremouw, W., 123
French, V., 14
Freud, S., 15, 25
Fricker-Elhai, A. E., 232
Friman, P. C., 20, 107, 169, 170, 214
Frosh, S., 22
Fuligni, A. J., 147
Funderburk, B., 64, 137, 177, 235

Gallagher, N., 65
Gansle, K. A., 202
Garcia, J. L. A., 145
Garcia-Coll, C., 143
Gardner, F., 236
Garner, P., 138
Gilmore, S. K., 39
Glogower, F., 38, 131
Glynn, T., 88
Goldsmith, D., 142
Goldstein, G. L., 134
Gone, J. P., 140, 150
Gonella, J., 70
Gonzalez, Z., 147
Gordon, B. N., 159
Gordon, T., 17, 69, 73, 74, 77, 79
Gottlieb, L. N., 49
Gottman, J. M., 77
Greenberg, M. T., 221
Greene, D., 108
Greening, T., 16
Gresham, F. M., 196, 202, 239
Griest, D. L., 52, 56, 241
Gringlas, M. B., 22
Grossman, D., 49
Grove, D., 122
Gunnar, M. R., 99–100
Gutkin, T. B., 125

Hager, W., 78
Haggerty, R. J., 29
Hails, S., 174
Hall, C. S., 16, 17
Hall, E. T., 141, 142
Hall, M. R., 141, 142
Hamden, L., 203
Hamlet, C. C., 235

Hammersly, G. A., 129
Hammond, M., 49, 230
Hancock, L., 41, 46, 120, 203
Hanf, C., 42, 51, 58
Hann, D. M., 23
Hansen, D. J., 130, 131
Harkness, S., 22, 142
Hart, B., 22
Harwood, M. D., 239
Harwood, R. L., 146, 147
Haugaard, J., 23
Hawkins, R. P., 202, 203
Hayes, S. C., 159, 236
Haynes, S. N., 236
Hazan, C., 23
Head, M. R., 200, 243
Heise, E., 78
Helm, G., 174
Hembree-Kigin, T. L., 26, 31, 59, 66,
    124, 136, 160, 182, 191, 197,
    200, 203, 232
Hemme, J. M., 234
Henderlong, J., 108
Henderson, K., 190
Herbert, M., 45, 125, 132, 133, 136, 238
Hernstein, R. J., 107
Herron, R., 86, 237
Herschell, A. D., 63, 65, 66
Hersen, M., 24, 71n, 72
Hill, S. A., 144, 145
Hintze, J. M., 205
Ho, D. Y. E., 148
Ho, M. K., 145, 151
Hoagwood, K., 190, 191, 243
Hobbs, S. A., 56, 129, 234
Hoff, E., 22, 144
Hoffman, E., 81
Hoghughi, M., 14, 229
Hojat, M., 70
Holden, G. W., 14, 17, 18, 20, 21
Hollingsworth, T., 49, 84
Hollon, S. D., 29, 30, 160
Honig, W. K., 97
Hood, K. K., 64
Horn, M., 24, 25, 219
Horvath, D. L., 22
Houlihan, D., 235

Houts, A. C., 169, 170
Hudson, A., 235
Hughes, J. R., 49
Huh, K., 135
Humphreys, L., 56, 113, 234
Hupp, S. D. A., 239
Hursh, D. E., 202

Innocenti, M. S., 135
Irvine, A. B., 191, 228
Iwata, B., 99

Jackson, M. D., 82
Jankowiak, W., 148
Jarrett, R. B., 236
Jason, L. A., 135
Jensen, W. R., 127
Johnson, B. T., 118
Johnson, S., 120
Johnson, S. M., 134
Johnston, J. M., 19
Jones, F. H., 123
Jones, K. M., 169, 170
Jones, M. L., 64
Jones, R. R., 25, 26, 32, 88, 93, 136,
    160, 177, 203, 225
Joseph, G. E., 108

Kanarek, R. B., 174
Kanoy, K., 159
Kaufman, N., 228
Kavanagh, K., 40, 221, 226, 227, 228,
    232
Kazak, A. E., 135
Kazdin, A. E., 70, 109, 190, 195, 237
Kelleher, C., 243
Kelley, M. L., 114, 177
Kelly, M. J., 39
Kerwin, M. L. E., 20
Khanna, F., 170
King, H. E., 56
Kirkpatrick, M. A., 214
Kitayama, S., 141, 146
Klein, K., 52
Klinnert, M. D., 39, 72, 134
Klugness, L., 209
Knight, G. P., 147

Knutson, N. M., 229
Kohn, A., 108
Kolpacoff, M., 49, 84
Koskinen, P. S., 182
Kotchick, B. A., 143, 155, 230
Kotler, J. S., 57, 234
Kratochwill, T. R., 177, 189, 190,
    195–196, 196
Krebs, L., 81
Kubany, E. S., 77
Kuerschner, S., 235
Kuhn, B. R., 166
Kuipers, H., 18
Kumpfer, K. L., 26, 29, 31, 82, 160, 220,
    229
Kupst, M. J., 134
Kusche, C., 221

Lam, M., 147
Landesman Ramey, S., 3, 14
Larzelere, R. E., 18, 20
Lauritzen, P., 78
Laursen, B., 22, 144
Lawson, A. B., 141
LeBlanc, L. A., 214
Lee, H. E., 135
Lemanek, K., 134
Lepper, M. R., 108
Lerman, D. C., 109
Lerner, R. M., 17
Levant, R. F., 78
Levine, A., 24, 177
Levine, E. S., 144
Levine, M., 24, 177
Leyendecker, B., 146
Liebert, R. M., 170
Linscheid, T. R., 174
Lipson, K., 232
Long, E. S., 134
Long, N., 14, 52, 229
Long, P., 56
Lowry, M. A., 131
Luiselli, J. K., 94, 160
Lundquist, L. M., 130

MacMillan, V. M., 131
Magen, R. H., 118

Peterson, R. F., 77
Pfadt, A., 214
Phillips, M., 135
Piaget, J., 17
Piazza, C. C., 174
Pincock, C., 174
Pincus, D. B., 198, 238
Pine, J., 160
Polaha, J., 214
Poling, A., 107
Polster, R. A., 160
Popkin, M. H., 83
Post, R. A., 214
Powers, S. W., 64
Prince, K., 144
Puckering, C., 22
Pugh, G., 135

Quant, B., 233

Raajpoot, U. A., 143
Ramchandani, P., 233
Rapoff, M. A., 134
Rapp, J. T., 134
Rathvon, N., 205
Reavis, H. K., 127
Reid, J. B., 3, 14, 23, 25, 26, 32, 39, 40,
        88, 93, 99–100, 136, 160, 177,
        200, 203, 220, 221, 224, 225,
        226, 229, 241, 242–243
Reid, M. J., 177, 230
Reiss, S., 108
Resetar, J. L., 180
Reyno, S. M., 232
Rhode, G., 127
Richard, D. S., 77
Richardson, D., 174
Riley-Tillman, T. C., 243
Ringeisen, H., 190
Rinn, R. C., 78
Risley, T. R., 22, 94
Ritchie, M. H., 69
Roberts, M., 197
Roberts, M. W., 56, 64, 113, 234
Robinson, E. A. 58, 64, 122, 199
Robinson, M. P., 82

Robinson, P. W., 82
Rogers, T. R., 56
Rogoff, B., 142
Rolider, A., 125
Romero, A. J., 141
Rose, S. D., 118
Rothbaum, F., 17
Routh, D. K., 159
Rudolph, K. D., 21, 135
Ruggiero, K. J., 232
Ruma, P. R., 86
Rzasa, T., 120

Samuel, P., 174
Sanders, M. R., 27, 87, 88, 131, 136,
        233, 237
Santelli, B., 233
Sattler, J. M., 196
Saunders, M., 225
Schaefer, C. E., 26, 160, 183
Schauss, S., 121, 135
Schlinger, H. D., 97
Schneiger, A., 228
Schoenwald, S. K., 191, 243
Scholmerich, A., 147
Schrepferman, L., 40
Schroeder, C. S., 159
Schuchmann, L. F., 86, 237
Schuhmann, E., 64
Schulman, J. L., 134
Schultz, L. A., 39, 72, 134
Schulze, P. A., 147
Scott, S., 230
Sedlar, G., 232
Seideman, R. Y., 151
Seligman, M. E. P., 220
Shapiro, E. S., 196
Sheperis, C. J., 239
Sheridan, S. M., 177, 180
Shernoff, E. S., 189, 190
Shriver, M. D., 26, 114, 180, 190, 196,
        199, 243
Sidman, M., 109
Sims, H., 121
Skinner, B. F., 19, 20, 94
Sloop, E. W., 38, 131
Slough, N. M., 222

Smith, D. W., 232
Smith, P. K., 23
Smolkowski, K., 191, 228
Sneed, T. J., 160
Snyder, J. J., 23, 25, 40, 99, 229, 241, 242
So, S., 108
Spaccarelli, S., 49
Sprott, J. E., 150, 154
Staddon, J. E. R., 97
Steege, M. W., 236
Stein, H. T., 16
Stevens, T. M., 134
Stewart, D. A., 170
Stewart-Brown, S., 49
Stokes, T. F., 121, 130
Stoolmiller, M., 99
Stoyva, J. M., 134
Strain, P. S., 108
Strand, P. S., 177
Strauss, M. A., 64
Streisand, R., 135
Stuart, R. B., 140, 141
Sue, D., 145, 149
Sue, D. W., 145, 149
Super, C. M., 22, 142
Suran, B. G., 134
Sweeney, L., 64, 234
Sweitzer, M., 78
Szmania, S. J., 142

Tarbox, R. S. F., 214
Tardif, T., 22, 144
Taylor, E. T., 46
Taylor, H. A., 174
Taylor, T. K., 49, 82
Tercyak, K. R., 135
Teti, D. M., 18, 21
Thompson, R. W., 86
Thompson, V. L., 145
Tiano, J. D., 195
Tiedemann, G., 56, 57
Timmer, S. G., 230, 232
Tisdelle, D. A., 119
Tollison, J. W., 170
Touyz, S., 64, 234
Tremblay, G. C., 209

Trivette, C. M., 135
Tseng, V., 147, 148, 149
Tseng, W. S., 140
Tully, I., 88
Turk, D. C., 119
Turnbull, A., 233
Turner, K., 88

Urdan, T., 108
Urquiza, A. J., 230, 232
Utting, D., 135

Valdez, C. R., 233–234
Valleley, R. J., 160, 180
Van Der Veer, R., 18
Van Dijken, S., 18
Van Houten, R., 125
Van Ijzendoorn, M., 18
Van Londen, A., 170
Van Londen-Barentsen, M. W., 170
Van Son, M. J., 170
VandenBos, G. R., 24, 25
Venning, H. B., 209
Vigilante, V. A., 113, 177
Vincent, J., 235
Volmink, J., 138
Vorndran, C. M., 109

Wade, S. M., 3, 14
Wahler, R. G., 23, 113, 177
Walle, D. L., 129
Walter, H. I., 39
Wampold, B. E., 190, 191
Warzak, W. J., 117, 118, 126, 161, 214, 239
Watson, T. S., 190, 196, 236, 243
Webster-Stratton, C., 26, 30, 42, 43, 45, 46, 48, 49, 84, 120, 125, 132, 133, 136, 160, 177, 193, 203, 222, 230, 233, 238
Weidinger, D., 166
Weinraub, M., 22
Weiss, B., 190
Weiss, L., 136
Weissberg, R. P., 220
Weisz, J. R., 190
Wells, K. C., 56, 160, 170, 230

SUBJECT INDEX

Academic problems, 180–183

Active listening, 45, 75–76, 77–78, 79, 80–81, 83, 89

Active Parenting program, 83–84

Active targeted teaching, 4

Adam (case study on enuresis), 170

Additive effects, of program components, 235

Adherence. *See* Treatment adherence

Adler, Alfred, 16, 79, 81, 82, 83

Administration on Developmental Disabilities, x

Adolescence, problems common in, 183–187

Adolescence Transitions Program (ATP), 221, 226–228

ADVANCE treatment (The Incredible Years) 136

African American culture, and parenting, 143–145, 152

and Parent–Child Interaction Therapy, 64

Aggression
as Living With Children target, 33
from punishment, 109

American Psychological Association, on empirical support, 29

Analogies, practitioner's use of, 126–127

Antecedents, 94, 94–97, 118
and empirically supported parent training programs, 112–113

Applied behavior analysis, 20, 94, 195–196

Aristotle, 14

Asian American culture, and parenting, 148–150, 152

Assessment, comprehensive, 196–198
in case examples, 204–205, 208–209, 213
in family check-up (Adolescence Transitions Program), 227

285

Assessment, comprehensive (*continued*)
    and identification of target problem, 199
    questions on culture in, 152
Assessment methods, research needed on, 236
Assumptions, of practitioners, 6
Attachment theory, 18
    in Parent–Child Interaction Therapy, 58, 63
Attends, in Helping the Noncompliant Child program, 53, 57
Attention, differential, 112
    in case examples, 205
    and feeding problems, 175
Attention-deficit/hyperactivity disorder (ADHD), case example on, 204–208
Attention reduction, and classroom behavior problems, 178
Attributes, of parenting, 20–21
Authoritarian parenting style, 21
Authoritative parenting style, 21
Aversive control, 99
    and bringing about silence, 129
    time-out as, 114
    See also Punishment
Avoidance, 98–99
Awareness training, 132

Barkley's Defiant Child program, 237
BASIC Early Childhood program, 42.
    See also Incredible Years BASIC program
Bavolek, Stephen, 85
"Behavior," 19
Behavioral analysis, 8, 93–94
    antecedents in, 94–97
    consequences in, 97
        conditions affecting, 105–108
        and extinction, 100–101
        punishment, 101–103 (*see also* Punishment)
        as reinforcement, 97–100 (*see also* Reinforcement)

    and parents as conditioned reinforcers or punishers, 103–105, 111
Behavioral consultation service delivery, 195
Behavioral family interventions, 27
Behavioral interventions, 94
Behavioral parenting programs, Gordon's rejection of, 74
Behavioral play therapy, 60, 65
    sample session outline on, 59
Behavioral problems in classroom, 177–180
Behavioral skills training (BST), 8, 138, 238
    components of, 118–123, 128
    and monitoring of children's behavior, 200
    review of behaviors as first step in, 133
    and sleep problems, 169
Behavioral theory (behaviorism), 18–20, 27
    in history of parent training, 24, 25
    and parent responsiveness, 21
    and Systematic Training for Effective Parenting, 81
Behavior assessment, functional, 236
Behavior Coding System, 52
Behavior contract, 35, 239
    in case example, 211
Behavior management, teaching general principles of, 131
Behavior rating forms, 198
Bias
    cultural, 140
    selection, 41
Bowlby, John, 18
Boys Town National Resource and Training Center, 86
BST. See Behavioral skills training
"Bug-in-the-ear" device (Parent–Child Interaction Therapy), 60, 62, 63, 67, 122

Case examples
    on child problems other than noncompliance, 165–166

academic problems, 180–183

classroom behavior problems, 177–180

feeding problems, 174–176

problems common in adolescence, 183–187

sleep problems, 166–169

toileting problems, 169–173

on evidence-based practice, 204

attention deficit, 204–208

stealing, 208–212

toileting, 212–216

Catching child being good, 43–44, 110, 111, 115, 122, 130

Catching parent being good, 122, 138

Central Michigan University, and Parent–Child Interaction Therapy, 66

Chaining of skills, 119

Characteristics of parenting, 20–21

Child behavior, positive affecting of, 4

Child Behavior Checklist, 198

Child care, in African American community, 144

Child development

Freud's stage theory of, 15–16

research on models of, 241–243

See also at Developmental

Child-directed interactions, 75

Child-directed play, 60, 111, 124

Child-focused approach, 25

Child guidance clinics, 24

Child noncompliance. See Noncompliance

Child participation, in Helping Noncompliant Child program, 55

Child Problem Inventory, Eyberg, 198

Child problems other than noncompliance, 165–166

and framework for developing interventions, 161–165, 187

academic problems, 180–183

classroom behavior problems, 177–180

feeding problems, 174–176

problems common in adolescence, 183–187

sleep problems, 166–169

toileting problems, 169–173

lack of empirically supported programs for, 160, 187

and Parent–Child Interaction Therapy, 65

and parent training programs, 160–161, 187

research on parent training for, 238

and research protocols, 194

Children, 183

Child's Game, 52–53, 57, 143

Choice, as affecting consequences, 105, 107–108

Classroom behavior problems, 177–180

Client characteristics, 194–195. See also Parent training

Cline, Foster, 84

Clinical expertise, 191

Clinics, child guidance, 24

Clothing, assessment questions on, 153

Coding System, Parent–Child Interaction, 59

Coercion theory or model, 51, 236, 241–242

Coercive family process (cycle), 25–26, 32, 99–100

escalating cycle of negative reinforcement in, 114

and social reinforcers, 35

Cognitive–behavioral theories, and behavioral approach, 20

Cognitive theories, 17–18

Collaborative approach to parent training, 133, 192

in The Incredible Years, 45, 47, 48

Commands, 112–113

in case examples, 206

"do" commands (Helping the Noncompliant Child program), 53

"don't" vs. "do" commands, 113

in European American culture, 143

in framework for developing interventions, 164

and classroom behavior problems, 179

Experience, of practitioner, 191
Experimental analysis of behavior, 20, 93–94
Experimental control, 70, 72
Experimental design, 71
Expert model and role, 133, 192
    in European American culture, 143
Extended family, 13
    in African American community, 144, 152
        church members and ministers as, 145
    and Native American culture, 151
External validity, 72
Extinction, 100–101
    in case examples, 206, 210, 215
    and empirically supported parent training programs, 111–12, 115
    in framework for developing intervention, 162, 163
        academic problems, 181
        classroom behavior problems, 178
        feeding problems, 175
        problems of adolescence, 185
        sleep problems, 167
        toileting problems, 171
    and negative punishment, 102
Extinction burst, 100, 101, 178, 233
    predicting, 128
Eyberg, Sheila, 58, 59
Eyberg Child Problem Inventory, 198

Fading of intervention, 203
    in case examples, 208, 212, 216
Families (Patterson), 33, 41
Family
    in Asian culture, 148, 152
    assessment questions on, 153
    extended family, 13
        in African American community, 144, 145, 152
        and Native American culture, 151
    in Latino culture, 146–147, 152
    and Native American culture, 151, 152
    See also Parent

Family check-up (FCU), in Adolescence Transition Program, 227
Family coordinators (FC), in FAST Track program, 222
Family Effectiveness Training (video), 79
Family Effectiveness Training program, 74
Family Management Curriculum (FMC), 228
Family resource center (FRC), in Adolescence Transition Program, 227
Family rules, in Parent Effectiveness Training, 76
Family variables, 22–23
FAST Track program, 57, 220, 221–224
Fay, Charles, 84
Fay, Jim, 84
Feedback
    as behavioral skill training component, 119, 121–123
    in case examples, 206, 207, 210, 212, 215, 216
    flexibility in, 192
    in framework for developing intervention, 163, 164
        academic problems, 181, 182
        classroom behavior problems, 178, 179
        feeding problems, 175, 176
        problems of adolescence, 185, 186
        sleep problems, 167, 168
        toileting problems, 171, 172
    and frequency of visits, 130
    in Living With Children program, 37
    in Parent–Child Interaction Therapy, 58, 62
Feeding problems, 174–176
Fidelity, 239
Flexibility, need for in use of programs, 90, 128, 136–137, 192
FMC (Family Management Curriculum), 228
Folk beliefs, assessment questions on, 153

and classroom behavior problems, 178

and feeding problems, 175

and problems of adolescence, 185

and sleep problems, 167

and toileting problems, 171

in The Incredible Years, 44

use of by itself, 112

"I" messages, 45, 76, 77–78, 80–81, 83, 89

Immediacy, as affecting consequences, 105, 106

Incentive programming, in The Incredible Years, 44, 47

Incentives, in parent training, 128, 134

Incredible Years, The: A Trouble-Shooting Guide for Parents of Children Aged 3–8 (Webster-Stratton), 47

supplemental parental-risk treatment with, 136

Incredible Years BASIC program, The, 30–31, 42–50, 67, 68

and group format, 234

nondirective play in, 43, 111

research needed on, 230

and school practice, 193

and treatment of child problems other than noncompliance, 238

video demonstration in, 46, 47, 48, 49, 50, 127

Indicated prevention programs, 220

Individualism, in European American culture, 141–142

Ineffective parenting behaviors, 14

Information sources, on parenting, 3–4

Institute of Medicine, on empirical support, 29

Instruction

as behavioral skill training component, 118–119

in case examples, 206, 207, 210, 211, 212, 215, 216

flexibility in, 192

in framework for developing intervention, 163, 164

academic problems, 181, 182

classroom behavior problems, 179

feeding problems, 175, 176

problems of adolescence, 185, 186

sleep problems, 167, 168

toileting problems, 171, 172

Instructional control, 183

Integrity, 239

Interaction of parent and child, 23, 25–26

coding system for, 59

observation of, 236

research on mechanisms of, 40

and social learning, 42

Interaction skills, parent-directed, 61

Internet, program material posted on, 89

Interventions

behavioral family, 27

fading of, 203

in case examples, 208, 212, 216

identification and development of, 201

in case examples, 205, 207, 209, 214

vs. prevention, 219–220

Interview, parent, 197

Intrinsic motivation, vs. reinforcement, 108

Jerry (case example of toileting), 212–214, 216

Job card grounding, 239

Julio (case study on problems of adolescence), 184, 187

Kathleen (case example on stealing), 208–209, 211–212

Kimberly (case study on academic problems), 180, 182

Language, careful choice of, 125–127

Latino American culture, and parenting, 145–148, 152

Leader's guide (Active Parenting program), 83

Munroe-Meyer Institute, x
Myth of uniformity, 141

Native American culture, and parenting, 150–151
Natural consequences, 44, 45
    in explanation of procedures, 126
    in Systematic Training for Effective Parenting, 80, 83
Negative punishers, 101
    and extinction, 102
Negative reinforcement, 98–99
    and coercive family process, 25–26, 99–100
    and toileting problems, 173
Negotiation, and adolescents, 187
Noncompliance, 159
    behavioral definition of, 199
    and other child problems, 159–160, 165
    and parent training, 26
    with treatment regimen (enuresis), 173
Nondirective behaviors
    with children during play, 60, 111
    with parents, 133
Nurturing Parenting programs, 85

Observation rooms, 122
    in Parent–Child Interaction Theory, 60
Oklahoma City-County Health Department, and Parent–Child Interaction Therapy, 66
Oregon Health Sciences University, 58
Oregon Research Institute (ORI), 30, 32
Oregon Social Learning Center (OSLC), 31, 224, 232, 241, 244
Outcome data, 203
Outcomes, prediction of, 128, 128–130
Outcomes measured in evaluation of programs, 71, 72

Parent(s), 14
    acquaintance with research on, 6
    as conditioned reinforcers and punishers, 103–105, 111

importance of, 3
    in Latino culture, 146–147
    as overreporting positive outcomes, 39
    as unmotivated or resistant, 118 (*see also* Parent motivation)
Parental behaviors, and child's problem behaviors, 199
Parent–child interaction, 23, 25–26
    coding system for, 59
    observation of, 236
    research on mechanisms of, 40
    and social learning, 42
Parent–Child Interaction Coding System, 59
Parent–Child Interaction Therapy (Hembree-Kigin & McNeil), 59
Parent–Child Interaction Therapy (PCIT), 30, 31, 58–66, 68
    and Asian American social–relational goals, 148
    and attachment theory, 18
    charts for, 127
    and child problems other than noncompliance, 160, 238
    criteria for parent skills training in, 200
    and group format, 234
    nondirective play in, 60, 111
    and order of interactions, 235
    progress criteria in, 234
    research needed on, 230
        and comparisons among programs, 237
Parent–child relationship, 115
    in coercive family process, 25–26, 99–101
    and reinforcers, 103–105
Parent Daily Report (Living With Children program), 34, 37, 40
Parent education, vs. parent training, 8
Parent Effectiveness Training (PET) program, 17, 69, 73–79
Parenting, 14, 27
    abundant information on, 3–4
    acquaintance with research on, 6
    and culture, 154

application of behavioral principles in, 110–115
and punishment role, 109
and reinforcing consequences, 105
assessment in, 197 (*see also* at Assessment)
and framework for developing interventions, 161, 163–164
Helping the Noncompliant Child, 50–58, 67–68 (*See also* Helping the Noncompliant Child program)
The Incredible Years, 30–31, 42–50, 67, 68 (*see also* Incredible Years BASIC program, The)
and interdependence in family relationships, 148
Living With Children, 30, 32–41, 68 (*see also* Living With Children program)
modifications to, 137, 154
Parent–Child Interaction Therapy, 58–66, 68 (*see also* Parent–Child Interaction Therapy)
and programs with less than full empirical support, 90
research needed on, 230–237
restricted problem sample for, 194
See also Evidence-based practice
Parent training programs with less than full empirical support, 69–70, 88–89, 237
Active Parenting, 83–84
caveats in consideration of, 89–90
Common Sense Parenting, 85–87, 237
criteria for evaluation of, 70–73
and empirically supported programs, 90
Love and Logic, 84
Nurturing Parenting, 85
Parent Effectiveness Training, 69, 73–79
Putting Kids First, 84–85

Systematic Training for Effective Parenting, 69, 79–83
Triple P Positive Parenting, 87–88, 89, 237
PATHS (Promoting Alternative Thinking Strategies) curriculum, 221
Patterson, Gerald, 25, 31–32, 42
and academic problems, 180
and child problems other than noncompliance, 160
and coercion model, 51, 58
and models of child behavior, 241
on parent training to address stealing, 209
and social learning, 42, 58, 87
See also Living With Children program
PCIT. *See* Parent–Child Interaction Therapy
Peer review, 70, 71
Permissive parenting style, 21
in Native American culture, 150
Personal responsibility, and Native American culture, 150
Phone calls, 37, 38, 130, 193, 201, 203, 214, 222, 228
Piaget, Jean, 17
Pinpointing process, in Living With Children program, 35, 36, 38
Plan for parent training, identification and development of, 201
in case examples, 205, 207, 209, 214
Plato, 14, 21
Point systems, 35, 38, 44, 111
in case example, 212
in explanation of procedures, 126
Positively affecting child behavior, 4
Positive punishers, 101
Positive reinforcement, 97–98, 98
initial unfavorable reaction to, 130
and toileting problems, 173
Practice, in parent training, 124–125
Practitioner support, research directions for, 231
Practitioners working with parents, 3
bases of clinical expertise in, 137
continuum of approaches for, 133

and feeding problems, 175
and problems of adolescence,
185, 186
and sleep problems, 167, 168
and toileting problems, 171, 172
and parent motivation, 123–125,
128
Reading problems, 180–183
Reason, limits of, 132–133
Referral
in case of conflict between treatment
and parents' culture, 154
and level of expertise, 192
Rehearsal
as behavioral skill training component, 119, 120–121
in case examples, 206, 207, 210, 211,
215, 216
flexibility in, 192
in framework for developing intervention, 163, 164
academic problems, 181, 182
classroom behavior problems,
178, 179
feeding problems, 175, 176
problems of adolescence, 185,
186
sleep problems, 167, 168
toileting problems, 171, 172
Reinforcement, 32, 97–99
in case examples, 205, 206, 210, 215
and coercive family process, 25–26,
99–100
and commands, 113
concerns about effects of (intrinsic
motivation), 108
and empirically supported parent
training programs, 111, 115
in framework for developing interventions, 162, 163, 164
academic problems, 181
classroom behavior problems, 178
feeding problems, 175
problems of adolescence, 185
sleep problems, 168, 169
toileting problems, 171
negative, 25–26, 98–200, 173

by parents, 103–105, 111
positive, 97–98, 98, 130, 173
and time-out, 242
Religion
in African American communities,
145
assessment questions on, 153
Reminders, 128, 130–131
Replication
of research on empirically based programs, 235
of treatment efficacy, 71, 72
Research, on parenting, 20–23
crucial variables in, 190–191
on efficacy vs. effectiveness, 189–190
and evidence-based practice, 6 (*see
also* Parent training programs,
empirically supported)
and practice, 195, 229–230
and client characteristics,
194–195
and dissemination, 243–244
on empirically supported parent
training programs,
230–237
on models of child development
and parenting, 241–243
on parent-training methodology,
231, 238–241
and practitioner characteristics,
191–192
scientific knowledge as improving, 241
and setting, 192–194
steps in evidence-based parent
training, 195–204
and treatment of problems other
than noncompliance, 231,
238
Research database, 73
Research design, 71, 72
Resources of parents, 128, 135–136,
233. *See also* Socioeconomic
status
Response induction, 130
Responsiveness, parent, 21
Restricted population sample, 195

Restricted problem sample, 194–195
Roger (case study on classroom behavioral problems), 177, 180
Rogers, Carl, 16
  and Thomas Gordon, 73–74
  and Systematic Training for Effective Parenting, 81
Role play
  in case examples, 212, 214, 215
  dolls in, 240
  in framework for developing intervention
    and classroom behavior problems, 179
    and feeding problems, 176
    and problems of adolescence, 185, 186
    and sleep problems, 168, 169
    and toileting problems, 171, 172
  humorous, 132
  in Living With Children program, 37
  in Parent–Child Interaction Therapy, 58, 62

Sample for research
  restricted population, 195
  restricted problem, 194–195
Sanders, Matthew, 87
School
  and academic problems, 180–183
  and classroom behavioral problems, 177–180
School settings, 192, 193, 233–234
Selected prevention strategies, 220
Self-management skills, for parents (The Incredible Years), 45, 49
Service delivery model, parent training as, 26
  problem solving, 10, 195
Setting of research and practice, 192–194
  generalization of (clinic to home), 121, 130
  home as, 124–125
    and analogues to home, 197

  in low-income areas, 233
  for programs
    Helping the Noncompliant Child, 51
    The Incredible Years, 42
    Living With Children, 33
    Parent–Child Interaction Therapy, 59
    Parent Effectiveness Training, 74
    Systematic Training for Effective Parenting, 80
  research needed on, 231, 241
  school settings, 192, 193, 233–234
Signals, discriminative stimuli as, 96–97
Single-parent family, 23
Skills training, behavioral. See Behavioral skills training
Skill teaching
  and effort, 107
  in Helping the Noncompliant Child program, 54
Skinner, B. F., 19
Sleep problems, 166–169
Social aggression, as Living With Children target, 33
Social attention
  in differential attention, 112
  and feeding problems, 175
Social customs, assessment questions on, 153
Socialization, 13–14
  and attachment, 18
Social Learning Approach to Family Intervention (Patterson et al.), 33–34, 40
Social learning theory or model, 42
  and behavioral approach, 20
  and Parent–Child Interaction Theory, 58
Social reinforcement, removal of, 112
Social validity, 72
Social workers, in child guidance clinics, 24
Sociocultural variables, 22

Socioeconomic status (SES)
  and need for services, 195
  as parenting variable, 22, 144
    and parent training success, 232,
      233
Spanking
  and bringing about silence, 129
  and concerns about punishment, 109
  and culture, 144, 152
  disapproval of
    in Helping the Noncompliant
      Child program, 54
    in The Incredible Years, 44
    in Parent–Child Interaction Ther-
      apy, 61, 63–64
Spirituality, in African American communities, 145, 152
Standing rules, 54
Stealing, case example on, 208–212
STEP. See Systematic Training for
  Effective Parenting
Stereotypic thinking, 140, 154
Stimuli, discriminative, 94, 95, 96–97,
  113, 115
Stimulus control
  in case examples, 206, 210, 215
  in framework for developing inter-
    vention, 162, 164
    academic problems, 181, 182–183
    classroom behavior problems, 179
    feeding problems, 175
    problems of adolescence, 186
    sleep problems, 167
    toileting problems, 172
Style, parenting, 21
Systematic Training for Effective Par-
  enting (STEP), 16, 69, 79–83

Tangible incentives, in parent training,
  134
Target problem behavior and goal, operational definition of, 198–200
  in case examples, 205, 209, 213–214
Technology, as effort-reducing, 134–135
Theories of human behavior and parenting, 15

behavioral, 18, 27
  in history of parent training, 24,
    25
  and parent responsiveness, 21
developmental and cognitive, 17–18
  and parent responsiveness, 21
humanistic, 16–17
psychodynamic, 15–16
  and attachment theory, 18
  in history of parent training, 24
Time
  in European American culture, 142
  and Native American culture, 151,
    152
Time-out, 109, 113–115, 137, 242
  in case examples, 207, 211, 212, 216
  in Common Sense Parenting, 86
  in European American culture, 143
  in framework for developing inter-
    vention, 164
    and feeding problems, 176
  in Helping the Noncompliant Child
    program, 53–54
  in The Incredible Years, 44, 47
  learning to use, 119
  in Living With Children program,
    35, 36
  in Native American culture, 150
  in Parent–Child Interaction Ther-
    apy, 58, 61, 63–64, 67
  as punisher, 102
  and reissuance of command, 61, 114
  research directions for, 231
  in Triple P Positive Parenting Pro-
    gram, 87, 88
  in unfavorable housing setting, 233
Toileting problems, 169–173
  case example on, 212–214, 216
Token reinforcement programs, 35, 137
  and sleeping problems, 168–169
  and toileting problems, 171
Training of practitioner, ix, 191
Transfer, of skills to home setting, 121.
  See also Generalization
Translating research into practice,
  243

ABOUT THE AUTHORS

Mark D. Shriver, PhD, is an associate professor of pediatrics and psychology at the Munroe-Meyer Institute for Genetics and Rehabilitation and the University of Nebraska Medical Center. Dr. Shriver specializes in the treatment of a diverse population of children with a wide variety of behavioral health conditions, educational problems, and developmental disabilities. His research and clinical interests include management of challenging behaviors at home and school, academic assessment and intervention for children with disabilities, and parent training. He has extensive clinical experience in training parents to address child problems in the home. He is also director of the Academic Evaluation and Intervention Clinic at the Munroe-Meyer Institute. This clinic trains parents in academic interventions to improve the academic performance of children with disabilities. He regularly consults with early childhood education and special education agencies, Head Start programs, after-school programs, and school-age education and special education programs on behavioral and academic problems experienced by children in the classroom. He has numerous publications in peer-reviewed journals. He is coeditor of the *Journal of Evidence-Based Practices for Schools* and serves on the editorial boards of four other journals.

Keith D. Allen, PhD, is a professor of pediatrics and psychology at the Munroe-Meyer Institute for Genetics and Rehabilitation and the University of Nebraska Medical Center. Dr. Allen specializes in the treatment of children with behavioral health conditions and developmental disabilities. His research and clinical interests include management of pain and stress-related disorders in children; parent training; and management of challenging behaviors in school, medical, and dental settings. He has served as a consultant to school districts on the development of appropriate interventions for children with learning and behavioral disabilities. He has worked for over 20 years to improve behavioral technology for managing children undergoing invasive medical and dental treatment. Dr. Allen has extensive experience with training parents as change agents and has published recently on problems with adherence to treatment recommendations. Dr. Allen is codirector of the Nebraska Internship Consortium in Professional Psychology, one of the largest predoctoral intern training consortiums in the United States, and he recently received an Outstanding Teacher Award for excellence in education. Dr. Allen has over 80 publications and book chapters on interventions with children with behavioral health concerns. He currently serves on five editorial boards of peer-reviewed journals related to the behavioral health of children.